Thyroid Toxicity

Edited By

Javier Del Pino

Toxicology and Pharmacology Department,
Veterinary School,
Complutense University of Madrid,
Ciudad Universitaria s/n,
Madrid 28040, Spain

Maria Jesus Diaz

Toxicology and Pharmacology Department,
Veterinary School,
Complutense University of Madrid,
Ciudad Universitaria s/n,
Madrid 28040, Spain

&

Maria Teresa Frejo

Toxicology and Pharmacology Department,
Veterinary School,
Complutense University of Madrid,
Ciudad Universitaria s/n,
Madrid 28040, Spain

CONTENTS

FOREWORD

Thyroid hormones are very important for everyday's life since they control basal metabolic rate and oxygen consumption by the organism, but are still more important for the role they play in development of the central nervous system that is, in addition, an irreversible process. So all situations that could interfere with its normal function, and more specifically during the prenatal and immediately after birth periods, are extremely important.

The ebook entitled "Thyroid Toxicity" by Del Pino et al proposes a very interesting and practical approach to the most frequent substances that could play a role interfering on its physiological activity. The book starts explaining the physiology of the thyroid system, exerted through thyroid hormones (THs), which acting through nuclear receptors present a wide variety of functions affecting metabolism, growth and maturation.

Thyroid hormones are essential in early fetal life and immediately after birth to promote normal brain development. Two different periods can be separated in the process of brain differentiation. The first takes place during pregnancy in which the hormones of the mother are responsible for brain differentiation in the fetus and another postnatal period reaching two or three years of age in which the hormones of the baby play a very important role. These two periods are absolutely crucial for the normal neurological development of the child and if not enough hormones are available in this period the brain could be permanently affected. All the alterations that could appear in this time window are irreversible so any further treatment with thyroid hormones will not solve the neurological defects.

Thyroid hormones are also responsible for growth from very early in the fetal period until sexual maturation. Alterations on hormone levels through this period, on the contrary to the previous one, is reversible, thus if a 6 year old child starts being treated with the lacking hormones the situation could be recovered and the child would reach a normal stature.

Deficiencies and/or elevations in thyroid hormone levels may cause many clinical signs and symptoms, being the most important the deficiencies found in prenatal and immediately postnatal periods since they lead to mental retardation, low stature and in some cases also seizures and deafness. These alterations are irreversible, as mentioned before. During adult age, a slowing down of all the systems (nervous, cardiovascular, plasma lipids, *etc.*) can appear with the reduction of hormones or by the contrary an increase in neural processing together with tachycardia and diarrhea and a permanent feeling of high temperature can appear when an increase is present.

Thyroxin is one of the most frequently used drugs all over the world. Normally thyroid hormones are used in the treatment of hypothyroidism or goiter, but also cases of drug over-dosage have been reported (iatrogenic thyrotoxicosis). A special chapter of this book is focused on the prevalence, the consequences and the treatment of this complication when the hormone has been used for non-appropriate L-thyroxin treatment, like for obesity, or also following the ingestion of thyroid hormone contaminated beef with or after accidental thyroid hormones ingestion.

Endocrine disruptors (ED) are gaining notoriety for the havoc they wreak on human body systems. EDs may affect the well being of several populations thus, a reasonable information policy about their health effects is of socio-economic relevance. The safety of some food additives, pesticides and of some UV screens, should lead to political activities to direct the proper use of these compounds. Information made available to consumers will help them make balanced decisions about their risks of exposure to these chemicals. However, exposure to EDs is unavoidable.

ED's should be sorted according to their high production volume and to the different types of exposure to humans. In this regard, ED's may:

Pollute the environment and are taken up by humans via unwanted and unidentified incorporation through the air, through dermal contact or through the food chain. These are most of the "classical ED's". These ED's probably have effects in the brain, the cardiovascular system and the bone, and some of them might be exerted through interferences with the thyroid.

Be intentionally administered to humans, but unwillingly incorporated. To these group belong certain cosmetics. Some absorbers of ultraviolet (UV) light present in perfumes, nail lacquer, after shaving lotions or other compounds and used as stabilizers, have been shown to display estrogenic and limited antiandrogenic properties as well as thyroid influences.

Be deliberately and willingly administered to humans. Synthetic chemicals and plant-derived products included in some functional foods are eaten by humans in order to obtain some advantages. However, many of them exert not only estrogenic, but also antiestrogenic, antiandrogenic, antithyroidal and antiglucocorticoid activities. Furthermore, in this regard, flavonoids derived from soya interfere with thyroid hormone synthesis, release and binding to the transporter protein in the blood, i.e. transthyretin.

Several natural and synthetic compounds are known to interfere with thyroid hormone binding proteins in serum, thus modulating free hormone concentrations and disrupting thyroid hormone homeostasis. Among the EDs tested so far genistein, a major isoflavonoid of soy containing food products as well as some similar compounds as daidzein and glyceitin are potent inhibitors of thyroxine binding to transthyretin. Furthermore, another polyphenolic nutrient, xanthohumol, contained in hops and some beer products also interferes with thyroid hormone distribution and transport in serum leading to altered thyroid homeostasis, increased elimination of thyroid hormones by the urine and lead to goitrogenesis by depletion of thyroid hormone and iodine stores in the body. Thus natural compounds contained in our nutrition, specifically interfere with T4 binding to transthyretin, therefore shifting T4 to thyroglobulin (TBG) and albumin binding. As transthyretin has different distribution space and target tissues compared to TBG and albumin, EDs might alter thyroid hormone homeostasis and tissue availability.

Mutual interference of different hormone axes have been found, such as the steroid and thyroid hormone axis. Some EDs, active in the steroid axis, interfere with thyroid hormone related endpoints such as malic enzyme in the liver, which is an important information for future screening and testing programs on EDs in the hormone field. Thus many experiments already provide data for the necessary risk assessment with respect to multiorganic effects of EDs.

The focus of many studies about one important ED namely Polichlorinated Biphenils (PCBs) has been centered mainly on how the exposure to them is able to increase metabolic disorders not only in the offspring, but also in the mother. Very recently a paper has been published in which PCB congeners could activate the expression of an enzyme that altered the structure of other PCB molecules which in turn could activate the thyroid hormone receptor, a much unexpected situation. This was first observed in experimental animals, but then also in human placental tissue. In a subset of placentas, where no PCBs were detected, thyroid hormones correlated with thyroid response genes in the placenta, but when PCBs were present, this correlation did not existed: This is the paradigm of an endocrine disruptor.

A large number of compounds such as pesticides, drugs, heavy metals, cosmetics, industrial chemicals and natural compounds have been shown to also interfere with thyroid homeostasis by acting on different regulation points of thyroid hormone metabolism, binding to thyroid receptors or altering gene transcription regulated through thyroid hormones. There is special concern about thyroid disruptors because even small changes in thyroid homeostasis may adversely affect human health, especially during critical periods of vulnerability such as development, as has been mentioned before, but also during senescence or in sensitive population groups.

UV filters are high production volume chemicals used for protection of human skin as well as for protection of products (UV absorbers) against UV irradiation. As demonstrated by recent chemical-analytical studies (e.g., sewage treatment plants, lake water), UV filters are released into the environment in significant amounts. The endocrine activity demonstrated for some of these compounds thus raises important questions of human and environmental health on the one hand, and on technical and economic aspects on the other hand.

In view of the release of UV filters into the environment, such evaluations should not be limited only to human toxicity versus sun protection, but also include the environmental relevance. So far, only a fraction of the UV filters and UV absorbers used has been tested for endocrine activity, and only very few of them have been studied for long-term toxicity, the basis for risk assessment. Monitoring data are missing in humans and limited to a few isolated data in wildlife.

A major finding from these experiments has been the effects of UV-screens on the thyroid hormone axis. These effects are probably independent from their also demonstrated estrogenic action. As these compounds are contained not only in sunscreens and various cosmetics but also as UV protectants for various products of daily life, the potential negative effects need to be further studied not only in animal experiments and also specially their interference with the human thyroid hormone axis requires attention since, especially in children, it reaches relevant concentrations.

Regulatory agencies and policy should react to make sure that these substances may not be harmful to wildlife and humans.

The studies available were supposed to provide new information as to whether the UV screens and the topical application of the stabilizer present in many cosmetics might be harmful to human health since they exert (anti)estrogenic, (anti)androgenic, (anti)thyroidal, or (anti)adrenal effects on humans.

However, the prerequisite for such an effect would be the absorption of the substances through the skin. As it appears now OMC and 4-MBC do not penetrate in appreciable amounts through the skin when commercially available preparations were used. This was obviously not the case, but the evident accumulation in lakes, rivers or wastewater is also including additional concerns for human health.

Even if a sufficient safety margin should be found for human use of an individual chemical, the problem of environmental contamination, *i.e.*, contribution to the mixture of EDs, would remain.

Several groups have investigated thyroid hormone related endpoints, such as hepatic deiodinase activity in livers of rats treated for several generations with UV screens.

Livers from parent rats exposed to UV filters and their offspring of both genders were analysed for type I 5'deiodinase activities. Significant alterations after UV-screen exposure of rats, which are compatible with altered thyroid weights and altered serum thyroid hormone levels, were found as well as a second generation effect. Increasing doses of 4-MBC decreased hepatic type I 5'-deiodinase in males.

Several chapters deal with these problems and with other environmental exposures that are associated with thyroid dysfunction in subjects with autoimmune thyroid disease and some are clearly identified as inducing thyroid autoimmunity. These chapters give some clues to the understanding of the relationship between environment and the genetic background. This should help in identifying patients at risk and may provide therapeutic options for the future.

A specific group of pathogens, toxins and substances of biological origin, which may cause a disruption of the thyroid system either directly or indirectly through the systemic effects they induce, are called BSATs. The thyroiditis results in inflammation of the thyroid gland that can sometimes degenerate into destructive thyrotoxicosis. A chapter refers to the main agents that induce thyroid disruption and the known mechanisms through which these effects are induced.

The thyroid effects of some drugs, such as amiodarone and lithium have been known for many years, but novel antineoplastic agents introduced more recently have become the focus of intense attention over the past few years. The corresponding chapter summarizes our current knowledge on drugs capable of altering thyroid function or structure, with attention to the underlying mechanisms.

Metals such as Cd, Pb, Cr, Mn, Hg and Cu are known to induce thyroid toxicity in humans and animals. On the other hand, other metals are essential for the proper function of thyroid system such as Se, Zn and Fe among others, and their deficiency has been related to thyroid disruption. This is the subject of another interesting chapter of this book.

Experimental evidence has shown the ability of multiple pesticides to affect thyroid homeostasis. By interfering with the deiodination of TH leading to increased T3 degradation; or by binding to TH-binding proteins and thus altering circulating TH levels; it may mimic TH action or may also interfere with thyroid function.

Overall, experimental and epidemiological studies indicate that the induction of hypothyroidism is the general effect from pesticide exposure, supporting that this situation causes a decrease in TH activity. Given the important role of TH on metabolism and brain development, exposure to even low doses of thyroid-disrupting pesticides may contribute to increase the risk of thyroid disease and irreversible neurodevelopmental disorders.

The thyroid gland is almost unique since it can be affected by both external and internal radiation wherein administration of radioactive iodide specifically affects the thyroid gland. One of the chapters focus on both types of radiation and the changes that can be seen acutely and chronically in the thyroid after it has been subjected to irradiation. In addition, the neoplastic potential of radiation exposure on thyroid follicular epithelium is presented and illustrated.

Currently there is a significant increase in consumption of new types of foods called functional foods, especially soy, which could lead to a reduced availability of iodine and thus to goitrogenic effects. Also, the use of dietary supplements, which are widespread today, can cause thyrotoxicosis since some of them may contain fraudulently added active thyroid hormones in addition to minerals and dietary elements. Furthermore, plant supplements, which are consumed worldwide, may contain many components that could alter the normal functioning of the thyroid system due to their phytochemical components. Thus, the increasing use of plant supplements presents a particular challenge to health care of patients due to the high risk of potential interactions of these plants with thyroid function. For example high intake of plant foods from the Cruciferae family has been shown to induce goitrogenic effects in certain populations with reduced availability of iodine in their diet.

The metabolism of cyanogenic plants like cassava, sorghum, bamboo, lima bean, which are important sources of carbohydrates for many populations, releases thiocyanate that has been proved to have also goitrogenic properties.

Food additives used to preserve flavor or enhance taste and appearance could also induce disruption of the thyroid system. Nitrite and nitrate salts are added to cured meats such as bacon, sausage and ham to prevent the growth of bacteria spores and to add color and flavor. Nitrate salts are natural components of plants, found in high concentrations in leafy vegetables such as lettuce and spinach and in some root vegetables such as beets, and are also a contaminant in drinking water. Nitrate salts are of particular interest because they might cause thyroid cancer. Dye additive to foods such as erythrosine possess a negative effect on thyroid function in some cases.

Foods are composed of a variety of natural compounds with nutritional effects. However, some of them may also possess anti-nutritional and thyreotoxic effects, such as glucosinolates. Currently, functional foods have been incorporated as sources of nutrients to our diet in order to meet certain nutritional requirements. However, their effects on the thyroid gland are unknown and should be determined in order to perform a complete risk assessments of these foods. Food supplements, are another source of nutrients, especially minerals and trace elements such as iodine and zinc that are necessary for the proper functioning of the thyroid gland, but if its use is not controlled, it might induce thyroid alterations. Finally, during food processing different chemical compounds such as nitrates and erythrosine can be used, which could also induce harmful effects on the thyroid. A special chapter discusses the different foods and supplements.

Some natural flavonoids are known to inhibit TPO activity, the key enzyme for thyroglobulin iodination and iodothyronine coupling in thyroid hormone synthesis. A model of stable expression of human TPO in a human thyroid carcinoma cell line FTC-133 has been established, which allows functional analysis of TPO activity. Using enzymatic active membrane preparations of these TPO expressing cells the effects of ED on TPO inhibition has been analyzed. Several of the EDs concentration dependently inhibited TPO. An important novel observation is that iodide can prevent inactivation of TPO by EDs. This might have major implications with respect to EDs exposure, as many regions of Europe and the whole work still have inadequate iodide supply and intake, which might increase the risk of EDs exposure with respect to inhibition of TPO, the key enzyme of thyroid hormone biosynthesis. These observations might again have relevance in our societies, where soy intake increases and might interfere with availability of adequate thyroid hormone supply.

Taken together the book is a very interesting piece of evidence, that we are surrounded by a high amount of substances that may interfere among others with thyroid function, and that this interference could be responsible for a number of possible alterations of our normal functions since the thyroid gland plays a very important role in keeping a normal function of our body.

Jesus A.F. Tresguerres
Professor of Physiology and Endocrinology
Medical School
University Complutense Madrid
Spain

PREFACE

Thyroid hormones are involved in numerous physiological processes as regulators of metabolism, bone remodeling, cardiac function and mental status. Moreover, thyroid hormones are of special importance in fetal development, more particularly, the development of the brain. Thus, maintenance of normal thyroid functioning is essential for psychological, biochemical, immunological, endocrinal and physiological wellbeing of the body as well as correct development. To our knowledge this ebook is the first monograph on thyroid toxicity. Thyroid Toxicity gathers all information about the toxic effects of different kind of compounds on thyroid system and the molecular mechanisms through which they induced these effects.

This e-book answers various important questions such as the mechanism through which various compounds induce toxicity on thyroid gland, induce endocrine disruption and especially how they affect body and brain development and brain function. Aside from learning key concepts that may be overlooked while scanning literature, the reader will benefit from gems of information scattered throughout the book.

Javier Del Pino
Toxicology and Pharmacology Department,
Veterinary School,
Complutense University of Madrid,
Ciudad Universitaria s/n,
Madrid
Spain

CONTRIBUTORS

Alberto Cique Moya	Enviromental Health and NBQ Service, Instituto de Medicina Preventiva de la Defensa, Ministerio de Defensa, Madrid, Spain.
Carmen Freire	National School of Public Health, Oswaldo Cruz Foundation (FIOCRUZ), Rio de Janeiro, Brazil; University of Granada, Granada, Spain; Biomedical Research Centre Network for Epidemiology and Public Health (CIBERESP), Spain.
Giuseppe Barbesino	Thyroid Unit, Massachusetts General Hospital, Harvard Medical School. Harvard University, Boston, MA, USA.
Immacolata Cristina Nettore	Department of Molecular and Clinical Endocrinology and Oncology, University of Naples Federico II, Naples, Italy.
Javier Del Pino	Toxicology and Pharmacology Department, Veterinary School, Complutense University of Madrid, Spain.
Jimena Garcia Lobo	Pharmacology Department, Health Sciences School, Alfonso X University, Madrid, Spain.
Margarita Lobo Alonso	Toxicology and Pharmacology Department, Veterinary School, Complutense University of Madrid, Spain.
Maria Jesus Diaz Plaza	Toxicology and Pharmacology Department, Veterinary School, Complutense University of Madrid, Spain.
Maria Jose Anadon Baselga	Toxicology and Legal Medicine Department, Medicine School, Complutense University of Madrid, Spain.
Maria Teresa Frejo Moya	Toxicology and Pharmacology Department, Veterinary School, Complutense University of Madrid, Spain.
Marjorie Safran	Department of Medicine, Division of Endocrinology, University of Massachusetts Health Center, Worcester, MA, USA.
Miguel Andres Capo Marti	Toxicology and Pharmacology Department, Veterinary School, Complutense University of Madrid, Spain.
Paolo Emidio Macchia	Department of Molecular and Clinical Endocrinology and Oncology, University of Naples Federico II, Naples, Italy.
Paula Moyano Cires	Toxicology and Legal Medicine Department, Medicine School, Complutense University of Madrid, Spain.
Virginia A. LiVolsi	Department of Pathology & Laboratory Medicine, University of Pennsylvania, Perelman School of Medicine, Philadelphia, PA, USA.
Zubair W. Baloch	Department of Pathology & Laboratory Medicine, University of Pennsylvania, Perelman School of Medicine, Philadelphia, PA, USA.

Thyroid Toxicity

First published in 2016.

Editors: Javier Del Pino, Maria Jesus Diaz and
Maria Teresa Frejo

ISBN (eBook): 978-1-68108-221-9

ISBN (Print): 978-1-68108-222-6

BENTHAM SCIENCE Bentham eBooks

CHAPTER 1

The Thyroid System

Javier Del Pino[1,*], Paula Moyano[2] and María Teresa Frejo[1]

[1]Departament of Toxicology and Pharmacology, Veterinary School, Complutense University of Madrid, Madrid, Spain and [2]Departament of Toxicology and Legal Medicine, Medical School, Complutense University of Madrid, Madrid, Spain

Abstract: The thyroid gland, one of the largest endocrine glands in the body, synthesizes thyroid hormones (THs), which present a wide variety of functions affecting metabolism, growth and maturation, and other organ-specific effects. From a metabolic perspective, thyroid hormones increase oxygen consumption and heat generation. Moreover, they increase protein catabolism, promote gluconeogenesis, increase utilization of glucose and promote lipid metabolism. With regard to other organ-specific effects, thyroid hormones influence cardiac function by increasing heart rate, myocardial contractility, blood volume, and cardiac output while decreasing peripheral vascular volume. They stimulate the production of cytokines, growth factors and other factors to stimulate bone development and growth. In addition, thyroid hormones also promote increased motility in the gastrointestinal system and increase adrenergic activity and sensitivity in the central nervous system. Because they also promote cell differentiation, growth and maturation, thyroid hormones are essential in early fetal life to promote normal growth and brain development. Deficiencies and elevations in thyroid hormone levels may cause many clinical signs and symptoms. This chapter discusses the anatomy and physiology of the thyroid gland and the thyroid disorders that could be induced, especially, by toxic substances.

Keywords: Hyperthyroidism, hypothyroidism, thyroid functions, thyroid gland, toxicity.

INTRODUCTION

The discovery of the thyroid gland, and elucidation of its structure, action and pathologies have been developed by different researchers, mainly in the 19th and 20th centuries. However, mention to the thyroid gland and its diseases can be found in documents of ancient Greek, Indian and Egyptian medicine [1].

Goiter has always been a disease of great appeal to the general population because of its extended prevalence. Mentions to goiter have been found in documents

*Corresponding author Javier Del Pino: Department of Toxicology and Pharmacology, Complutense University of Madrid, Madrid, Spain; E-mail: jdelpino@pdi.ucm.es

Javier Del Pino, Maria Jesus Diaz and Maria Teresa Frejo (Eds)

dating from 2700 B.C. [2]. In Indian Ayurvedic medicine (1400 B.C.), goiter was described in detail and was called 'galaganda'. This type of medicine classified thyroid diseases into three types; "Vataja (hyperthyroidism), Kaphaja (hypothyroidism) and Medaja (thyroidal cyst)" and described their symptoms [1].

The thyroid gland gets its name from the Greek word "θυρεοειδής", or shield-shaped, due to its lobed shape similar to a shield. This term was described by Galen between 130-200 B.C. [3]. One of the first descriptions of the thyroid gland in Greek medicine was given by Hippocrates and Plato, who characterized it. They reported that this gland has a spongy nature and is accountable for lubricating the respiratory tract. However, Galen asserted that the spongy constitution of this gland was more fitted for absorption rather than secretion [1].

Surgical treatment of goiter was first described in the 6th century by Aetius [4]. Later, Roger Frugardi in 1170 described the surgical procedure to treat goiter, though it was a dangerous procedure with extremely high mortality rates. However, in the 19th century, due to advances in anesthesia, antisepsis and in controlling hemostasis, mortality rates were reduced. Surgeries performed by CA Theodor Billroth (1829-1894) and Theodor Kocher (1841-1917) were successful [5].

Leonardo Da Vinci depicted the thyroid gland in 1511 during his anatomical research, and although he knew its exact anatomical constitution, he could not comprehend its role and postulated that it was formed to fill the gap between muscles of the neck and to keep the trachea away from the sternum [1, 5].

In 1656, Thomas Wharton found the exact anatomical organization of the thyroid gland and showed that secretion is the gland's primary function. He described that the thyroid gland was responsible for heating the thyroid cartilage, which is normally cold due to its superficial position, lubricating the neck and to giving shape and grace to the neck [1, 5]. Later, Morgagni, reported the two lobes and isthmus of the thyroid gland, and Thomas Wilkinson King, in 1833, described the thyroid colloid, and its importance [1].

The first person to use iodine as a treatment for goiter was Coindet of Geneva, who successfully prescribed hydriodate of potash or 'tincture of iodine'. In 1833, Boussingault recommended salt iodization to prevent goiter. Chatin found in 1850 that iodine treatment may be used to prevent endemic goiter and cretinism. He associated these diseases with iodine deficit, and suggested iodine supplementation in drinking water, using mineral water springs. He proved in 1835 that salt sent from goiter-free regions to regions with endemic goiter decreased the incidence of goiter. David Marine found in 1907 that iodine is necessary for thyroid function [1].

In 1896 Bauman showed the presence of iodine in the gland and in 1914 Kendall isolated and crystallized thyroxine (T4), the first hormone that could be purified and chemically synthesized in 1927 by Harington and Barger [1].

With the use of radioactive iodine isotopes, the presence of triiodothyronine (T3) in the gland and extrathyroidal tissues was demonstrated by Gross and Pitt-Rivers, and Roche, Michel and Lissitzky in 1952. They showed not only that T3 is formed directly in the gland, but also outside of it as a metabolite of T4, and that T3 was probably the most active form intracellularly [5].

Recently, thanks to advances in molecular biology, progress has been made in understanding the interaction between thyroid hormones (THs) and their cellular receptors as well as the consequences of these interactions in organs, systems and the whole organism [5].

THYROID GLAND

The thyroid gland, one of the largest endocrine glands in the body, is located underneath the larynx and anterior to the upper part of the trachea. It is an odd and asymmetric gland that consists of two lateral lobes connected by a narrow band of thyroid tissue called the isthmus that overlies the region from the second to fourth tracheal cartilages (Fig. **1**) [6-8].

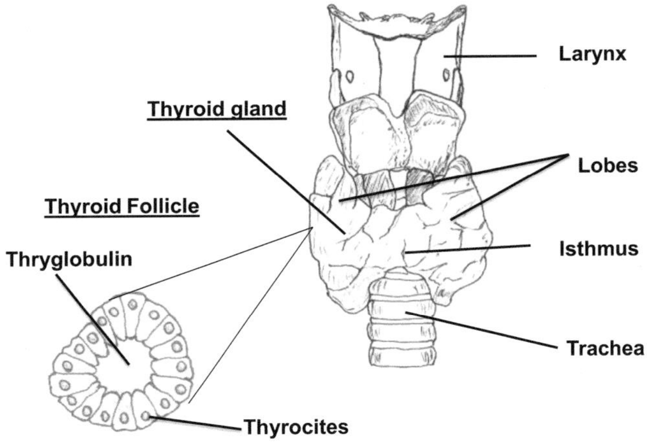

Figure 1: Thyroid grand and follicle.

The thyroid gland is highly vascularized and innervated. It is irrigated by two superior thyroid arteries that arise from the branches of the external carotid artery, each one of which provides three branches to the thyroid gland (inter, extern and posterior) and by two inferior thyroid arteries that come from the thyrocervical trunk, each one of them providing three branches to the thyroid gland (inferior, posterior and deep). In addition, sometimes there is a middle or Neubauer thyroid artery that arises from the aorta or the innominate artery. From the gland the veins form a plexus from which three groups of veins arise; the first one is the superior vein, which serves as tributary to the internal jugular vein directly or by draining into the thyrolinguofacial trunk. In the second group, the inferior thyroid veins drain into the internal jugulars and into the brachiocephalic trunk. In the third group, the medial thyroid veins drain into the internal jugular. The lymphatic vessels, around the thyroid gland form a thyroidal plexus. The descendent lymphatic vessels separate from it, ending in ganglia situated in front of the trachea and above the thymus, and the ascendant lymphatic vessels that end in prelaryngeal nodes, and in part in the lateral neck nodes. Finally, the innervation of the thyroid gland comes both from the simpatico cervical nerves and from the superior recurrent laryngeal nerves [9, 10].

The lobes of the thyroid are integrated by follicles of varying size (20-250 μm) that are the functional units of the thyroid gland. They are empty, spherical structures that contain a substance called colloid produced by the thyrocytes, the major constituent of which is a large glycoprotein called thyroglobulin. The follicular cells are cuboidal to low columnar (under conditions of normal iodine intake) and their secretory polarity is directed toward the lumen of the follicles. An extensive grid of interfollicular capillaries procures the follicular cells with a rich blood supply. Follicular cells have extensive sections of rough endoplasmic reticulum and a large Golgi apparatus in their cytoplasm for synthesis and packaging of substantial amounts of proteins (*e.g.*, thyroglobulin) that are then transported into the follicular lumen. The interface between the luminal side of the follicular cells and the colloid is changed by several microvillus projections [6, 9].

The thyroid gland secretes two major hormones, T4 and T3, of which T4 is more abundant, but T3 is the most potent and is considered to be the principal thyroid hormone. Thyroid hormones are required for the normal performance of a variety of physiological actions affecting virtually every organ system in the body. Regulation of thyroid hormone secretion occurs through the hypothalamic-pituitary-thyroid (HPT) axis. Unlike other endocrine glands, which secrete their hormones once they are produced, the thyroid gland stores considerable amounts of the thyroid hormones in the colloid until the body needs them. Deficiency of thyroid hormones, caused by a variety of conditions, results in many pathophysiological processes, some of which have potentially serious outcomes if they are not treated [6, 7, 11].

THYROID SYSTEM DEVELOPMENT

The first endocrine gland to arisen in embryonic development is the thyroid gland. The development of a functional thyroid system depends on the embryogenesis, differentiation and maturation of the thyroid gland, together with the development of the HPT axis and thyroid hormone metabolism, which results in the regulation of TH function, production, and secretion [12].

Fetal thyroid maturation can be divided into two phases (Fig. **2**). The first one takes place during the first trimester of gestation, in which anatomic development and embryogenesis of the HPT axis occurs. The maturation of the HPT axis, which includes hormone production and control, takes place in the second phase [6]. The human thyroid gland begins to develop in the third week of gestation [13]. Around 24 days after insemination, the thyroid gland starts to emerge from a little solid mass of endoderm, which forms a thickened pouch known as the thyroid primordium, situated in the floor of the primordial pharynx and at the end of the foramen cecum. As the embryo grows, the developing thyroid gland descends through the tissues of the neck, but persist united to the foramen cecum by a small tube named the thyroglossal duct, which degenerates and withdraws by the seventh week of gestation. By gestation day (GD) 45-50, the thyroid gland tissues arise and relocate to their final location, covering both sides of the lower portion of the larynx and the upper portion of the trachea [6, 10, 13, 14].

From GD 70, the thyroid gland is both functional and mature. By the end of the first trimester, when histological differentiation of the thyroid and pituitary glands has taken place, both T4 and thyroid stimulating hormone (TSH) can be determined in fetal tissue, iodine can be concentrated and T4 can be synthesized by the thyroid gland, and the pituitary tissue can synthesize TSH [6, 15-17]. From GD 29 in thyroid follicle cells and after maturation of thyroid follicle cells, thyroglobulin (TBG), the precursor protein upon which thyroid hormones are synthetized and stored, is present [18]. Fetal serum TBG levels are detected from gestation week 11, and increase until birth [19]. Albumin is the quantitatively most significant T4-binding protein in the first trimester, and further increasing levels of albumin have an impact on T4 binding until gestation week 41 [20].

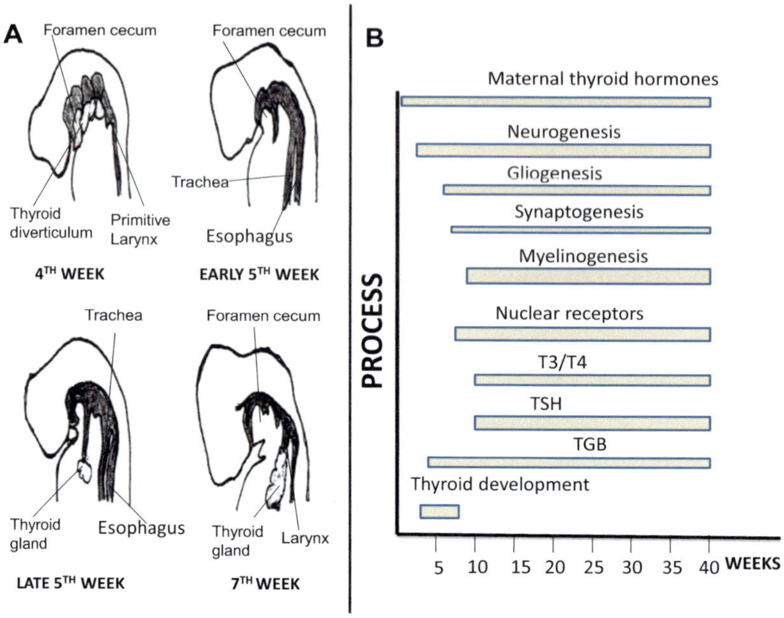

Figure 2: Thyroid development. A) Thyroid development from 4th to 7th week. B) Timeline of human thyroid system and brain development from conception to birth. Adapted from Kirsten [6] and from Howdeshell [13].

The fetal HPT axis is structurally complete at the end of the first trimester, and its maturation continues into the second trimester [6]. Before reaching 18 weeks of pregnancy, the HPT axis is relatively inactive and fetal thyroid hormone production is low. However, during the second half of gestation, the HPT endocrine pathway starts to be functional under the influence of increasing serum TSH levels, and generates increasing amounts of T3 and T4 [21]. Therefore, initial growth and development of the thyroid seems to be independent of TSH, as TSH secretion can only be measured after 10-12 weeks of gestation [20, 22]. Fetal serum TSH levels increase gradually, so that at 40 weeks of pregnancy, they are higher than adult levels [6, 15]. In contrast, fetal T3 levels are non-detectable or rather low until gestation week 20 and are lower at term than adult values, due to placental and hepatic inner-ring deiodination of T4 to reverse T3 [12, 23]. Increased TH synthesis is due, partly, to an increase in thyroid gland follicular cell uptake of iodide after gestation weeks 18-20 and subsequent maturation of the HPT axis. The auto-regulation of iodide uptake by the fetal thyroid gland develops during weeks of gestation 36-40 [14]. After delivery, there is a spectacular increase in the potential of the liver to convert T4 to T3 that results in a significant increase in T3 levels. A gradual increase in T4 also takes place, reaching adults levels at 36 weeks pregnancy [6, 24].

Fetal HPT axis development is independent of the maternal axis. In this regard, the placenta is not only impermeable to TSH, but poses a barrier to the THs that limits T4 and T3 transfers from the mother to the fetus [6]. Moreover, although both thyrotropin-releasing hormone (TRH) and iodine freely cross the placenta, maternal TRH has little effect on the fetal HPT system since there is very little TRH in maternal circulation and most of it is degraded within the placenta. Fetal TRH levels are high due to increased synthesis of TRH by the placenta and selected fetal tissues, specifically the pancreas. The placenta is also penetrable to antithyroid drugs that can disrupt fetal and neonatal thyroid function [6, 21].

There is growing data showing that THs act on embryological and fetal tissues early in development. Thyroid hormones and associated receptors are already found in human fetal tissues prior to the synthesis and secretion of fetal THs [22, 25]. During the first trimester, an adequate supply of maternal THs must be sustained to ensure normal development, as evidenced by impaired psychomotor development and visuospatial processing in offspring born to mothers with low serum levels of free T4 [12]. Also, deiodinase enzymes are expressed in the early brain before the thyroid gland develops to tightly control T3 levels [17].

BIOLOGICAL FUNCTIONS

Thyroid hormones are regulators of development, metabolism, and other organ-specific effects (Fig. **3**) [26]. From a metabolic perspective, they increase basal metabolic rate (BMR) and regulate thermogenesis [26]. BMR, which is defined as the measure of oxygen consumption during rest [6], is the primary source of energy expenditure in humans, and reductions in it can result in obesity and weight gain [27]. THs stimulate BMR by increasing adenosine triphosphate (ATP) production and by generating and maintaining ion gradients, which leads to an increase in oxygen consumption and heat production [28-30]. The Na^+/K^+ gradient across the cell membrane and the Ca^{2+} gradient between the cytoplasm and sarcoplasmic reticulum are altered by THs. This alteration requires ATP consumption to maintain the gradient [29, 31, 32]. THs maintain BMR by uncoupling oxidative phosphorylation in mitochondria [29], or decreasing the activity of transport molecules that introduce reducing equivalents into the mitochondria [33, 34]. THs also stimulate metabolic cycles involving fat, glucose, and protein catabolism and anabolism, but these are small contributions to BMR [29].

Thyroid hormones regulate plasma glucose levels, insulin sensitivity, and carbohydrate metabolism through their actions in the liver, white adipose tissue, skeletal muscle, and pancreas [35]. THs increase glycolysis, gluconeogenesis, glucose absorption from the intestine and the use of glucose by the cells [6]. In this regard, T3 treatment has been reported to induce an increase in genes that regulate glycogenolysis and gluconeogenesis in liver [36]. Moreover, treatment with T4 has been observed to increase alanine transport into hepatocytes, increasing production of metabolic intermediates of the gluconeogenic pathway and finally conversion of alanine into glucose [29].

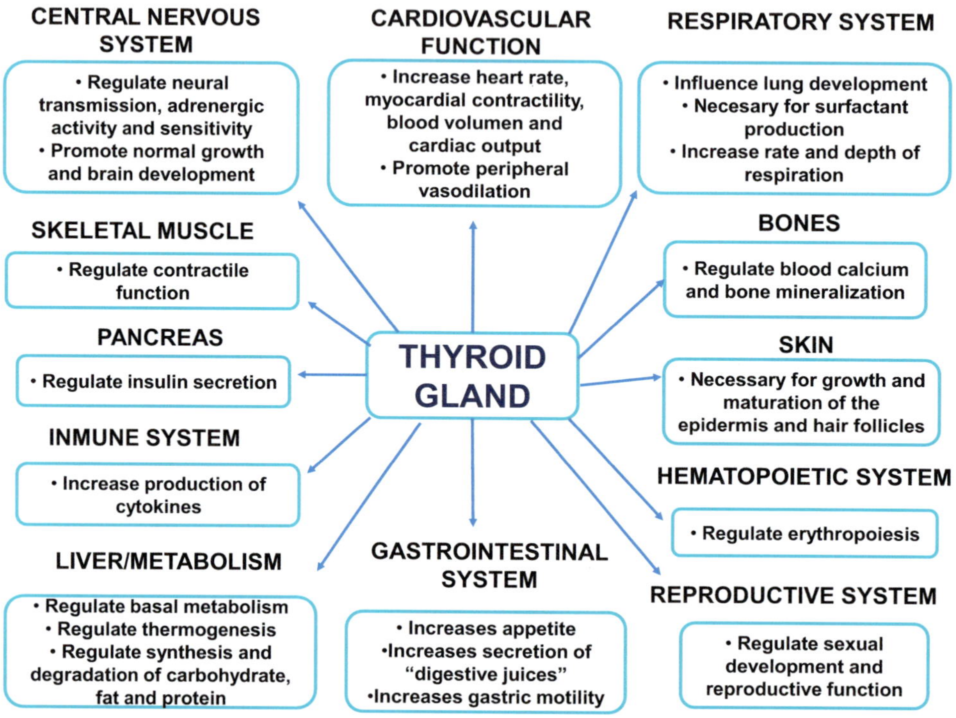

Figure 3: Main biological functions of thyroid hormones [6].

Lipid metabolism is regulated by THs through liver-specific actions of T3, TRβ, and nuclear hormone receptor crosstalk. THs stimulate both lipogenesis and lipolysis, although when their levels are increased, the net effect is fat loss [37]. In addition, THs regulate cholesterol synthesis through multiple mechanisms. THs increase uptake of cholesterol [38], which has been reported to be a major pathway of T4-mediated cholesterol lowering after T4 treatment of patients with hypothyroidism [39]. In addition, THs also reduce cholesterol through non-LDL receptor-mediated pathways [40].

Calcium and water balance are also influenced by THs. Hypercalcemia occurs and water is kept in the extracellular compartments in hypothyroid conditions, while in hyperthyroidism urinary and fecal calcium excretion are promoted. Moreover, bone demineralization takes place, and there is an efflux of calcium from the bones, which results in elevated serum ionized calcium and phosphate levels and decreased circulating levels of 1,25-dihydroxyvitamin D. These effects lead to decreased intestinal calcium absorption and a negative calcium balance [6].

In addition, an association between weight and thyroid status has been reported. In this regard, a positive association between serum TSH levels and body weight change in both men and women has been found [41, 42]. Moreover, given the influence of central regulation of THs on orexigenic neuropeptides [43], variable control of the HPT axis with altered leptin levels also could be liable for this metabolic irregularity [29]. Furthermore, it has been shown that T3 or T4 treatment of hypothyroid patients produced significant weight loss and reduction in total cholesterol and apolipoprotein B, only with T3 treatment [44].

With regard to other organ-specific effects, thyroid hormones influence cardiac function by increasing heart rate, myocardial contractility, blood volume, and cardiac output while decreasing peripheral vascular volume [26]. Skeletal muscle has been reported to be a thyroid hormone target for contractile function, recovery, and transport as well as for metabolism and glucose disposition [45, 46]. Thyroid hormone stimulation induces transition to fast-twitch fibers and transition to a faster myosin heavy chain (MHC) configuration. Moreover, THs have been described to stimulate the production of cytokines, growth factors and other factors to stimulate bone development and growth [26]. Thyroid hormones also promote increased motility in the gastrointestinal system and increase neural transmission and synaptic plasticity [6, 47].

THs are essential for normal growth and development. Body development, bone development and maturation, and tooth development and eruption are all under the control of THs. Skeletal development takes place through the combined action between THs and growth hormone, somatomedin, and other growth factors. THs also regulate bone formation indirectly through actions on the pituitary gland. Ossification and fusion of the cartilaginous growth plates lead to bone maturation and are also dependent on THs [6]. In addition, THs are required for normal brain development [48, 49]. In the nervous system, THs regulate cell migration and differentiation of neurons, oligodendrocytes, astrocytes and microglia [48, 50].

Finally, there is evidence that THs influence sexual development, reproductive role and correlated molecular mechanisms and pathways [51]. In this regard, THs influence the synthesis and function of sex steroid hormones, but this interaction is bi-directional, resulting in the tight regulation of these effects [51]. During development, THs have been reported to be necessary for regular gonadal development and the production of normal sex ratios in different species. However, due to the contradictory results in these data commented above, further studies are required to clearly determine the effect of THs in gonadal differentiation.

THYROID PATHOLOGY

Thyroid hormones present a wide range of functions, thus their deficiencies and elevations may cause many clinical signs and symptoms. Depending on the severity of the disease, the signs and symptoms may be absent or fully developed [26, 52].

Thyroid disorders can be divided into two types depending on pathological lesions. The first type is diffuse thyroid lesions, which are associated with non-neoplastic disorders affecting the gland (hyperplasia and thyroiditis). The other type is nodular lesions which integrate those disorders that consist of neoplastic hyperplasia as well as benign and malignant tumors [9].

Thyroid disorders can be also classified depending on the effect on thyroid hormone levels. Hyperthyroidism occurs when there is an overproduction of THs and hypothyroidism results when there is an under production. These disorders are further categorized by the endocrine gland causing the disorder, being further classified as primary, secondary, or tertiary. Diseases categorized as primary arise from a disorder within the thyroid gland, while those categorized as secondary or tertiary arise from damage to the pituitary and hypothalamus gland, respectively [26].

Disorders of the thyroid gland mainly include hypothyroidism, hyperthyroidism and euthyroid sick syndrome. In addition, due to recent advances in highly sensitive assays for detecting TSH, disorders may also be categorized as overt or subclinical. Subclinical disorders are identified before the signs and symptoms appear in the patient and before thyroid hormone levels are abnormal. The only abnormality seen in subclinical disorders is an alteration in TSH values. TH levels will be normal in these cases. Overt cases present with clinical signs and symptoms and abnormalities in TSH and TH levels [26, 53].

Euthyroid Sick Syndrome

'Sick euthyroid syndrome' or 'non-thyroidal illness syndrome' (NTIS) is characterized by decreased serum T3 and T4 concentrations, increased serum reverse T3 (rT3) concentrations and unaltered or inappropriately low serum TSH, indicating profoundly altered negative feedback in the pituitary and hypothalamus, but absence of thyroid disease symptoms (Docter *et al.* 1993) [54]. This alteration is particularly common in hospitalized patients and is often due to alterations in the concentration of hormone binding proteins, the actions of certain drugs, effects of non-thyroidal illnesses, or peripheral resistance to THs. The thyroid laboratory parameter appears to return to normal after patients recover from these illnesses. Therefore, assessments of thyroid status should be performed when illnesses subside, unless deemed necessary for a patient outcome [26].

The ultimate effects of the observed changes in local TH metabolism on tissue function during illness are currently unknown. However, the common view is that while changes observed during the acute phase of illness are beneficial they may become deleterious during prolonged critical illness, making the stage and severity of illness a major determinant of NTIS [26, 54].

Hyperthyroidism

Hyperthyroidism occurs when there is an excessive production of thyroid hormones and may be caused by a variety of conditions. The term thyrotoxicosis is used to describe the clinical state of high thyroid hormone concentrations. The most common cause of hyperthyroidism (thyrotoxicosis) is Grave's disease (70%-80%). Grave's disease represents an autoimmune disorder where the antibodies produced are directed against the TSH receptors in the thyroid gland causing an overproduction of T3 and T4. Grave's disease has a low prevalence rate in the population (0.3%-0.6%) and occurs more frequently in women. Thyroiditis, which causes transient hyperthyroidism as a result of the release of stored THs, multinodular goiter and thyroid adenoma are the other most common causes of hyperthyroidism. The other causes only represent 5%-8% of the cases and it is very uncommon for it to be due to the xenobiotic exposure [9, 55].

When hyperthyroidism is overtly expressed, signs and symptoms will likely be presented in conjunction with decreased TSH and increased T3 and T4 concentrations. In cases of subclinical hyperthyroidism, thyroid hormones are in the normal range, and only the TSH level is abnormal. Treatment for hyperthyroidism may involve the use of antithyroid drugs to inhibit the production of thyroid hormones or surgical thyroidectomy or radioactive iodine to reduce the hyper-functioning thyroid tissue [26, 56].

Typically, hyperthyroid patients suffer from nervousness, anxiety, irritability, mood swings, talk rapidly, and are gaunt and restless. Moreover, they present heat intolerance, sweating, palpitations, insomnia and warm fine skin. Prominent eyes or a stare may also be present. Hyperthyroidism causes an acceleration of general activity. This condition makes the heart beat much faster (tachycardia), which could lead to arrhythmias, especially in the elderly. In addition, an increase in the blood pressure and decreased peripheral vascular resistance are also common [9, 55].

The increase in THs produces an increase in the BMR and heat production. Patients tend to eat more, but often lose weight. Apart from fat loss, patients often lose muscle mass. Both glucose absorption and production are increased as well as insulin release, but hyperthyroidism impairs glucose tolerance. Both the synthesis and clearance of cholesterol and triglycerides are increased, with the latter predominating [57, 58].

Gastrointestinal motility is increased and absorption of nutrients is decreased. These effects together with the increased food intake could lead to diarrhea. In addition, dyspnea is also observed due to the increase in the BMR, CO_2 production, increased sensibility to hypoxemia and hypercapnia. Hyperthyroidism increases red blood cell mass, but the increase in the plasma volume could induce pseudoanemia. Moreover, due to the malabsorption of nutrients, it could also induce anemia due to vitamin B_9 or B_{12} deficiency [9, 55].

Calcium metabolism is affected reducing intestinal abortion and increasing urinary elimination. Bone resorption is increased, which increases calcium blood levels. In this regard, hyperthyroidism could induce osteoporosis. Neuromuscular effects, with muscle weakness, fatigue and hyperactive tendon reflexes with both accelerated contraction and relaxation phases are present in hyperthyroidism [9, 55].

Hypothyroidism

Hypothyroidism occurs when there are insufficient thyroid hormones available to the tissues. The majority of hypothyroid cases are primary (99%), meaning that they arise from a disorder of the thyroid gland itself such as conditions or treatments that destroy thyroid tissue or interfere with thyroid hormone production. To a much lesser extent they may be due to pituitary and/or hypothalamic disease that results in TSH and/or TRH deficiencies. Hypothyroidism could also be produced by a deficiency in T4 conversion to T3 or peripheral resistance to THs. Approximately 2%-15% of the population is afflicted with this disorder and it carries a gender bias seen more frequently in women [9, 52, 55, 59].

The main cause of hypothyroidism is a diet deficient in iodine, especially in developing countries. Autoimmune hypothyroidism is the most common cause of hypothyroidism in the adult, the incidence being higher in the elderly and women. Autoimmune thyroiditis, also known as Hashimoto's thyroiditis, is the most prevalent cause of autoimmune hypothyroidism in iodine-sufficient areas. Hashimoto's thyroiditis is caused by the autoimmune destruction of thyroid tissue leading to thyroid gland inflammation and reduced thyroid hormone production. Because this disorder is autoimmune in nature, it frequently occurs with other diseases that are also immune in nature and often presents with circulating antithyroid antibodies. Other possible causes of primary hypothyroidism are thyroid ablation or xenobiotic exposure to drugs, pesticides, cosmetics and industrial chemicals, among others. The main causes of secondary hypothyroidism are tumors, traumas, infiltrative processes and xenobiotic exposure, among others. Finally the main causes of tertiary hypothyroidism are craniopharyngioma, surgery and radiotherapy, among others [9, 55, 59-61].

When the disorder is overtly expressed, signs and symptoms will likely be presented in conjunction with elevated TSH and decreased T3 and T4 concentrations. In cases of subclinical hypothyroidism, signs and symptoms are not present, THs are in the normal range, and only the TSH level is abnormal. Treatment of patients with hypothyroidism involves oral replacement through the drug levothyroxine. Oral replacement of THs will reverse the laboratory finding and clinical signs and symptoms [26, 52].

An additional cause of hypothyroidism is neonatal hypothyroidism, also known as congenital hypothyroidism or cretinism. This disorder affects infants from birth and results from the complete absence of the thyroid gland (athyreosis) or it is secondary to defects in thyroid hormone synthesis. This disorder occurs in approximately 1 in 3500-4000 live births and if left untreated can lead to profound mental retardation [26].

Hypothyroidism slows the functional activities of the organism. Some symptoms of this condition are tiredness, fatigue, weight gain, drowsiness, decreased intestinal activity and constipation, increased extreme sensitivity to cold, swollen face, eyes and skin, brittle and thin nails and hair. Hypothyroidism is correlated with hypometabolism defined by diminished resting energy expenditure, weight gain, increased cholesterol values, reduced lipolysis, and lessened gluconeogenesis. Hypothyroidism is associated with non-alcoholic fatty liver disease (NAFLD) characterized by steatosis. In fact, increased TSH levels in hypothyroidism have been correlated with the grade of steatosis [9, 45, 62, 63].

Thyroid hormone deficiency also results in a decrease of blood pressure and could cause bradycardia, reduced systolic contractility, prolonged ventricular diastolic relaxation and increased systemic vascular resistance. Therefore, it produces a reduction of blood supply to the tissues. Other cardiac manifestations may include heart block, pericarditis, pericardial effusion, and rare cardiac tamponade. If hypothyroidism is not treated, it can cause heart failure [9, 55, 64, 65].

It also promotes weight gain and water retention, increases calcium absorption, mild anemia, decreases bone turnover, and prolongs the bone remodeling cycle, induces gastrointestinal dysfunction with constipation and decreased gut motility. The hypothyroid skin is generally pale with a tinge of yellowish discoloration accompanied with edema, most marked around the eyes and hands [9, 55].

In addition, hypothyroidism is usually associated with neuromuscular symptoms like stiffness, spams, bradykinesia, muscle weakness, cramps, aches and paresthesia. The more commonly affected nerves are the median nerve and cranial nerves II, V, VII and VIII. At the level of central nervous system, it could induce lethargy, depression, occasionally reversible dementia, memory impairment without other evidence of intellectual deficits. Cerebellar ataxia could also occur with gait disturbance, intention tremors and poor coordination [9, 55].

Deficits in THs all along the gestation and initial development can lead to cognitive damage and deep mental retardation in humans and other mammals. In hypothyroid subjects, cerebral and cerebellar growth and nerve myelination are seriously retarded. Overall, brain dimension and vascularity are diminished. During infancy, a lack or deficit of THs is devastating and leads to permanent, irreversible mental retardation, even when treated later in childhood. Moreover, a deficiency of THs after three to four years of life leads to retarded skeletal and bone maturation as well as retarded eruption of permanent teeth. Representatively, these children have immature skeletal proportions and facial features, and there is a reduction in epiphyseal growth and bone mineralization that results in the radiographic discovering of dysgenesis of the ossifying epiphyseal centers of the bone. It also produces sexual maturation delay in both genders [26, 66].

CONCLUDING REMARKS

The thyroid gland is a complex endocrine organ that has diverse functions and control over multiple organ systems and processes. It functions through an elaborate connection between the hypothalamus, pituitary, and the thyroid gland to maintain normal levels of circulating hormones. High and low levels of thyroid hormones can lead to abnormalities such as hypo- and hyperthyroidism that arise from a variety of causes with homeostasis impairment or developmental effects.

The population is exposed to many substances such as drugs, pesticides, metals, industrial chemicals, natural or novel foods among others that could alter the thyroid system. The vast majority of these compounds induce hypothyroidism and a very few induce hyperthyroidism and even less of those induce subclinical alterations. Therefore, it is important to determine the effect on the thyroid system of these substance and their combinations, especially for those that produce hypothyroidism, in order to prevent the occurrence of these thyroid diseases through exposure.

CONFLICT OF INTEREST

The author confirms that author has no conflict of interest to declare for this publication.

ACKNOWLEDGEMENTS

Declared None.

REFERENCES

[1] Niazi AK, Kalra S, Irfan A, Islam A. Thyroidology over the ages. Indian J Endocrinol Metab 2011; 15(Suppl 2): 2230-8210.
[2] Langer P. History of goiter. In: Endemic Goiter. Vol 44. Geneva: WHO; 1960. pp. 9.
[3] Brunicardi FC, Schwartz SI. Schwartz´s principles of surgery 8 Ed. McGraw-Hill, Medical Publishing Division, 2005.
[4] Marketos S, Eftychiadis A, Koutras DA. Thyroid diseases in the Byzantine era. J R Soc Med 1990; 83(2): 111-113.
[5] Escobar RF, Bernal J, Obregón MJ, Escobar HF, Morreale G. Fisiología del Tiroides. In: Tresguerres JAF, Aguilar E, Devesa J, Moreno B. Eds. Tratado de Endocrinología Básica y Clínica. Vol. II. Madrid: Spain; Síntesis Publisher, 2000.
[6] Kirsten D. The thyroid gland: physiology and pathophysiology. Neonatal Netw 2000; 19: 11-26.
[7] Rhoades R, Tanner GA. Medical Physiology. Lippincott Williams & Wilkins, 2003.
[8] Hung W. Clinical Pediatric Endocrinology. Mosby Year Book, 1992.
[9] Falk SA. Thyroid Disease: Endocrinology, Surgery, Nuclear Medicine, and Radiotherapy. Lippincott-Raven, 1997.
[10] Troncone L, Shapiro B, Satta MA, Monaco F. Thyroid Diseases: Basic Science, Pathology, Clinical and Laboratory Diagnoses. Taylor & Francis, 1993.
[11] Patton KT, Thibodeau GA. The Human Body in Health & Disease, Elsevier/Mosby, 2014.
[12] Patel J, Landers K, Li H, Mortimer RH, Richard K. Thyroid hormones and fetal neurological development. J Endocrinol 2011; 209: 1-8.
[13] Howdeshell KL. A model of the development of the brain as a construct of the thyroid system. Environ Health Perspect 2002; 110 (Suppl 3): 337-348.
[14] Moore KL, Persaud TVN, Torchia MG. The Developing Human: Clinically Oriented Embryology. Saunders/Elsevier, 2008.

[15] Harrell GB, Murray PD. Diagnosis and management of congenital hypothyroidism. J Perinat Neonatal Nurs 1998; 11(4): 75-83.

[16] Miculan J, Turner S, Paes BA. Congenital hypothyroidism: diagnosis and management. Neonatal Netw 1993; 12: 25-34.

[17] Obregon MJ, Calvo RM, Del Rey FE, de Escobar GM. Ontogenesis of thyroid function and interactions with maternal function. Endocr Dev 2007; 10: 86-98.

[18] Fisher DA. Fetal thyroid function: diagnosis and management of fetal thyroid disorders. Clin Obstet Gynecol 1997; 40: 16-31.

[19] Thorpe-Beeston JG, Nicolaides KH, McGregor AM. Fetal thyroid function. Thyroid 1992; 2: 207-217.

[20] Kratzsch J, Pulzer F. Thyroid gland development and defects. Best Pract Res Clin Endocrinol Metab 2008; 22: 57-75.

[21] Fisher DA. Thyroid function in premature infants. The hypothyroxinemia of prematurity. Clin Perinatol 1998; 5: 999-1014, viii.

[22] Calvo RM, Jauniaux E, Gulbis B, *et al.* Fetal tissues are exposed to biologically relevant free thyroxine concentrations during early phases of development. J Clin Endocrinol Metab 2002; 87: 1768-1777.

[23] Hume R, Simpson J, Delahunty C, *et al.* Human fetal and cord serum thyroid hormones: developmental trends and interrelationships. J Clin Endocrinol Metab 2004; 89: 4097-4103.

[24] Thorpe-Beeston JG, Nicolaides KH, Felton CV, Butler J, McGregor AM. Maturation of the secretion of thyroid hormone and thyroid-stimulating hormone in the fetus. N Engl J Med 1991; 324, 532-536.

[25] Kester M H, Martinez de Mena R, Obregon MJ, *et al.* Iodothyronine levels in the human developing brain: major regulatory roles of iodothyronine deiodinases in different areas. J Clin Endocrinol Metab 2004; 89: 3117-3128.

[26] Chiasera JM. Back to the basics: thyroid gland structure, function and pathology. Clin Lab Sci 2013; 26: 112-117.

[27] Refetoff S. Resistance to thyroid hormone: one of several defects causing reduced sensitivity to thyroid hormone. Nat Clin Pract Endocrinol Metab 2008; 4 (1): 1.

[28] Harper ME, Seifert EL. Thyroid hormone effects on mitochondrial energetics. Thyroid 2008; 18: 145-156.

[29] Mullur R, Liu YY, Brent GA. Thyroid hormone regulation of metabolism. Physiol Rev 2014; 94: 355-382.

[30] Silva JE. Thermogenic mechanisms and their hormonal regulation. Physiol Rev 2006; 86: 435-464.

[31] Clausen T, Van Hardeveld C, Everts ME. Significance of cation transport in control of energy metabolism and thermogenesis. Physiol Rev 1991; 71: 733-774.

[32] Ismail-Beigi F. Regulation of Na+,K(+)-ATPase expression by thyroid hormone. Semin Nephrol 1992; 12: 44-48.

[33] Fahien L A, Laboy JI, Din ZZ, *et al.* Ability of cytosolic malate dehydrogenase and lactate dehydrogenase to increase the ratio of NADPH to NADH oxidation by cytosolic glycerol-3-phosphate dehydrogenase. Arch Biochem Biophys 1999; 364: 185-194.

[34] Harper ME, Brand M D. The quantitative contributions of mitochondrial proton leak and ATP turnover reactions to the changed respiration rates of hepatocytes from rats of different thyroid status. J Biol Chem 1993; 268: 14850-14860.

[35] Crunkhorn S, Patti ME. 2008. Links between thyroid hormone action, oxidative metabolism, and diabetes risk? Thyroid 2008; 18: 227-237.

[36] Feng X, Jiang Y, Meltzer P, Yen PM. Thyroid hormone regulation of hepatic genes *in vivo* detected by complementary DNA microarray. Mol Endocrinol 2000; 14: 947-955.

[37] Oppenheimer JH, Schwartz HL, Lane JT, Thompson MP. Functional relationship of thyroid hormone-induced lipogenesis, lipolysis, and thermogenesis in the rat. J Clin Invest 1991; 87: 125-132.

[38] Lopez D, Abisambra Socarras JF, Bedi M, Ness GC. Activation of the hepatic LDL receptor promoter by thyroid hormone. Biochim Biophys Acta 2007; 1771: 1216-1225.

[39] Klein I, Danzi S. Thyroid disease and the heart. Circulation 2007; 116: 1725-1735.

[40] Goldberg I J, Huang LS, Huggins LA, *et al.* Thyroid hormone reduces cholesterol *via* a non-LDL receptor-mediated pathway. Endocrinology 2012; 153: 5143-5149.

[41] Knudsen N, Laurberg P, Rasmussen LB, *et al.* Small differences in thyroid function may be important for body mass index and the occurrence of obesity in the population. J Clin Endocrinol Metab 2005; 90: 4019-4024.

[42] Fox CS, Pencina MJ, D'Agostino RB, *et al.* Relations of thyroid function to body weight: cross-sectional and longitudinal observations in a community-based sample. Arch Intern Med 2008; 168: 587-592.

[43] Fliers E, Klieverik LP, Kalsbeek A. Novel neural pathways for metabolic effects of thyroid hormone. Trends Endocrinol Metab 2010; 21: 230-236.

[44] Celi FS, Zemskova M, Linderman JD, *et al.* 2011. Metabolic effects of liothyronine therapy in hypothyroidism: a randomized, double-blind, crossover trial of liothyronine *versus* levothyroxine. J Clin Endocrinol Metab 2011; 96: 3466-3474.

[45] Simonides WS, Thelen MH, van der Linden CG, Muller A, van Hardeveld C. Mechanism of thyroid-hormone regulated expression of the SERCA genes in skeletal muscle: implications for thermogenesis. Biosci Rep 2001; 21: 139-154.

[46] Simonides WS, van Hardeveld C. Thyroid hormone as a determinant of metabolic and contractile phenotype of skeletal muscle. Thyroid 2008; 18: 205-216.

[47] Noda M. Possible role of glial cells in the relationship between thyroid dysfunction and mental disorders. Front Cell Neurosci 2015; 9.

[48] Bernal J, Guadano-Ferraz A, Morte B. Perspectives in the study of thyroid hormone action on brain development and function. Thyroid 2003; 13: 1005-1012.

[49] Zoeller RT. Environmental chemicals impacting the thyroid: targets and consequences. Thyroid 2007; 17: 811-817.

[50] Horn S, Heuer H. Thyroid hormone action during brain development: more questions than answers. Mol Cell Endocrinol 2010; 315: 19-26.

[51] Duarte-Guterman P, Navarro-Martin L, Trudeau VL. Mechanisms of crosstalk between endocrine systems: regulation of sex steroid hormone synthesis and action by thyroid hormones. Gen Comp Endocrinol 2014; 203: 69-85.

[52] Kaplan LA, Pesce AJ. Clinical Chemistry: Theory, Analysis, Correlation. Mosby/Elsevier, 2010.

[53] U.S. Prevention Services Task Force. Screening for thyroid disease: recommendation statement. Ann Intern Med 2004; 140 (2): 125-127.

[54] De Vries EM, Fliers E, Boelen A. The molecular basis of the non-thyroidal illness syndrome. J Endocrinol 2015; 225: R67-R81.

[55] Albarrán AJ. Endocrinología, Editorial Medica Panamericana Sa de. 2010

[56] Bahn Chair RS, Burch HB, Cooper DS, *et al.* Hyperthyroidism and other causes of thyrotoxicosis: management guidelines of the American Thyroid Association and American Association of Clinical Endocrinologists. Thyroid 2011; 21: 593-646.

[57] Brent GA. Clinical practice. Graves' disease. N Engl J Med 2008; 358: 2594-2605.

[58] Motomura K, Brent GA. Mechanisms of thyroid hormone action. Implications for the clinical manifestation of thyrotoxicosis. Endocrinol Metab Clin N Am 1998; 27: 1-23.

[59] Ridgway EC. Modern concepts of primary thyroid gland failure. Clin Chem 1996; 42: 179-182.

[60] Duntas LH. Chemical contamination and the thyroid. Endocrine 2015; 48(1):53-64.

[61] Barbesino G. Drugs Affecting Thyroid Function. Thyroid 2010; 20(7): 763-770.

[62] Brent GA. Hypothyroidism and thyroiditis. In: Williams Textbook of Endocrinology, edited by Melmed SP, Larsen PR, and Kronenberg HM. Eds. Elsevier, 2012.

[63] Chung GE, Kim D, Kim W, *et al.* Non-alcoholic fatty liver disease across the spectrum of hypothyroidism. J Hepatol 2012; 57(1): 150-156.

[64] Grais IM, Sowers JR. Thyroid and the heart. Am J Med 2014; 127: 691698.

[65] Patil VC, Patil HV, Agrawal V, Patil S. Cardiac tamponade in a patient with primary hypothyroidism. Indian J Endocrinol Metab 2011; 15: S144-146.

[66] Martin RJ, Fanaroff AA, Walsh MC. Neonatal-perinatal Medicine: Diseases of the Fetus and Infant. Elsevier / Mosby, 2011.

CHAPTER 2

Endocrine Disruption

Javier Del Pino[1,*], Paula Moyano[2] and María José Anadon[2]

[1]*Departament of Toxicology and Pharmacology, Veterinary School, Complutense University of Madrid, Madrid, Spain and* [2]*Departament of Toxicology and Legal Medicine, Medical School, Complutense University of Madrid, Madrid, Spain*

Abstract: The thyroid system controls several developmental processes and participates in many physiological functions such as metabolic regulation, energy homeostasis, bone remodeling, reproduction, cardiac function and mental status in both children and adults. Thyroid function is regulated through the interaction between the hypothalamus, the pituitary and the thyroid. A large number of compounds such as pesticides, drugs, heavy metals, cosmetics, industrial chemicals and natural compounds have been shown to disrupt thyroid system homeostasis by acting on diverse regulation points of thyroid hormones metabolism, binding to thyroid receptors or altering gene transcription regulated through thyroid hormones among other mechanisms involved. There is special concern about thyroid disruptors because even slight variations in thyroid homeostasis may negatively affect human health, particularly during critical periods of vulnerability such as development and senescence or in sensitive population groups. This chapter focusses on known disrupting mechanisms and key factors influencing them.

Keywords: Endocrine disruption, thyroid hormones.

INTRODUCTION

Initially, endocrine-disruptor (ED) was described by the U.S. Environmental Protection Agency (EPA) as "an exogenous compound that disrupts synthesis, secretion, transport, metabolism, binding action, or elimination of natural blood-borne hormones that are present in the organism and are responsible for homeostasis, reproduction, and developmental process" [1].

However, after accumulated evidence showed that mechanisms of action are much broader than originally recognized, EDs have been defined as "natural or synthetic compounds which through environmental or inappropriate developmental exposures disrupt the hormonal and homeostatic systems that enable the body to communicate with and respond to its environment" [2]. Thus, compounds that influence thyroid

[*]**Corresponding author Javier Del Pino:** Department of Toxicology and Pharmacology, Complutense University of Madrid, Madrid, Spain; E-mail: jdelpino@pdi.ucm.es

Javier Del Pino, Maria Jesus Diaz and Maria Teresa Frejo (Eds)

hormones metabolism, either by the hypothalamic-pituitary-thyroid (HPT) axis or directly through nuclear receptors, are denominated "thyroid disruptors" (TDs) [3]. The thyroid gland is highly dependent on dietary iodine intake for normal function, and thus may be especially vulnerable to exogenous disruption. In this regard, thyroid function could be altered by diet, through consumption of naturally occurring goitrogens such as goitrin or flavonoids in legumes and plants [4]. In addition, the thyroid system can be disrupted by drugs, metals, synthetic chemicals and their byproducts (more than 150 in all), plastics, plasticizers, pesticides, and fungicides (Table **1**) [2-6].

Table 1. Endocrine disruptors that alter thyroid function.

Industrial chemicals and byproducts (solvents/lubricants): Polychlorinated dioxins and furans (*PCDD/Fs (dioxins)*), Perchlorate, Polychlorinated biphenyls (PCBs) Polybrominated biphenyls (PBBs)
Plastics and plasticizers: Bisphenol A (BPA), tetrabromobisphenol A (TBBPA) and Phthalates
Pesticides: Alachlor, dicamba, carbamate, chlorpyrifos Dichlorodiphenyltrichloroethane (DDT), Fipronil Endosulfan, heptachlor, lindane, toxaphene
Fungicides: Amitriole, Vinclozolin, mancozeb
Sunscreen-Cosmetics: Benzophenone 2 and 3 Homosalate (HMS), 2-ethylhexyl 4-dimethylaminobenzoate (OD-PABA) and 4-aminobenzoic acid (PABA)
Heavy metals: Cadmium, mercury, lead
Polyphenols: isoflavones (soy), flavonoids (catechin, quercetin)

The thyroid gland is a vital organ because of the health of each organ and tissue requires an euthyroid condition and an optimally working HPT axis. Thyroid hormones (THs) are implicated in numerous physiological processes such as metabolic regulation, energy homeostasis, bone remodeling, cardiac function and mental condition. Therefore, preservation of regular thyroid function is critical for psychological and physiological wellbeing [7, 8]. The thyroid gland in adults, is normally able to compensate, by thyroid hyperplasia and goiter, for mild or moderate disruption of normal thyroid function [4]. Thyroid hormones are known to play an essential action in development of the fetus, regulating growth and differentiation of many tissues and organs, especially development of the central nervous system [6, 9, 10]. Throughout the earliest period of gestation, the fetus confides completely on transplacental transference of maternal THs and therefore, on regular maternal thyroid function, but maternal thyroid homeostasis keeps supporting considerably to fetal development throughout the remaining period of gestation [9, 11]. The disruption of the HPT axis during development can produce deep damage on mammalian brain development, leading to mental retardation and neurological deficiencies [12]. The impact of TDs on population could be based on timing, dose, and length of exposure time, synergy between compounds, as well as genetic and immune status, conditioning them to thyroid disease. This highlights that an important part of the population may be at risk or be more vulnerable to thyroid disruption.

THYROID HORMONE CONTROL AND METABOLISM

The thyroid system is controlled by the HPT axis (Fig. **1**). In this regard, Thyrotropin-releasing hormone (TRH), liberated from hypophysiotropic neurons situated in the medial and periventricular parvocellular subdivisions of the hypothalamic paraventricular nucleus, regulate the production and secretion of thyroid stimulation hormone (TSH) from the pituitary gland [13]. Moreover, TSH synthesis is also induced by the direct action of tetraiodo-L-thyronine (T4) and 3,3,5-triiodo-L-thyronine (T3) binding to thyrotropic cells [3]. TSH in turn stimulates the synthesis of thyroglobulin (Tg), thyroid peroxidase (TPO), sodium-iodide symporter (NIS) protein, production and release of T4 and T3 (Fig. **2**), which consequently produce negative feedback on both pituitary and hypothalamus [14, 15]. T4 and, to a minor degree, T3 are discharged into the sanguine fluid where they are transported by the TH delivery proteins thyroxin-binding globulin (TBG), transthyretin (TTR), and albumin [16]. Because of its appetent binding to blood proteins, T4 possesses a much longer half-life than T3.

T4 is converted to the active hormone T3 by monoiodothyronine deiodinase type I (DI1) in the liver, kidney and thyroid, contributing to the maintenance of circulating T3 levels and the clearance of plasma reverse T3 (rT3). Monoiodothyronine deiodinase type II (DI2) is the main T3-activating enzyme in target cells in the brain. In addition, monoiodothyronine deiodinase type III (DI3) eliminates an iodine atom from the tyrosyl ring which transforms either T4 to the inactive rT3 or T3 to the inactive diiodothyronine (T2) [17, 18]. These 3 types of monoiodothyronine deiodinases (DIs) control the local availability of T3 for cellular action, playing a crucial function in modulation of the physiological outcome of THs [19]. THs cross the plasma membranes using highly specific transporters, termed monocarboxylate transporter (MCT) 8 and 10, and organic anion-transporting polypeptide 1c1 (OATP 1c1), the last mentioned being critical for TH transport across the blood brain barrier (BBB) [20]. Since removal of TH take place after glucuronidation and sulfation, its biding with glucuronic acid, leads to the main metabolic pathway of TH metabolism [21].

Once inside the cell, thyroid hormones binds to the thyroid receptors (TRs) that are ligand-modulated transcription factors of the nuclear receptor superfamily [8]. Two genes, TRα and TRβ, codify for TRs, which by alternative promoter utilization and alternative splicing result in diverse TR isoforms and isotypes [15]. TRα1 and TRβ1 are the main forms to which THs bind [8]. These two isoforms present different spatial and temporal expressions and are also diversely expressed during growth. In this regard, TRα1 is especially profuse in the central nervous system (CNS), heart and immune system, whereas TRβ1 is preferentially expressed in the brain, liver, and kidney [10]. They both present analogous attraction for T3 (10^{-9} M–10^{-10} M) and transactivate target gene transcription in a concentration-dependent way [15].

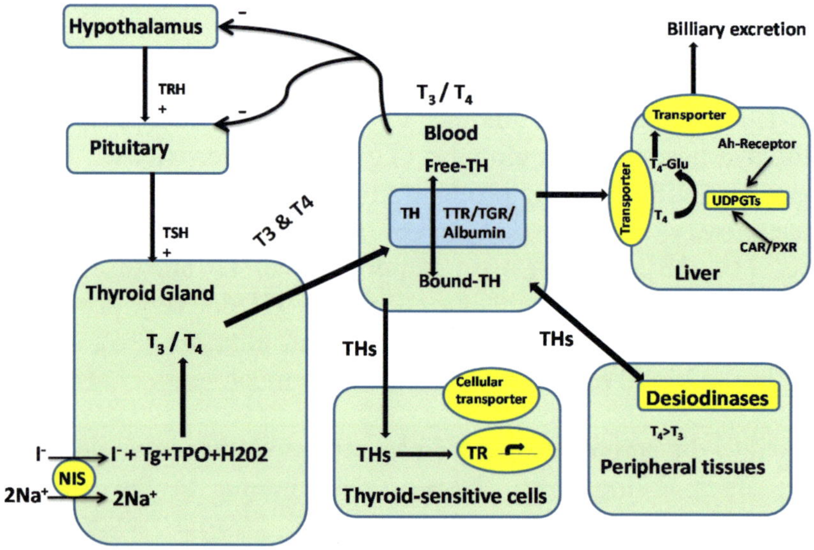

Figure 1: Hypothalamic–pituitary–thyroid axis. TRH, thyrotropin releasing hormone; TSH, thyroid stimulating hormone; T4, thyroxine; T3, triiodothyronine; I, iodine; UDPGT, uridine diphosphate glucuronyltransferase; TR, thyroid hormone receptor; TH, thyroid hormone; NIS, the sodium iodide synmporter; TPO, thyroperixidase; Gluc, glucose. Adapted from Miller and coworkers [25].

To regulate transcription, TR binds to a particular nucleotide sequence termed the TH-responsive element (TRE) that acts as a homodimer or heterodimer with other nuclear receptors, especially with the retinoid X receptor (RXR) [22]. Once this complex binds to a TRE in the promoter region of target genes, TR binds to a series of proteins, named co-activators or co-repressors, in a ligand-dependent manner, which regulate the transcription of these genes [21, 23]. Once TRs are unoccupied by T3, they enroll basal repressors, like the silencing mediator of the retinoid and thyroid hormone receptor (SMRT) and the nuclear receptor co-repressor (NCoR). These cofactors permit the supplementary enrollment of histone deacetylases, which rearrange the architecture of chromatin, and result in the inhibition of target genes at lessen levels than in the lack of the receptor. Counterwise, T3 binding to TRs produces conformational modifications that lead to co-repressor liberation, and consequent co-activator enrollment. These co-activators, such as those of the p160/SRC (steroid receptor co-activator) group, have intrinsic histone acetylase action and induce a molecular events that ends in the induction of target gene transcription [11, 24].

MECHANISMS OF ACTION OF THYROID DISRUPTORS

Thyroid-disrupting compounds (TDs) can target the system at various points such as iodine uptake, synthesis, secretion, transport, cellular uptake, peripheral inducing/repressing metabolism of THs by iodothyronine deiodinases, transcriptional activity of TRs and expression of TH-regulated genes [10, 25].

Inhibition of Iodine Uptake in the Follicular Thyroid Cells

Iodine uptake is promoted by the plasma membrane transport NIS, which concentrates it at levels 20-40 times greater than those presented in the blood, thus getting enough iodine concentration to produce adequate amounts of THs (Fig. **2**) [26]. Some TDs such as perchlorate, thiocyanate, bromate, and nitrate have been shown to contend with iodine for binding to the NIS transporter and hereby repress the capture of iodine into the follicular thyroid cell, inducing a decrease in the synthesis of T4 and T3 [3, 27, 28].

Inhibition of T3 and T4 Synthesis in the Thyroid Cells

T4 and T3 synthesis in thyroid cells requires iodide, hydrogen peroxide (H_20_2), the enzyme TPO, and Tg (Fig. **2**). TPO reduces the hydrogen peroxide so it can oxidize iodine, permitting iodide molecules to bind to the tyrosyl residues of the thyroglobulin molecule, forming mono- (MIT) and di-iodothyronine (DIT). Two DIT molecules produce T4; one DIT and one MIT produce T3 [3]. TSH induces

TPO synthesis and NIS transport protein, Tg, and H_2O_2 production, and the intra-thyroidal synthesis of T3 relative to T4 [3].

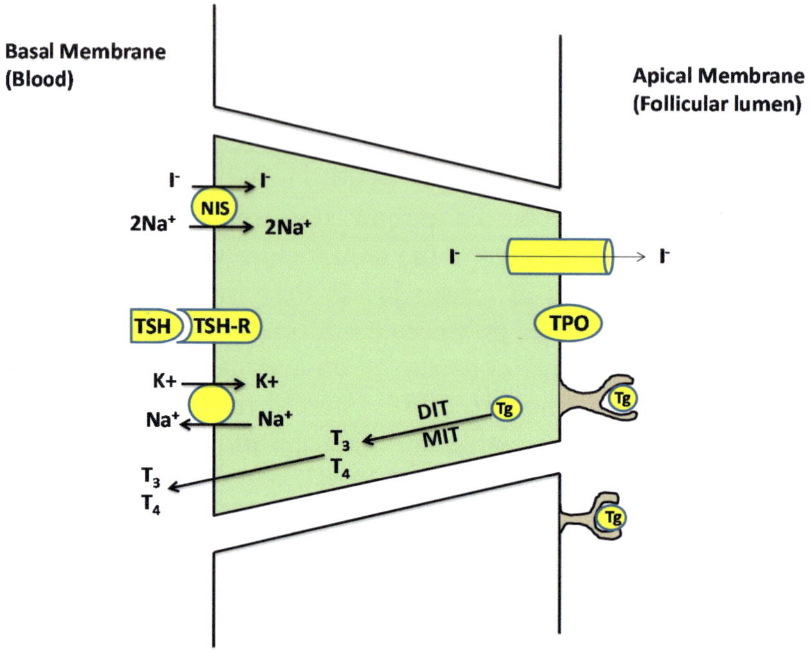

Figure 2: The thyroid follicle cell: iodine metabolism. Adapted from Boas and coworkers [9]. DIT, di-iodotyrosine; MIT, mono-iodotyrosine; Tg, thyroglobulin; T4, thyroxine; I, iodine; T3, triiodothyronine; TPO, thyroperoxidase; NIS, sodium-iodide symporter; TSH, thyroid-stimulating hormone; TSH-R, thyroid-stimulating hormone receptor.

Specific TDs such as ethylene thiourea, mancozeb, amitrole, benzophenone-2, and soy isoflavones have been shown to block TPO synthesis and preclude the synthesis of thyroglobulin, thus lessening production of T3 and T4 [29]. In addition, TRH and TSH, which regulate the synthesis of T4 and T3, could be altered by some TDs, inhibiting this function. The mechanism could be receptor-binding blockage or other mechanisms that impede TSH and TRH from performing their actions on upregulation of cellular metabolism and synthesis of T4 and T3 [30, 31].

Blockade of Thyroid Hormones Binding to Transport Proteins

THs are transported mainly bound to transport proteins (< 0.5% is transported free). TBG binds 75% of T4, TTR binds 20%, and albumin binds <5% of the remaining T4. Transport proteins keep a pool of T4 and T3 hormones in order to act in the amount necessary and at the specific time on each specific tissue, particularly in the

CNS [3]. TTR is the most important thyroid transport protein in the human nervous system, playing a critical role in maintaining the correct free T4 values in the extracellular environment of nervous tissue, which is detached of T4 homeostasis in the organism. TTR may could regulate the distribution of T4 through the BBB and promote maternal-to-fetal transport across the placenta [32]. PCBs, flame retardants, phthalates, and pentachlorophenol have been reported to bind to TTR. These compounds, when bound to TTR, may be carried to the fetus and fetal nervous system, with a consequent reduction in fetal nervous system T4 levels [30].

Alteration of Cellular Metabolism of THs

Particular thyroid disruptors (flame retardants, PCBs, bisphenol A and dioxin) have been determined to either block or induce cellular capture of THs, resulting in likely elevated biliary elimination of T4 and T3. Alteration of cellular uptake of THs could lead to variations in nuclear thyroid receptor activity, leading to disrupted gene transcription. PCBs, FD&C red #3, octyl methoxycinnamate (OMC), methoxychlor, lead and cadmium have been described to alter the function of the deiodinase enzymes [30]. The result of this action is to decrease peripheral synthesis of T3 [31].

On the other hand, THs are metabolized in the liver and kidneys by biding to sulfate or glucuronic acid mediated by sulfotransferase (SULT) isoenzymes or uridine diphosphophate glucuronosyltransferase (UDPGT) respectively [3]. Some thyroid disruptors (PCBs, triclosan, pentachlorophenol and dioxins) block the function of sulfotransferases, leading to lessened sulfation and abnormal regulation of peripheral T4 and T3 concentrations, as a result of the active role that these enzymes perform in cerebral, uterine, mammary, and intestinal TH regulation [30, 31]. Some thyroid disruptors (acetochlor, PCBs, dioxins and bisphenol A) also increase UDPGT hepatic catabolism [4], leading to augmented biliary excretion of T4 and T3 [31]. Constitutive androstane receptor (CAR) and pregnane X receptor (PXR) could be activated by endocrine disruptors inducing the expression of drug transporters and xenobiotic metabolizing enzymes, including UDPGTs and SULTs [33]. Thus, CAR/PXR stimulation by xenobiotics may indirectly lead to dysregulation of T4 and T3 levels.

Disruption of THs Transcriptional Process

Thyroid-disrupting chemicals can mimic or antagonize the action of T3 on control of TH target genes by different ways. In this regard, a few environmental chemicals such as some phthalates, hydroxylated polybrominated diphenyl ethers

(PBDEs), halogenated phenolic compounds, like PCBs and hydroxylated PCBs, have been shown to bind to TRs, and to alter their transcriptional activities [34-38]. Besides, it has been described that environmental compounds can selectively distinguish between TRα and TRβ [39] and produce this effect selectively.

TDs may induce their actions by fomenting the enrollment of coactivators by TRs, or by blocking the process induced by T3. Indeed, NH-3 is a synthetic selective TRβ1 antagonist that block TH function by inhibiting both coactivator and corepressor union, and seems to be an agonist in terms of corepressor liberation, and an antagonist in terms of coactivator binding [40]. Bisphenol-A (BPA) has been described to suppress TR-mediated transcription by enrolling the nuclear corepressor N-CoR to the TR [41]. The anti-thyroid drugs methimazole and propylthiouracil have been shown to significantly suppress transcriptional actions regulated by TR. These molecules block the function of T3 by promoting the enrollment of transcriptional corepressors and/or the separation of coactivators [42]. Also, 4-OH-PCB has been reported to eliminate TR/coactivator (SRC-1) complex regulated transactivation [43].

Disruption of the TH transcriptional process may implicate crosstalk with other nuclear receptors. In this sense, OH-PCB can in part separate the heterodimer RXR/TR from TRE, which could suppress the transcription of target genes [44]. It has been also described that peroxisome proliferator-activated receptors (PPARs) may block the transcriptional action of TRs by competing for RXR sequences with THs [45]. In this regard, it has been reported that PPAR disruptors such as phthalates might indirectly change TR transcriptional activity [46].

Finally, some compounds can also alter the expression of TRs. In this regard, T3-dependent activation has been reported to be significantly inhibited by phthalates through a decrease in the expression of TRβ1 [47]. Moreover, BPA was shown to reduce TRα and TRβ mRNAs levels, and also moderately suppress RXR gene expression [48].

Other Mechanisms

Regular thyroid function needs correct development of the thyroid gland itself and settlement of a well-functioning HPT axis. It is not yet patent, whether some TDs could alter thyroid actions by altering thyroid development, production of anti-thyroid antibodies or by interplay with other relevant compounds in thyroid metabolism such as iodine or selenium [22].

Cross-Species Extrapolation of Mechanism

There are many circumstances in which the results of a chemical in one species are analogous to those in another, which allows interspecies extrapolation of the harmful actions of TDs. However, species dissimilarities in the relationship between alterations in blood total T4 and downstream harmful results, perhaps regulated by differences in kinetics cannot be ruled out. Thus, species dissimilarities in the expression or architecture of particular functional proteins (*e.g.* receptors and enzymes) may alter the toxicity of particular substances in distinct species [25].

FACTORS INFLUENCING EFFECTS OF THYROID DISRUPTORS

Thyroid function could be altered by TDs depending on both the class of compounds and dose and length of exposure time. Discrete alterations of the thyroid system by TDs may be compensated without any adverse effect. However, serum THs levels are tightly modulated within a given individual and minor changes in them may have results on general health [49, 50]. Individual normal levels of THs could vary from normal population levels. Thus, a value within standard "normals" is not unavoidably normal for a specific person and therefore, the effects of TDs on the health of the population could be underestimated [25, 51]. In this regard, thyroid disruption is commonly produced non-linearly in a U-shaped or inverted-U dose-response curve [52], so pitiful amounts of TDs able to produce harmful effects that cannot be predicted by their actions at much higher doses; thus the level of exposure necessary to elicit thyroid disruption could be lower than expected [53].

TDs are not characterized by any structural similarity making it difficult to predict, from known TDs other compounds that may exert thyroid-disrupting activity [6]. Some TDs show structural similarity to THs, which may lead them to bind to TH protein carriers or receptors, blocking TH actions [4].

Other factors that should be considered in the effects of TDs is that the induction of THs metabolism by them could alter THs levels, thus their function. Moreover, some TDs need biological transformation to become active, which may be age- and species-dependent [4].

The geographical localization of the population is an important factor to be taken into account. Exposure to TDs could take place by nearby location to the site of release, but also at vast distances due to transport by meteorological processes. This is especially important for persistent compounds.

The lipophilicity of chemicals lets them pass the different barriers of the body, to be eliminated in milk, and predisposes them to being stored in lipophilic tissues, prolonging their effects in the body. Thus, some compounds are still contemplated as dangerous years after being banned or restricted [4].

There are persons within the overall population who are more at risk than others to exposure to TDs. Indeed, TDs affect genders differently, and thyroid disruption is more common in women, and thus, women should be contemplated as at higher risk if exposed [4]. Pregnant women, due to their elevated dependence from the thyroid gland, could be especially responsive to particular types of toxic agents that result in an additional risk to the thyroid gland such as perchlorate or compounds that induce liver metabolism of T4 [25]. Individuals of between 50–79 and $\geq$ 80 years of age present a 2-fold and 5-fold greater risk of hypothyroidism respectively, in contrast to those of 12–49 years of age [54]. On the other hand, a slightly low iodine diet may potentiate or trigger the results of thyroid disruption, particularly throughout periods of susceptibility such as development and adaptive challenges throughout illness [55]. Infants and children are more susceptible than adults to TDs due to the fact that they have a limited diet and they are differentiating and growing organisms with high metabolic requirements. Population with marginal thyroid dysfunction or a genetic inclination to autoimmune thyroid disease may suffer thyroid disease at low levels of TDs that would be harmless to others [4].

Exposure to TDs is especially important during critical periods. Indeed, THs present a decisive action throughout fetal development and any decompensation during this crucial period of susceptibility, in a window from the second trimester to 2 years of age in humans, could have tragic permanent results, especially on neurocognitive development [9, 56-58]. Throughout the first half of gestation, the fetus mainly relies on maternal T4 transplacental transference and defective maternal thyroid homeostasis could have a deleterious result on neurodevelopment of her offspring. The fetus is also more defenseless due to the incomplete development of its thyroid axis and detoxification mechanisms [4]. During gestation, endocrinological and physiological disruptions induce the maternal thyroid gland and lead to marked gestation-specific variations in TH levels. Therefore, thyroid actions assessments in newborns could lead to large variations that could hide any real effects of TDs. Thus, assessment of TSH particularly, but also TH levels, requires to consider gestational age, maternal height and weight and smoking habit [9].

Finally, many studies center their attention on one kind or one class of compounds. However, in normal situation, population is exposed to a composition of compounds that could theoretically have cumulative, synergistic, or antagonistic results on thyroid actions [4, 25, 29]. Therefore, exposure to chemical mixtures should be studied to determine the final effects that synergistic exposure may produce.

CROSSTALK BETWEEN THYROID HORMONES AND THE REPRODUCTIVE SYSTEM

THs present significant actions in vertebrate gonadal maturation and function. Recent research evidence suggests that THs interact with the reproductive system and their disruption is connected with harmful results on reproductive function [59-61]. In different vertebrate species, TH disruption has been related to sex steroid hormone disruption, infertility, and in males with impaired testicular function and spermatogenesis [22, 59, 62-65]. THs also regulate the reproductive system during its development and they are needed to balance gender ratios. Indeed, in different vertebrate species it has been reported that THs are needed for regular gonadal development and generation of regular gender ratios [65-71]. The results in these species indicate likely species dissimilarities and that there is a sensitivity window to the effects of THs.

The mechanism through which this crosstalk takes place is unknown. THs could affect both sex steroid production (enzymes) and function (receptors) during development and adulthood. These results could rely on dose, time, sex, reproductive stage, and species [22, 72-76]. T3 could affect sex steroid-related gene expression in the SNC and gonad, but the mechanism has not been determined. In this sense multiple putative TRE binding sites in some genes that regulate sex hormone levels have been found [77, 78]. T3/TRα could compete with steroidogenic factor-1 (SF-1) to bind to the SF-1 response element present in the Cyp19 promoter and inhibit expression of Cyp19 [79]. *In vitro* studies using mammalian cell lines have also shown that TR and estrogen receptor (ER) can compete for the same estrogen responsive element (ERE) in the promoter of the oxytocin receptor gene [80]. THs and sex steroids can also interact through membrane- induced mechanisms, adding many possible sites of interactions [81].

CONCLUDING REMARKS

Thyroid hormones are strongly involved in vertebrate physiology regulation in adults and body developmental control, especially central nervous system development. A large number of compounds have been reported to disrupt thyroid system homeostasis, and thus they could impair physiology and developmental processes. The alteration of TH signaling pathways in the developing human nervous system, could disturb the procedure of neural differentiation and possibly explain the notion that exposure to TDs is associated to cognitive deficits in humans. The mechanisms of action of TDs are complicated and, although TR independent mechanisms have been determined, there is absence of data about TR-related mechanisms, which means that there may be some compounds that are not currently recognized as TDs. A comprehensive survey of the immense number of environmental compounds to which the population is exposed is needed to determine if more compounds could also be TDs. Reliable biomarkers of thyroid disruption, which can inform of possible adverse effects that could occur at subclinical levels of alteration of THs are necessary, because the possible adverse effects induced could currently be underestimated. Many parameters substantially complicate the assessment of the risk of TDs. In this regard, the extensive variety of targets and the proof that many of them can be disrupted at the same time make it complicated to explain the effects observed. In addition, TDs can also disrupt cellular processes that alter various hormone-signaling pathways. Lastly, although the results of TDs are regularly less powerful than those of THs, it is also essential to keep in mind that humans are continuously exposed to numerous contaminants which can behave synergistically and result in effects that are different from those of the individual contaminants. A better understanding of these issues may result in modifications in public policy and consciousness, and make it possible to reduce adverse results for future generations.

CONFLICT OF INTEREST

The author confirms that author has no conflict of interest to declare for this publication.

ACKNOWLEDGEMENTS

Declared None.

REFERENCES

[1] Kavlock RJ, Daston GP, De Rosa C, *et al.* Research needs for the risk assessment of health and environmental effects of endocrine disruptors: a report of the U.S. EPA-sponsored workshop. Environ Health Perspect 1996; 104(Suppl 4): 715-740.

[2] Diamanti-Kandarakis E, Bourguignon JP, Giudice LC, *et al.* Endocrine-disrupting chemicals: an Endocrine Society scientific statement. Endocrine reviews 2009; 30(4): 293-342.

[3] Patrick L. Thyroid disruption: mechanism and clinical implications in human health. Alternative medicine review: a journal of clinical therapeutics 2009; 14(4): 326-346.
[4] Brucker-Davis F. Effects of environmental synthetic chemicals on thyroid function. Thyroid 1998; 8(9): 827-856.
[5] Barbesino G. Drugs affecting thyroid function. Thyroid 2010; 20(7): 763- 770.
[6] Duntas LH. Chemical contamination and the thyroid. Endocrine 2015; 48(1): 53-64.
[7] Bauer M, Whybrow PC. Thyroid hormone, neural tissue and mood modulation. World J Biol Psychiatry 2001; 2(2): 59-69.
[8] Oetting A, Yen PM. New insights into thyroid hormone action. Best Pract Res Clin Endocrinol Metab 2007; 21(2): 193-208.
[9] Boas M, Feldt-Rasmussen U, Main KM. Thyroid effects of endocrine disrupting chemicals. Mol Cell Endocrinol 2012; 355(2): 240- 248.
[10] Jugan ML, Levi Y, Blondeau JP. Endocrine disruptors and thyroid hormone physiology. Biochem Pharmacol 2010; 79(7): 939-947
[11] Hofmann PJ, Schomburg L, Kohrle J. Interference of endocrine d isrupters with thyroid hormone receptor-dependent transactivation. Toxicol Sci 2009; 110(1): 125-137.
[12] Bernal J. Pathophysiology of thyroid hormone deficiency during fetal development. J Pediatr Endocrinol Metab 2005; 18(Suppl 1): 1253-1256.
[13] Lechan RM, Fekete C. The TRH neuron: a hypothalamic integrator of energy metabolism. Prog Brain Res 2006; 153: 209-235.
[14] Duntas LH, Emerson CH. On the fortieth anniversary of thyrotropin- releasing hormone: the hormone that launched a new era. Thyroid 2009; 19(12): 1299-12301
[15] Zoeller RT, Tan SW, Tyl RW. General background on the hypothalamic- pituitary-thyroid (HPT) axis. Crit Rev Toxicol 2007; 37(1- 2):11-53.
[16] Richardson SJ. Cell and molecular biology of transthyretin and thyroid hormones. Int Rev Cytol 2007; 258:137-193.
[17] Bianco AC, Salvatore D, Gereben B, Berry MJ, Larsen PR. Biochemistry, cellular and molecular biology, and physiological roles of the iodothyronine selenodeiodinases. Endocr Rev 2002; 23(1): 38-89.
[18] Soldin OP, O'Mara DM, Aschner M. Thyroid hormones and methylmercury toxicity. Biol Trace Elem Res 2008; 126 (1-3): 1-12.
[19] Kohrle J. Thyroid hormone transporters in health and disease: advances in thyroid hormone deiodination. Best Pract Res Clin Endocrinol Metab 2007; 21(2):173-191.
[20] Visser WE, Friesema EC, Jansen J, Visser TJ. Thyroid hormone transport in and out of cells. Trends Endocrinol Metab 2008; 19(2):50-56.
[21] Lazar MA. Thyroid hormone receptors: multiple forms, multiple possibilities. Endocr Rev 1993; 14(2): 184-193.
[22] Duarte-Guterman P, Navarro-Martin L, Trudeau VL. Mechanisms of crosstalk between endocrine systems: regulation of sex steroid hormone synthesis and action by thyroid hormones. Gen Comp Endocrinol 2014; 203:69-285.
[23] Ahuja HS, Szanto A, Nagy L, Davies PJ. The retinoid X receptor and its ligands: versatile regulators of metabolic function, cell differentiation and cell death. J Biol Regul Homeost Agents 2003; 17(1): 29-45.
[24] Flamant F, Gauthier K, Samarut J. Thyroid hormones signaling is getting more complex: STORMs are coming. Mol Endocrinol 2007; 21(2): 321- 333.
[25] Miller MD, Crofton KM, Rice DC, Zoeller RT. Thyroid-disrupting chemicals: interpreting upstream biomarkers of adverse outcomes. Environ Health Perspect 2009; 117(7): 1033-1041.
[26] Dohan O, De la Vieja A, Paroder V, *et al.* (2003) The sodium/iodide Symporter (NIS): characterization, regulation, and medical significance. Endocr Rev 2003; 24(1): 48-77.
[27] De Groef B, Decallonne BR, Van der Geyten S, Darras VM, Bouillon R. Perchlorate *versus* other environmental sodium/iodide symporter inhibitors: potential thyroid-related health effects. Eur J Endocrinol 2006; 155(1): 17-25.
[28] Wolff J. Perchlorate and the thyroid gland. Pharmacol Rev 1998; 50(1): 89-105.
[29] Crofton KM. Thyroid disrupting chemicals: mechanisms and mixtures. Int J Androl 2008; 31(2): 209-223.

[30] Boas M, Feldt-Rasmussen U, Skakkebaek NE, Main KM. Environmental chemicals and thyroid function. Eur J Endocrinol 2006; 154(5): 599- 611.

[31] Santini F, Vitti P, Ceccarini G, *et al. In vitro* assay of thyroid disruptors affecting TSH-stimulated adenylate cyclase activity. J Endocrinol Invest 2003; 26(10): 950-955

[32] Ulbrich B, Stahlmann R. Developmental toxicity of polychlorinated biphenyls (PCBs): a systematic review of experimental data. Arch Toxicol 2004; 78(5): 252-268.

[33] Maglich JM, Watson J, McMillen PJ, Goodwin B, Willson TM, Moore JT. The nuclear receptor CAR is a regulator of thyroid hormone metabolism during caloric restriction. J Biol Chem 2004; 279(19): 19832-19838.

[34] Fritsche E, Cline JE, Nguyen NH, Scanlan TS, Abel J. Polychlorinated biphenyls disturb differentiation of normal human neural progenitor cells: clue for involvement of thyroid hormone receptors. Environ Health Perspect 2005; 113(7): 871-876.

[35] Ishihara A, Sawatsubashi S, Yamauchi K. Endocrine disrupting chemicals: interference of thyroid hormone binding to transthyretins and to thyroid hormone receptors. Mol Cell Endocrinol 2003; 199(1-2): 105-117.

[36] Kitamura S, Jinno N, Suzuki T, *et al.* Thyroid hormone-like and estrogenic activity of hydroxylated PCBs in cell culture. Toxicology 2005; 208(3): 377-387.

[37] Kojima H, Takeuchi S, Uramaru N, Sugihara K, Yoshida T, Kitamura S. Nuclear hormone receptor activity of polybrominated diphenyl ethers and their hydroxylated and methoxylated metabolites in transactivation assays using Chinese hamster ovary cells. Environ Health Perspect 2009; 117(8): 1210-1218.

[38] Jugan ML, Levy-Bimbot M, Pomerance M, Tamisier-Karolak S, Blondeau JP, Levi Y. A new bioluminescent cellular assay to measure the transcriptional effects of chemicals that modulate the alpha-1 thyroid hormone receptor. Toxicol *In Vitro* 2007; 21(6):1197-11205.

[39] Schriks M, Roessig JM, Murk AJ, Furlow JD. Thyroid hormone receptor isoform selectivity of thyroid hormone disrupting compounds quantified with an *in vitro* reporter gene assay. Environ Toxicol Pharmacol 2007; 23(3): 302-307.

[40] Lim W, Nguyen NH, Yang HY, Scanlan TS, Furlow JD. A thyroid hormone antagonist that inhibits thyroid hormone action *in vivo*. J Biol Chem 2002; 277(38): 35664-356670.

[41] Moriyama K, Tagami T, Akamizu T, *et al.* Thyroid hormone action is disrupted by bisphenol A as an antagonist. The Journal of clinical endocrinology and metabolism 2002; 87(11): 5185-5190.

[42] Moriyama K, Tagami T, Usui T, *et al.* Antithyroid drugs inhibit thyroid hormone receptor-mediated transcription. The Journal of clinical endocrinology and metabolism 2007; 92(3): 1066-1072.

[43] Iwasaki T, Miyazaki W, Takeshita A, Kuroda Y, Koibuchi N. Polychlorinated biphenyls suppress thyroid hormone-induced transactivation. Biochem Biophys Res Commun 2002; 299(3): 384-388.

[44] Miyazaki W, Iwasaki T, Takeshita A, Kuroda Y, Koibuchi N. Polychlorinated biphenyls suppress thyroid hormone receptor-mediated transcription through a novel mechanism. J Biol Chem 2004; 279(18): 18195-18202.

[45] Juge-Aubry CE, Gorla-Bajszczak A, Pernin A, *et al.* Peroxisome proliferator-activated receptor mediates cross-talk with thyroid hormone receptor by competition for retinoid X receptor. Possible role of a leucine zipper-like heptad repeat. J Biol Chem 1995; 270(30): 18117-18122.

[46] Desvergne B, Feige JN, Casals-Casas C. PPAR-mediated activity of phthalates: A link to the obesity epidemic? Mol Cell Endocrinol 2009; 304(1- 2): 43-48.

[47] Sugiyama S, Shimada N, Miyoshi H, Yamauchi K. Detection of thyroid system-disrupting chemicals using *in vitro* and *in vivo* screening assays in Xenopus laevis. Toxicol Sci 2005; 88(2): 367-374

[48] Iwamuro S, Yamada M, Kato M, Kikuyama S. Effects of bisphenol A on thyroid hormone-dependent up-regulation of thyroid hormone receptor alpha and beta and down-regulation of retinoid X receptor gamma in Xenopus tail culture. Life sciences 2006; 79(23): 2165-2171.

[49] Auso E, Lavado-Autric R, Cuevas E, Del Rey FE, Morreale De Escobar G, Berbel P. A moderate and transient deficiency of maternal thyroid function at the beginning of fetal neocorticogenesis alters neuronal migration. Endocrinology 2004; 145(9): 4037-4047.

[50] Lavado-Autric R, Auso E, Garcia-Velasco JV, *et al.* Early maternal hypothyroxinemia alters histogenesis and cerebral cortex cytoarchitecture of the progeny. J Clin Invest 2003; 111(7): 1073-1082.

[51] Andersen S, Pedersen KM, Bruun NH, Laurberg P. Narrow individual variations in serum T(4) and T(3) in normal subjects: a clue to the understanding of subclinical thyroid disease. J Clin Endocrinol Metabol 2002; 87(3): 1068-1072.
[52] vom Saal FS, Welshons WV. Large effects from small exposures. II. The importance of positive controls in low-dose research on bisphenol A. Environ Res 2006; 100(1): 50-76.
[53] Vandenberg LN, Colborn T, Hayes TB, *et al.* Hormones and endocrine-disrupting chemicals: low-dose effects and nonmonotonic dose responses. Endocrine reviews 2012; 33(3): 378-455.
[54] Aoki Y, Belin RM, Clickner R, Jeffries R, Phillips L, Mahaffey KR. Serum TSH and total T4 in the United States population and their association with participant characteristics: National Health and Nutrition Examination Survey (NHANES 1999-2002). Thyroid 2007; 17(12): 1211- 23.
[55] Kohrle J. (2008) Environment and endocrinology: the case of thyroidology. Ann Endocrinol (Paris) 2008; 69(2): 116-122.
[56] Berbel P, Mestre JL, Santamaria A, *et al.* Delayed neurobehavioral development in children born to pregnant women with mild hypothyroxinemia during the first month of gestation: the importance of early iodine supplementation. Thyroid 2009; 19(5): 511-519.
[57] Pop VJ, Brouwers EP, Vader HL, Vulsma T, van Baar AL, de Vijlder JJ Maternal hypothyroxinaemia during early pregnancy and subsequent child development: a 3-year follow-up study. Clin Endocrinol (Oxf) 2003; 59(3): 282-288.
[58] Porterfield SP. Thyroidal dysfunction and environmental chemicals- potential impact on brain development. Environ Health Perspect 2000; 108(Suppl 3):433-438.
[59] Dittrich R, Beckmann MW, Oppelt PG, *et al.* Thyroid hormone receptors and reproduction. J Reprod Immunol 2011; 90(1): 58-66.
[60] Wajner SM, Wagner MS, Maia AL. Clinical implications of altered thyroid status in male testicular function. Arq Bras Endocrinol Metabol 2009; 53(8): 976-982.
[61] Zoeller RT. Environmental neuroendocrine and thyroid disruption: relevance for reproductive medicine? Fertil Steril 2008; 89(2 Suppl): e99- e100.
[62] Jiang JY, Imai Y, Umezu M, Sato E. Characteristics of infertility in female hypothyroid (hyt) mice. Reproduction 2001; 122(5): 695-700.
[63] Krassas GE, Poppe K, Glinoer D. Thyroid function and human reproductive health. Endocrine reviews 2010; 31(5): 702-755.
[64] Maran RR. Thyroid hormones: their role in testicular steroidogenesis. Arch Androl 2003; 49(5): 375-388.
[65] Wagner MS, Wajner SM, Maia AL. The role of thyroid hormone in testicular development and function. J Endocrinol 2008; 199(3): 351-365.
[66] Bernhardt RR, von Hippel FA, Cresko WA. Perchlorate induces hermaphroditism in threespine sticklebacks. Environ Toxicol Chem 2006; 25(8): 2087-96
[67] Buchholz DR, Paul BD, Fu L, Shi YB. Molecular and developmental analyses of thyroid hormone receptor function in Xenopus laevis, the African clawed frog. Gen Comp Endocrinol 2006; 145(1): 1-19.
[68] Cooke PS, Holsberger DR, Witorsch RJ, *et al.* Thyroid hormone, glucocorticoids, and prolactin at the nexus of physiology, reproduction, and toxicology. Toxicol Appl Pharmacol 2004; 194(3): 309-335.
[69] Decuypere E, Kühn ER. Thyroid hormone physiology in galliformes: Age and strain related changes in physiological control. American Zoologist 1988; 28(2): 401-415
[70] Goleman WL, Urquidi LJ, Anderson TA, Smith EE, Kendall RJ, Carr JA. Environmentally relevant concentrations of ammonium perchlorate inhibit development and metamorphosis in Xenopus laevis. Environ Toxicol Chem 2002; 21(2): 424-430.
[71] Sharma P, Patino R. Regulation of gonadal sex ratios and pubertal development by the thyroid endocrine system in zebrafish (Danio rerio). Gen Comp Endocrinol 2013; 184: 111-119
[72] Allan ER, Habibi HR. Direct effects of triiodothyronine on production of anterior pituitary hormones and gonadal steroids in goldfish. Mol Reprod Dev 2012; 79(9): 592-602.
[73] Hapon MB, Gamarra-Luques C, Jahn GA. (2010) Short term hypothyroidism affects ovarian function in the cycling rat. Reprod Biol Endocrinol 2010; 8: 14.
[74] Morais RD, Nobrega RH, Gomez-Gonzalez NE, *et al.* Thyroid hormone stimulates the proliferation of Sertoli cells and single type A spermatogonia in adult zebrafish (Danio rerio) testis. Endocrinology 2013; 154(11): 4365-4376.

[75] Nelson ER, Allan ER, Pang FY, Habibi HR. Thyroid hormone and reproduction: regulation of estrogen receptors in goldfish gonads. Mol Reprod Dev 2010; 77(9): 784-794.

[76] Sechman A. The role of thyroid hormones in regulation of chicken ovarian steroidogenesis. Gen Comp Endocrinol 2013; 190: 68-75.

[77] Flood DE, Fernandino JI, Langlois VS. Thyroid hormones in male reproductive development: evidence for direct crosstalk between the androgen and thyroid hormone axes. Gen Comp Endocrinol 2013; 192: 2-14.

[78] Pezzi V, Panno ML, Sirianni R, *et al*. Effects of tri- iodothyronine on alternative splicing events in the coding region of cytochrome P450 aromatase in immature rat Sertoli cells. J Endocrinol 2001; 170: 381-393.

[79] Catalano S, Pezzi V, Chimento A, *et al*. Triiodothyronine decreases the activity of the proximal promoter (PII) of the aromatase gene in the mouse Sertoli cell line, TM4. Mol Endocrinol 2003; 17: 923-934.

[80] Vasudevan N, Ogawa S, Pfaff D. Estrogen and thyroid hormone receptor interactions: physiological flexibility by molecular specificity. Physiol Rev 2002; 82: 923-944.

[81] Zhang D, Trudeau V.L. Integration of membrane and nuclear estrogen receptor signaling. Comp Biochem Physiol A Mol Integr Physiol 2006; 144: 306-315.

CHAPTER 3

Environmental Autoimmune Thyroid Diseases

Marjorie Safran*

Department of Medicine, Division of Endocrinology, University of Massachusetts Health Center, Worcester, MA, USA

Abstract: Autoimmune thyroid diseases are the most common autoimmune endocrine disorders. Expression of thyroid dysfunction is dependent upon the interaction of genetic factors and environmental exposures. The genes identified so far account for only a small portion of genetic susceptibility for autoimmune thyroid disease. A number of environmental exposures are associated with exposing thyroid dysfunction in subjects with autoimmune thyroid disease and some are clearly identified as inducing thyroid autoimmunity although this is actually less common. Understanding the relationship between environment and the genetic background should help in identifying patients at risk and may provide therapeutic options for the future.

Keywords: Graves' disease, hashimoto's thyroiditis, thyroid autoimmunity.

INTRODUCTION

Autoimmune thyroid diseases (AITD) - Graves' disease (GD) and Hashimoto's thyroiditis (HT) - are the most common autoimmune endocrine diseases with a complex etiology involving genetic and environmental factors. From a genetic standpoint, there are multiple genes ranging from MHC class to non-MHC immune regulatory genes to thyroid specific genes that infer susceptibility to AITD [1]. Environmental exposure interaction, likely through epigenetic mechanisms, modulates the expression of the disease. From twin studies, it appears that the genetic background accounts for only about 70-80% of the disease susceptibility, with environmental triggers or exposures accounting for the remaining 20-30% [2].

There are multiple genes identified that infer susceptibility to AITD. These include MHC class genes, general immune modulatory genes and genes specific to the thyroid [1, 3, 4]. HLA-DR3 was the first gene identified as associated with GD in Caucasian populations, while the association with HT is less strong.

*Corresonding author Marjorie Safran: Department of Medicine, Division of Endocrinology, University of Massachusetts Health Center, Worcester, MA, USA; E-mail: marjorie.safran@umassmemorial.org

Conversely, the presence of DR1 and 8 seems to be protective of HT. Other HLA loci have been implicated in different populations.

The immune regulatory genes such as CD40, CTLA-4, PTPN22, FOXP3 and CD23 are associated with AITD in different ways, some of which are disease specific, some population specific and some age specific. For example, CD40, plays a critical role in B lymphocyte differentiation and the CC allele in a C/T polymorphism of the Kozak sequence is associated with GD in Caucasians, Japanese and Koreans [5], but not in Taiwanese [6]. CTLA-4 functions to suppress T cell activation and an AT repeat in its 3'UTR, which decreases CTLA-4 inhibitory activity, is linked to AITD, while two other SNP variations in the gene are associated with GD [5, 7]. The roll of CTLA-4 appears to be present across multiple populations. Polymorphisms in FOXP3, a Treg cell marker, are associated with Graves' disease in Caucasians younger than 30, but not in the Japanese population [8].

Two thyroid specific genes are associated with AITD: the thyroglobulin gene and the TSH receptor gene. Thyroglobulin is the major protein in the thyroid and antibodies to thyroglobulin are present in 75% of patients with HT. Polymorphisms in the thyroglobulin protein are associated with an increased risk for GD [9, 10]. The TSH receptor gene was initially found to be associated with GD by whole genome linkage studies and more recently non-coding SNPs seem to confer this association [11]. Recently SNP polymorphisms in the TSH receptor gene were associated with HT in a Chinese population [12].

All told, it is estimated that the genes identified account for <10% of the heritability of AITD leaving room for many more susceptibility genes to be identified [4, 13-16]. In addition, little is known about how specific environmental factors interact with these genes to increase the expression of AITD [4]. A number of environmental exposures have been associated with AITD in both human and animal studies. These include exposures such as infections, stress, iodine intake, smoking, drugs such as amiodarone, and interferon (IFN) and more recently the use of immunomodulatory agents such as alemtuzumab. It is generally unclear whether these environmental exposures trigger the autoimmune response *de novo* or whether they enhance expression of an ongoing autoimmune process [17]. The relationship between environmental exposures and expression of autoimmune thyroid dysfunction will be explored.

IODINE

One of the first environmental factors associated with AITD was iodine. It has long been recognized that the expression of AITD differs in areas of iodine deficiency *vs* areas of adequate iodine or excess [18-20]. Thyroid antibodies and HT are more common in areas of iodine sufficiency [21, 22]. Even mild iodine repletion in Denmark increased the incidence of hypothyroidism in an area with previous moderate iodine deficiency (urinary iodine = 45 microg/liter), but not in an area of moderate iodine deficiency (urinary iodine = 61 microg/liter) [23]. However, the prevalence of thyroid autoantibodies is increased even in the area of moderate iodine deficiency [24]. In a small town in Italy, subjects were evaluated 15 years after instituting iodination of salt. Beneficial effects included a decrease in goiter, non-autoimmune hyperthyroidism in the older population and thyroid autonomy in the population < age 45, but there was an increase in subclinical hypothyroidism, thyroid antibodies and HT, particularly in the younger population [25]. Research into the mechanism of iodine induced thyroid autoimmunity suggested unmasking of a cryptic epitope on thyroglobulin with resultant increase in AbTg, but not TPO-Ab [26]. In an animal model of spontaneous autoimmune thyroiditis, excess iodine in the drinking water increased the incidence of thyroiditis from 50% to 90% in adult NOD.H2h4 mice [27]. The effects of iodine on thyroid autoimmunity may be transient [28]. In a study from Germany, patients with goiter and negative antibodies were randomized to receive 0.5 mg iodine daily or levothyroxine for 6 months. Six of 31 subjects in the iodine treated group developed high anti-microsomal and anti-thyroglobulin antibody levels, four with hypothyroidism and two with hyperthyroidism. The two hyperthyroid subjects normalized after withdrawal of iodine as well as two of four hypothyroid subjects while the remaining two hypothyroid patients continued to have elevated autoantibodies and hypothyroidism.

SELENIUM

Selenium in the form of selenocysteine is an important component of thyroid deiodinases, enzymes critical to the metabolism of thyroid hormones and also an essential element in glutathione peroxidases and thioredoxin reductaces, important in protection from oxidative damage [29]. AITD is more prevalent in areas of selenium deficiency. In some [30-33], but not all studies [34], 6-12 month supplementation with selenium decreases anti-TPO antibody levels which rebound to previous levels after stopping. An improvement in the decreased thyroid echogenicity seen on ultrasound in patients with HT was shown with selenium supplementation [34]. However, there is no effect on thyroid hormone levels or thyroid hormone replacement doses [32, 34]. In addition, there is little data to demonstrate the long-term effects of selenium on disease expression.

INFECTIOUS AGENTS

Various infectious agents have been suspected in the pathogenesis of AITD including Yersinia enterocolitica, hepatitis C, congenital rubella infection and parvovirus B19 through mechanisms such as molecular mimicry, polyclonal T cell activation or MHC class II antigen induction [35-37].

Yersinia was one of the first infectious agents associated with AITD. Early studies suggested a significantly higher prevalence of antibodies to Yersinia in patients with GD than in controls [38]. Initial studies identified TSH binding sites on Yersinia that were recognized by immunoglobulin from patients with GD [39]. This, along with identification of amino acid homologies between Yersinia proteins and the TSH receptor suggests molecular mimicry as one of triggers for AITD in susceptible patients [40]. More recent studies continue to note increased evidence for infection in women with first or second-degree relatives with AITD [35], in subjects with GD, and in the effected twin in pairs discordant for GD [41]. However, the presence of these antibodies was not a risk factor for the development of AITD in a 5 year prospective study [42, 43]. In contrast with the findings for GD, there was no difference in the rate of Yersinia infection in antibody positive twins *vs* the antibody negative twins when twins were discordant for the presence of thyroid antibodies [44].

Hepatitis C virus (HCV) is the infection most associated with the development of AITD. While it is clearly shown that treatment of HCV with IFN increases the prevalence of both GD and HT [37], there is significant data that even untreated HCV increases both the presence of anti-thyroid antibodies and clinical disease [37, 45]. HCV infection induced poly-clonal B-lymphocyte expansion, commonly observed in a high proportion of patients with HCV infection, is responsible for the production of different autoantibodies and immune-complexes, such as mixed cryoglobulins [46]. The burst of chemokines and cytokines induced by HCV can stimulate auto-reactive lymphocytes in susceptible patients resulting in the development of organ specific and systemic autoimmune disorders one of which is thyroiditis [47]. In clinical studies, children with HCV were more likely to have thyroid antibodies or non-autoimmune subclinical hypothyroidism [48]. Adult patients with chronic hepatitis C were more likely to have hypothyroidism, anti-thyroglobulin antibodies, and anti-thyroid peroxidase antibodies than controls from both iodine deficient and sufficient areas or patients with chronic hepatitis B [49].

Looking at the question from the other direction, Hammerstad and coworkers studied 47 patients with high thyroid antibodies, including 13 with subclinical hypothyroidism, 17 with overt hypothyroidism, and found significant increases in IFN-α/β-inducible myxovirus resistance protein 1 (myxovirus resistance protein A; MxA) in all three groups compared to controls, suggesting the possibility of viral infection [50]. Most recently, Blackard was able to show that HCV could directly infect a human thyroid cell line *in vitro* leading to increased expression of the proinflammatory cytokine IL-8, thus raising the possibility of direct HCV infection of thyrocytes *in vivo* as a link between HCV infection and the induction of thyroid autoimmunity [51, 52].

MEDICATIONS

A number of medications have been associated with the development of AITD. These include amiodarone, lithium, and the immune modulatory drugs such as IFNα, interleukin-2 (IL-2) and highly active anti-retroviral therapy (HAART). With some drugs, the increased expression of thyroid dysfunction appears to be unmasking of underlying autoimmune disease, while other drugs directly cause a breakdown in the recognition of self-antigens through different mechanisms [17].

Amiodarone, a drug used in the treatment of cardiac arrhythmias, has diverse effects on thyroid function that are secondary to its high iodine content and also direct effects on the thyroid [53]. It is a potent inhibitor of type I 5'deiodinase, the enzyme that metabolizes thyroxine (T4) to the metabolically active hormone triiodothyronine (T3), decreases thyroid hormone entry into cells and has direct cytotoxic effects on the thyroid. Clinically, amiodarone associated hyperthyroidism is seen more frequently in areas of low iodine intake, while amiodarone associated hypothyroidism occurs more often in areas of iodine sufficiency [54]. Hypothyroidism occurs more frequently in patients who are positive for anti-thyroid peroxidase or anti-microsomal antibodies [55], but this appears to represent the increased susceptibility to thyroid dysfunction in patients with thyroid autoantibodies, rather than the induction of autoimmunity by amiodarone itself [56].

Lithium therapy is also associated with an increased risk of hypothyroidism in thyroid antibody positive subjects [57]. Much of the effect of lithium is secondary to its ability to decrease thyroid hormone synthesis and release and to decrease metabolism of T4 to T3 by inhibiting type I 5'deiodinase resulting in a high incidence of goiter and hypothyroidism in lithium treated subjects. While there is little evidence that lithium increases the expression of thyroid antibodies, one study did demonstrate a reduced number of cytotoxic/suppressor T-cells in lithium treated subjects *vs* a control group of patients with affective disorders treated with other drugs leaving open the possibility of a direct effect on immune function [58].

The evidence for the effect of immune modulatory drugs on induction of autoimmunity is much more robust [59]. IFN is used in the treatment of a number of malignant and non-malignant disorders including HVC, carcinoid tumors, hairy cell leukemia and Kaposi's sarcoma to name a few. It works by binding to receptors that activate multiple signaling pathways including JAK-STAT, Crk, insulin receptor substrate and MAP kinase resulting in activation of proinflammatory cytokines, increased MHC class I antigen expression on cells, including thyrocytes and decreased T-cell regulatory function [37]. Both the development of autoimmune antibodies and clinical disease has been seen with IFN treatment including AITD, type I diabetes, and systemic lupus erythematosus (SLE) among others [59]. Induction of clinical thyroid dysfunction is seen in up to 6% of patients treated with IFN, which can be both autoimmune and non-immune in etiology [37]. In those who develop non-autoimmune disease, it is postulated that IFN has direct tissue toxicity [60].

The presence of thyroid autoantibodies prior to treatment definitely increases the risk for developing thyroid dysfunction with IFN therapy. However, there also appears to be induction of de-novo thyroid autoimmunity with IFN. In a prospective study by Custro and coworker, 15% of 56 IFN treated thyroid antibody negative patients developed thyroid autoimmunity with 78% of those developing thyroid dysfunction [45]. It is interesting that those who did develop thyroid antibodies shared some of the autoimmune thyroid susceptibility genes previously described [7, 37]. The most common manifestation of IFN induced AITD is HT that may be reversible in some cases after withdrawal of the medication. GD is less often observed, but does not usually remit when therapy is stopped [17, 59].

Alemtuzumab is a monoclonal antibody that targets CD-52 on both T and B cells, resulting in their depletion. It is used in the treatment of multiple sclerosis (MS) [61] and as preparation for allogeneic stem cell transplantation [59]. In an early study of patients treated for MS with 5 days of alemtuzumab, 30% developed GD at 6-31 months post treatment [62]. This was confirmed in phase 3 trials with the drug where GD developed a mean of 32 months after treatment [63]. The effect appears to be treatment specific, since AITD developed in 23% of MS patients treated with 2-3 annual cycles of alemtuzumab *vs* only 3% of patients treated with interferon-β1a [64]. A much lower incidence of HT is noted (7% *vs.* 22% with

GD) [65]. Alemtuzumab associated AITD appeared rarely when used for other disorders such as combined with maintenance immunosuppression in renal transplantation, rheumatoid arthritis or as therapy for B-cell chronic lymphocytic leukemia, possibly secondary to maintenance immunosuppression, a lower female: male ratio of subjects and high death rate [59]. However, it has been noted in 11% of patients treated for vasculitis and when used as preparation for allogeneic stem cell transplantation in patients with sickle cell disease, 3 of 26 patients developed thyroid dysfunction; one with hypothyroidism 10 months after treatment, 2 with GD 3 years later [66].

The mechanism postulated for alemtuzumab-induced autoimmunity is that of immune reconstitution [67]. Alemtuzumab induces a profound long lasting lymphopenia with CD4+ and CD8+ T cells reduced by 60-70% for up to 18 months. CD8+ T-cells recover sooner than CD4+ memory T-cells that suppress autoimmunity. Thus it appears that autoimmunity is augmented when there is an imbalance between CD8+ stimulation and CD4+ inhibition resulting in the onset of GD between 6 months to years after therapy.

Similar to the proposed mechanism of alemtuzumab induced AITD, HAART induced AITD appears in the reconstitution phase [67]. Although other autoimmune disorders are noted in untreated HIV infected patients, thyroid dysfunction is usually non-immune in origin. However, as HAART decreases HIV replication CD4+ counts begin to increase. In the first 2-3 months, memory CD4+ cells are released from lymphoid tissue and later naïve CD4+ T-cells slowly recover. GD occurs 1-2 years after initiation of HAART and is recognized in 2-3% of patients.

OTHER FACTORS

Other exposures factors such as smoking, alcohol, vitamin D, stress and environmental toxins have been implicated in the development of AITD.

Smoking

Smoking has multiple interesting effects on the thyroid (reviewed in [68]). Smokers have lower TSH levels and increased thyroid hormone levels as compared to control subjects. There is an increased incidence in smokers of GD, autoimmune thyroid ophthalmopathy, and an increased risk of Graves' opthalmopathy after treatment with 131-iodine. In contrast, population studies identified a ~50% decreased risk for hypothyroidism in current smokers, but not former smokers, that is speculated to be secondary to AITD since thyroid antibodies appear less frequently in smokers *vs* non-smokers. A prospective study in the Netherlands followed more than 500 women who were relatives of patients with AITD [69]. All were antibody negative and euthyroid at the onset. Over a 5-year observation, the only risk factor identified for seroconversion, was cessation of smoking. Seroconversion and a general increase in TSH occurred 2-3 years after patients stopped smoking. This effect appears to be transient and as it was no longer present in subjects who stopped smoking more than 3 years prior to the identification of HD [70]. The mechanism for nicotine's effect on AITD seems to be autoimmune in nature. Nicotine appears to be anti-inflammatory [71], but there is also evidence that it has a profound effect on the gut microbiome [72], suggesting that this could indirectly be the mechanism for the relationship between smoking cessation and the incidence of AITD [73]. Thus smoking seems to have an adverse effect on the expression of GD and a beneficial effect on the incidence of HD.

Alcohol

In contrast to the divergent effect of smoking on GD *vs* HT, alcohol consumption appears to decrease the risk of developing both HT [74] and GD [75] with OR of 0.46 and 0.56 for >1 and >2 alcoholic drinks per week *vs* non-drinkers, respectively. In the 5 year prospective Amsterdam AITD study, alcohol consumption was not associated with the development of thyroid antibodies, but was less common in subjects who developed overt hypothyroidism as compared to those who remained euthyroid [76]. Moderate alcohol use may have a beneficial effect on the immune system as compared to excess alcohol or abstinence [77], but appears to have more of an effect on progression of AITD, rather than *de novo* expression of autoimmunity.

Miscellaneous

Other factors that have been associated with AITD are vitamin D, stress, environmental toxicants such as polyaromatic hydrocarbons, and radiation, but data is either minimal or conflicting [4, 17, 78]. For example vitamin D receptors are present on many immunocompetent cells. In a large observational study in Korea, a slightly lower mean 25(OH)D level was noted in women with anti-TPO antibodies, and the prevalence of TPO-Ab varied from 21% in vitamin D deficient subjects to 13% in vitamin D sufficiency [4]. However, again, this may just not be causative, since vitamin D levels were not identified as a risk factor in the development of thyroid autoantibodies in the prospective Amsterdam AITD study

[69]. Stress was also not a causative agent in this study. Most data on the effect of polyaromatic hydrocarbons, such as polychlorinated biphenyls (PCBs) and polyhalogenated biphenyls (PBBs) and organopesticides demonstrate that they have an effect on thyroid hormone action either by reacting at the thyroid hormone receptor or altering thyroid hormone metabolism, but there is little evidence that they effect autoimmunity [4, 11, 78, 79]. Radiation is more likely to cause destructive hypothyroidism (as in treatment with external radiation for Hodgkin's disease) or thyroid nodularity and cancer (as seen with the atomic bomb in Japan and Chernobyl), but a few studies have demonstrated an increase in thyroid antibodies that appear to dissipate over time suggesting they represented a reaction to neoantigens presented on irradiated thyroid cells rather than the development of innate autoimmunity [17, 78].

CONCLUDING REMARKS

Overall, a number of environmental exposures are associated with the presence of AITD. In the case of iodine, which is critical for thyroid hormone synthesis, increasing intake does appear to both increase the presence of thyroid autoantibodies and the expression of hypothyroidism in subjects with underlying AITD. Smoking is associated with a decreased prevalence of HT and an increased incidence with cessation. For a number of medications associated with AITD, such as amiodarone and lithium, it appears the drugs unmask underlying autoimmunity. This differs from the immune modulatory drugs that are more likely to induce *de novo* thyroid autoimmunity. Thus we can see increased thyroid autoimmune dysfunction in subjects after various environmental exposures, some of which induce thyroid autoimmunity *de novo* while others change progression of disease in already susceptible subjects. From a clinical standpoint, this should increase our awareness of possible thyroid dysfunction in patients who are susceptible to these complications. In the future, understanding the interaction between the environmental factors and underlying genetics should lead to new treatment options for AITD.

CONFLICT OF INTEREST

The author confirms that author has no conflict of interest to declare for this publication.

ACKNOWLEDGEMENTS

Declared None.

REFERENCES

[1] Hasham A, Tomer Y. Genetic and epigenetic mechanisms in thyroid autoimmunity. Immunol Res 2012; 54(1-3): 204-213.

[2] Hansen PS, Brix TH, Iachine I, Kyvik KO, Hegedus L. The relative importance of genetic and environmental effects for the early stages of thyroid autoimmunity: a study of healthy Danish twins. Eur J Endocrinol 2006; 154(1): 29-38.

[3] Tomer Y, Huber A. The etiology of autoimmune thyroid disease: a story of genes and environment. J Autoimmun 2009; 32(3-4): 231-239.

[4] Effraimidis G, Wiersinga WM. Mechanisms in endocrinology: autoimmune thyroid disease: old and new players. Eur J Endocrinol 2014; 170(6): R241-52.

[5] Jacobson EM, Tomer Y. The CD40, CTLA-4, thyroglobulin, TSH receptor, and PTPN22 gene quintet and its contribution to thyroid autoimmunity: back to the future. J Autoimmun 2007; 28(2-3): 85-98.

[6] Hsiao JY, Tien KJ, Hsiao CT, Hsieh MC. A C/T polymorphism in CD40 gene is not associated with susceptibility and phenotype of Graves' disease in Taiwanese. Endocr J 2008; 55(3): 477-484.

[7] Tomer Y. Genetic susceptibility to autoimmune thyroid disease: past, present, and future. Thyroid 2010; 20(7): 715-725.

[8] Ban Y, Tozaki T, Tobe T, *et al.* The regulatory T cell gene FOXP3 and genetic susceptibility to thyroid autoimmunity: an association analysis in Caucasian and Japanese cohorts. J Autoimmun 2007; 28(4): 201-207.

[9] Ban Y, Tozaki T, Taniyama M, *et al.* Multiple SNPs in intron 41 of thyroglobulin gene are associated with autoimmune thyroid disease in the Japanese population. PLoS One 2012; 7(5): e37501.

[10] Maierhaba M, Zhang JA, Yu ZY, *et al.* Association of the thyroglobulin gene polymorphism with autoimmune thyroid disease in Chinese population. Endocrine 2008; 33(3): 294-299.

[11] Eschler DC, Hasham A, Tomer Y. Cutting edge: the etiology of autoimmune thyroid diseases. Clin Rev Allergy Immunol 201; 41(2): 190-197.

[12] Liu L, Wu HQ, Wang Q, Zhu *et al.* Association between thyroid stimulating hormone receptor gene intron polymorphisms and autoimmune thyroid disease in a Chinese Han population. Endocr J 2012; 59(8): 717-723.

[13] Tomer Y, Hasham A, Davies TF, *et al.* Fine mapping of loci linked to autoimmune thyroid disease identifies novel susceptibility genes. J Clin Endocrinol Metab 2013; 98(1): E144-52.

[14] Brown RS, Lombardi A, Hasham A, *et al.* Genetic analysis in young-age-of-onset Graves' disease reveals new susceptibility loci. J Clin Endocrinol Metab 2014; 99(7): E1387-91.

[15] Muhali FS, Song RH, Wang X, *et al.* Genetic variants of BANK1 gene in autoimmune thyroid diseases: a case-control association study. Exp Clin Endocrinol Diabetes 2013; 121(9): 556-560.

[16] Muhali FS, Zhou-jiao Z, Wang Y, *et al.* Lack of association of IRF5 gene polymorphisms with autoimmune thyroid disease: a case-control study. IRF5 gene and AITD. Ann Endocrinol (Paris) 2014; 75(1): 19-24.

[17] McLachlan SM, Rapoport B. Breaking tolerance to thyroid antigens: changing concepts in thyroid autoimmunity. Endocr Rev 2014; 35(1): 59-105.

[18] Vanderpump MP, Tunbridge WM, French JM, *et al.* The incidence of thyroid disorders in the community: a twenty-year follow-up of the Whickham Survey. Clin Endocrinol (Oxf) 1995; 43(1): 55-68.

[19] Laurberg P, Pedersen KM, Hreidarsson A, Sigfusson N, Iversen E, Knudsen PR. Iodine intake and the pattern of thyroid disorders: a comparative epidemiological study of thyroid abnormalities in the elderly in Iceland and in Jutland, Denmark. J Clin Endocrinol Metab 1998; 83(3): 765-769.

[20] Papanastasiou L, Vatalas IA, Koutras DA, Mastorakos G. Thyroid autoimmunity in the current iodine environment. Thyroid 2007; 17(8): 729-739.

[21] Foley TP Jr. The relationship between autoimmune thyroid disease and iodine intake: a review. Endokrynol Pol 1992; 43 Suppl 1: 53-69.

[22] Lind P, Langsteger W, Molnar M, Gallowitsch HJ, Mikosch P, Gomez I. Epidemiology of thyroid diseases in iodine sufficiency. Thyroid 1998; 8(12): 1179-1183.

[23] Pedersen IB, Laurberg P, Knudsen N, *et al.* An increased incidence of overt hypothyroidism after iodine fortification of salt in Denmark: a prospective population study. J Clin Endocrinol Metab 2007; 92(8): 3122-3127.

[24] Pedersen IB, Knudsen N, Carle A, *et al.* A cautious iodization programme bringing iodine intake to a low recommended level is associated with an increase in the prevalence of thyroid autoantibodies in the population. Clin Endocrinol (Oxf) 2011; 75(1): 120-126.
[25] Aghini L.F, Fiore E, Tonacchera M, *et al.* The effect of voluntary iodine prophylaxis in a small rural community: the Pescopagano survey 15 years later. J Clin Endocrinol Metab 2013; 98(3): 1031-1039.
[26] Latrofa F, Fiore E, Rago T, Antonangeli L, Montanelli L, Ricci D, *et al.* Iodine contributes to thyroid autoimmunity in humans by unmasking a cryptic epitope on thyroglobulin. J Clin Endocrinol Metab 2013; 98(11): E1768-74.
[27] Burek CL, Talor MV. Environmental triggers of autoimmune thyroiditis. J Autoimmun 2009; 33(3-4): 183-189.
[28] Kahaly GJ, Dienes HP, Beyer J, Hommel G. Iodide induces thyroid autoimmunity in patients with endemic goitre: a randomised, double-blind, placebo-controlled trial. Eur J Endocrinol 1998; 139(3): 290-297.
[29] Duntas LH. Selenium and the thyroid: a close-knit connection. J Clin Endocrinol Metab 2010; 95(12): 5180-5188.
[30] Gartner R, Gasnier BC. Selenium in the treatment of autoimmune thyroiditis. Biofactors 2003; 19(3-4): 165-170.
[31] Turker O, Kumanlioglu K, Karapolat I, Dogan I. Selenium treatment in autoimmune thyroiditis: 9-month follow-up with variable doses. J Endocrinol 2006; 190(1): 151-156.
[32] Mazokopakis EE, Papadakis JA, Papadomanolaki MG, *et al.* Effects of 12 months treatment with L-selenomethionine on serum anti-TPO Levels in Patients with Hashimoto's thyroiditis. Thyroid 2007; 17(7): 609-612.
[33] Karanikas G, Schuetz M, Kontur S, *et al.* No immunological benefit of selenium in consecutive patients with autoimmune thyroiditis. Thyroid 2008; 18(1): 7-12.
[34] Nacamulli D, Mian C, Petricca D, *et al.* Influence of physiological dietary selenium supplementation on the natural course of autoimmune thyroiditis. Clin Endocrinol (Oxf) 2010 Oct; 73(4): 535-539.
[35] Tomer Y, Davies TF. Infection, thyroid disease, and autoimmunity. Endocr Rev 1993; 14(1) :107-120.
[36] Lehmann HW, Lutterbuse N, Plentz A, *et al.* Association of parvovirus B19 infection and Hashimoto's thyroiditis in children. Viral Immunol 2008; 21(3): 379-383.
[37] Tomer Y. Hepatitis C and interferon induced thyroiditis. J Autoimmun 2010; 34(3): J322-6.
[38] Shenkman L, Bottone EJ. Antibodies to Yersinia enterocolitica in thyroid disease. Ann Intern Med 1976; 85(6): 735-739.
[39] Heyma P, Harrison LC, Robins-Browne R. Thyrotrophin (TSH) binding sites on Yersinia enterocolitica recognized by immunoglobulins from humans with Graves' disease. Clin Exp Immunol 1986; 64(2): 249-254.
[40] Benvenga S, Santarpia L, Trimarchi F, Guarneri F. Human thyroid autoantigens and proteins of Yersinia and Borrelia share amino acid sequence homology that includes binding motifs to HLA-DR molecules and T-cell receptor. Thyroid 2006; 16(3): 225-236.
[41] Brix TH, Hansen PS, Hegedus L, Wenzel BE. Too early to dismiss Yersinia enterocolitica infection in the aetiology of Graves' disease: evidence from a twin case-control study. Clin Endocrinol (Oxf) 2008; 69(3): 491-496.
[42] Strieder TG, Tijssen JG, Wenzel BE, Endert E, Wiersinga WM. Prediction of progression to overt hypothyroidism or hyperthyroidism in female relatives of patients with autoimmune thyroid disease using thc Thyroid Events Amsterdam (THEA) score. Arch Intern Med 2008; 168(15): 1657-1663.
[43] Effraimidis G, Tijssen JG, Strieder TG, Wiersinga WM. No causal relationship between Yersinia enterocolitica infection and autoimmune thyroid disease: evidence from a prospective study. Clin Exp Immunol 2011; 165(1): 38-43.
[44] Hansen PS, Wenzel BE, Brix TH, Hegedus L. Yersinia enterocolitica infection does not confer an increased risk of thyroid antibodies: evidence from a Danish twin study. Clin Exp Immunol 2006; 146(1):32-38.
[45] Custro N, Montalto G, Scafidi V, *et al.* Prospective study on thyroid autoimmunity and dysfunction related to chronic hepatitis C and interferon therapy. J Endocrinol Invest 1997; 20(7): 374-380.
[46] Fallahi P, Ferrari SM, Politti U, Giuggioli D, Ferri C, Antonelli A. Autoimmune and neoplastic thyroid diseases associated with hepatitis C chronic infection. Int J Endocrinol 2014; 2014: 935131.

[47] Calvaruso V, Craxi A. Immunological alterations in hepatitis C virus infection. World J Gastroenterol 2013; 19(47): 8916-8923.
[48] Indolfi G, Stagi S, Bartolini E, *et al.* Thyroid function and anti-thyroid autoantibodies in untreated children with vertically acquired chronic hepatitis C virus infection. Clin Endocrinol (Oxf) 2008; 68(1): 117-121.
[49] Antonelli A, Ferri C, Pampana A, *et al.* Thyroid disorders in chronic hepatitis C. Am J Med 2004; 117(1): 10-13.
[50] Hammerstad SS, Jahnsen FL, Tauriainen S, *et al.* Inflammation and increased myxovirus resistance protein A expression in thyroid tissue in the early stages of Hashimoto's thyroiditis. Thyroid 2013; 23(3): 334-341.
[51] Akeno N, Blackard JT, Tomer Y. HCV E2 protein binds directly to thyroid cells and induces IL-8 production: a new mechanism for HCV induced thyroid autoimmunity. J Autoimmun 2008; 31(4): 339-344.
[52] Blackard JT, Kong L, Huber AK, Tomer Y. Hepatitis C virus infection of a thyroid cell line: implications for pathogenesis of hepatitis C virus and thyroiditis. Thyroid 2013; 23(7): 863-870.
[53] Bogazzi F, Tomisti L, Bartalena L, Aghini-Lombardi F, Martino E. Amiodarone and the thyroid: a 2012 update. J Endocrinol Invest 2012; 35(3): 340-348.
[54] Martino E, Safran M, Aghini-Lombardi F, *et al.* Environmental iodine intake and thyroid dysfunction during chronic amiodarone therapy. Ann Intern Med 1984; 101(1): 28-34.
[55] Martino E, Aghini-L.F, Mariotti S, *et al.* Amiodarone iodine-induced hypothyroidism: risk factors and follow-up in 28 cases. Clin Endocrinol (Oxf) 1987; 26(2): 227-237.
[56] Safran M, Martino E, Aghini-Lombardi F, Bartalena L, Balzano S, Pinchera A, *et al.* Effect of amiodarone on circulating antithyroid antibodies. BMJ 1988; 297(6646): 456-457.
[57] Kibirige D, Luzinda K, Ssekitoleko R. Spectrum of lithium induced thyroid abnormalities: a current perspective. Thyroid Res 2013; 6(1): 3-6614-6-3.
[58] Wilson R, McKillop JH, Crocket GT, *et al.* The effect of lithium therapy on parameters thought to be involved in the development of autoimmune thyroid disease. Clin Endocrinol (Oxf) 1991; 34(5): 357-361.
[59] Kong YC, Wei WZ, Tomer Y. Opportunistic autoimmune disorders: from immunotherapy to immune dysregulation. Ann N Y Acad Sci 2010; 1183: 222-236.
[60] Akeno N, Smith EP, Stefan M, *et al.* IFN-alpha mediates the development of autoimmunity both by direct tissue toxicity and through immune cell recruitment mechanisms. J Immunol 2011; 186(8): 4693-4706.
[61] Jones DE, Goldman MD. Alemtuzumab for the treatment of relapsing-remitting multiple sclerosis: a review of its clinical pharmacology, efficacy and safety. Expert Rev Clin Immunol 2014; 10(10): 1281-1291.
[62] Coles AJ, Wing M, Smith S, *et al.* Pulsed monoclonal antibody treatment and autoimmune thyroid disease in multiple sclerosis. Lancet 1999; 354(9191): 1691-1695.
[63] Tsourdi E, Gruber M, Rauner M, Blankenburg J, Ziemssen T, Hofbauer LC. Graves' disease after treatment with Alemtuzumab for multiple sclerosis. Hormones (Athens) 2015; 14(1): 148-153.
[64] CAMMS223 Trial Investigators, Coles AJ, Compston DA, Selmaj KW, Lake SL, Moran S, *et al.* Alemtuzumab *vs.* interferon beta-1a in early multiple sclerosis. N Engl J Med 2008; 359(17): 1786-1801.
[65] Daniels GH, Vladic A, Brinar V, *et al.* Alemtuzumab-related thyroid dysfunction in a phase 2 trial of patients with relapsing-remitting multiple sclerosis. J Clin Endocrinol Metab 2014; 99(1): 80-89.
[66] Williams KM, Dietzen D, Hassoun AA, Fennoy I, Bhatia M. Autoimmune thyroid disease following alemtuzumab therapy and hematopoietic cell transplantation in pediatric patients with sickle cell disease. Pediatr Blood Cancer 2014; 61(12): 2307-2309.
[67] Weetman A. Immune reconstitution syndrome and the thyroid. Best Pract Res Clin Endocrinol Metab 2009; 23(6): 693-702.
[68] Wiersinga WM. Smoking and thyroid. Clin Endocrinol (Oxf) 2013; 79(2): 145-151.
[69] Effraimidis G, Tijssen JG, Wiersinga WM. Discontinuation of smoking increases the risk for developing thyroid peroxidase antibodies and/or thyroglobulin antibodies: a prospective study. J Clin Endocrinol Metab 2009; 94(4): 1324-1328.

[70] Carle A, Bulow Pedersen I, Knudsen N, *et al*. Smoking cessation is followed by a sharp but transient rise in the incidence of overt autoimmune hypothyroidism - a population-based, case-control study. Clin Endocrinol (Oxf) 2012; 77(5): 764-772.

[71] Filippini P, Cesario A, Fini M, Locatelli F, Rutella S. The Yin and Yang of non-neuronal alpha7-nicotinic receptors in inflammation and autoimmunity. Curr Drug Targets 2012; 13(5): 644-655.

[72] Biedermann L, Zeitz J, Mwinyi J, Sutter-Minder E, Rehman A, Ott SJ, *et al*. Smoking cessation induces profound changes in the composition of the intestinal microbiota in humans. PLoS One 2013; 8(3): e59260.

[73] Mori K, Nakagawa Y, Ozaki H. Does the gut microbiota trigger Hashimoto's thyroiditis? Discov Med 2012; 14(78): 321-326.

[74] Carle A, Pedersen IB, Knudsen N, *et al*. Moderate alcohol consumption may protect against overt autoimmune hypothyroidism: a population-based case-control study. Eur J Endocrinol 2012; 167(4): 483-490.

[75] Carle A, Bulow PI, Knudsen N, *et al*. Graves' hyperthyroidism and moderate alcohol consumption: evidence for disease prevention. Clin Endocrinol (Oxf) 2013; 79(1): 111-119.

[76] Effraimidis G, Tijssen JG, Wiersinga WM. Alcohol consumption as a risk factor for autoimmune thyroid disease: a prospective study. Eur Thyroid J 2012; 1(2): 99-104.

[77] Romeo J, Warnberg J, Nova E, Diaz LE, Gomez-Martinez S, Marcos A. Moderate alcohol consumption and the immune system: a review. Br J Nutr 2007; 98 Suppl 1: S111-5.

[78] Brent GA. Environmental exposures and autoimmune thyroid disease. Thyroid 2010; 20(7): 755-761.

[79] Pearce EN, Braverman LE. Environmental pollutants and the thyroid. Best Pract Res Clin Endocrinol Metab 2009; 23(6): 801-813.

CHAPTER 4

Biological Select Agents and Toxins (BSAT)

Alberto Cique Moya[1,*], Miguel Andrés Capo Marti[2] and Javier Del Pino[2]

[1]*Environmental Health and NBC Service. Defense Preventive Medicine Institute. Ministry of Defense, Madrid, Spain and* [2]*Departament of Toxicology and Pharmacology, Veterinary School, Complutense University of Madrid, Madrid, Spain*

Abstract: Biological Select Agents and Toxins (BSATs) are a specific group of pathogens, toxins and substances of biological origin that pose not only a severe threat to human, plant, and animal health, but also have the potential to be used deliberately to cause disease, prompt fear, or destroy agricultural or animal products as biological warfare or bioterrorism agents. BSATs may cause a disruption of the thyroid system either directly or indirectly through the systemic effects they induce. Bioregulator agents, toxins and microbiological infections, which could induce acute, subacute or chronic thyroiditis, among others, could cause thyroid functional alteration. The thyroiditis induced through colonization of thyroid gland by these pathogen agents (induced mainly by virus or bacteria) or as a particular manifestation of a systemic disease, results in inflammation of the thyroid gland that can sometimes degenerate into destructive thyrotoxicosis. Otherwise, the possibility of their use as terrorist or criminal agents makes it necessary to know and recognize the implications arising from the intended use of these agents on the thyroid system. This chapter will refer to the main agents that induce thyroid disruption and the known mechanisms through which these effects are induced.

Keywords: Biological warfare agents, biorregulators, bioterrorism agents, thyroiditis.

INTRODUCTION

Warfare agents have been classically classified as chemical and biological warfare agents. The first group includes choking, blister, blood, nerve and riot control agents. Blood agents (hydrogen cyanide, cyanogen chloride and arsine) and their metabolites have been reported to present direct effects on the thyroid system in animal models and observations of exposed workers. They alter thyroid hormones levels by inhibiting uptake and utilization of iodine in the thyroid gland [1, 2].

Thyroid disruption has been also reported in populations affected in incidents where nerve agents have been spread like sarin or other compounds such as some

*Corresponding author Alberto Cique Moya:** Environmental Health and NBC Service. Defense Preventive Medicine Institute. Ministry of Defense, Madrid, Spain; E-mail: aciquemo@et.mde.es

Javier Del Pino, Maria Jesus Diaz and Maria Teresa Frejo (Eds)

blister agents, like lewisite, and more particularly its arsenic residues [3]. In addition, the iodine generated in nuclear explosions (Hiroshima or Nagasaki), in incidents at nuclear plants (Chernobyl) or in terrorist attacks with dirty bombs emitting radioactive iodine, has been reported to disrupt the thyroid system. For this reason, Nuclear Emergency Plans include administering potassium iodide to the population in order to limit the risk of damage to the thyroid gland from radioactive iodine fixation [4, 5]. Furthermore, other chemical substances not included in the list of chemical warfare agents, could also be used in terrorist attacks and may also induce thyroid disruption. For example, dioxins, whose effect on the thyroid system has been described from the Seveso disaster in Italy where thousands of people were affected and even today continue to suffer the consequences of such accidents [6], could be used to this aim.

Biological warfare agents are known as biological select agents and toxins (BSATs) which include a specific group of pathogens, toxins and substances of biological origin that pose not only a severe threat to the health of humans, plants, and animals, but also have the potential to be used deliberately to cause disease, prompt fear, or destroy agricultural or animal products as biological warfare or bioterrorism agents. The BSAT list is published as part of the US Code of Federal Regulations (42 CFR 73.3) and are subject to special security requirements (Table **1A** and **1B**) [7].

BSATs have been used as weapons of biological warfare for centuries [8-10]. For example, the Mongols during their war with the Genoese in the 14th century used the dead bodies of plague victims and threw them over the city wall of Caffa in an effort to infect the city's inhabitants. British forces fighting in the French and Indian War, in the late 18th century (1763), gave blankets which were supposed to be infected with Variola major virus (smallpox) to Native Americans to reduce their number. The use of biological agents as an act of terrorism is commonly a more recent phenomenon, from which stands out the mailing of the anthrax letters in 2001 that led to several human fatalities and produced great anxiety in the United States population. Moreover, fear that terrorist groups such as al-Qaeda and others might acquire and use biological weapons have risen continuously since 2001.

Biological agents are grouped into three groups according to the ease of dissemination in the environment, transferability, impact on the community and requirements in diagnostics [11, 12]:

- Group A: includes those biological agents easily disseminable or transmissible from person to person. Agents causing high mortality and morbidity are included in this group. If they were disseminated, this would provoke high psychological and sociological impact on society. Special protocols for identification and treatment are required. This group includes variola major (smallpox); *Bacillus anthracis* (anthrax); *Yersinia pestis* (plague); *Clostridium botulinum toxins* (botulism); *Francisella tularensis* (tularaemia); filoviruses, - Ebola hemorrhagic fever, - Marburg hemorrhagic fever; and arenaviruses, - Lassa (Lassa fever), - Junin (Argentine hemorrhagic fever) and related viruses.

- Group B: includes the biological agents that are moderately easy to disseminate. Their dissemination would cause moderate morbidity and mortality. They require special diagnostic protocols. This group includes *Coxiella burnetti* (Q fever); Brucella species (brucellosis); *Burkholderia mallei* (glanders); *Rickettsia prowazekii* (Typhus fever) alphaviruses, - Venezuelan encephalomyelitis, - eastern and western equine encephalomyelitis; Ricinus communis (ricin toxin from castor beans); epsilon toxin of *Clostridium perfringens*; and *Staphylococcus* enterotoxin B, and "food- or waterborne pathogens" (*Salmonella species - Shigella dysenteriae - Escherichia coli* O157:H7 - *Vibrio cholerae - Cryptosporidium* - Noroviruses).

- Group C: brings together those agents producing emerging diseases, whether genetically manipulated or not. They present relative ease of production and dissemination. They have high morbidity and their dissemination would cause a major impact on public health. This group includes Nipah virus, Hantaviruses, tick-borne hemorrhagic fever viruses, tick-borne encephalitis viruses, yellow fever, and multidrug-resistant tuberculosis.

BSATs may cause a disruption of thyroid system directly or indirectly through induction of their systemic effects. Midspectrum agents (bioregulators and toxins) [13-16] and biological warfare agents, which could induce acute, subacute or chronic thyroiditis [17], among others, could cause thyroid functional alteration. The possibility of their use as terrorist or criminal agents makes it necessary to know and recognize the implications arising from the intended use of these agents on the thyroid system.

Table 1A. Regulated select agents and toxins. Adapted from Kastenmayer and coworkers [7].

Regulated By CDC	Regulated by USDA (animal pathogens)
Bacteria	***Bacteria***
Botulinum neurotoxin-producing species of *Clostridium*	*Ehrlichia ruminantium*
Coxiella burnetii	*Mycoplasma mycoides subsp. Mycoides small colony*
Francisella tularensis	*Mycoplasma capricolum subsp. capripneumoniae*
Rickettsia prowazekii	***Viruses***
Rickettsia rickettsii	African horse sickness virus
Yersinia pestis	African swine fever virus
Fungi	Akabane virus
Coccidioides posadasii	Avian influenza virus (highly pathogenic)
Coccidioides immitis	Blue tongue virus
Viruses	Camel pox virus
B virus (Macacine herpesvirus)	Classical swine fever virus
Crimean-Congo hemorrhagic fever virus	Foot-and-mouth disease virus
Eastern equine encephalitis virus	Goat pox virus
Ebola virus	Japanese encephalitis virus
Lassa fever virus	Lumpy skin disease virus
Marburg virus	Malignant catarrhal fiver virus
Monkeypox virus	Menangle virus
Reconstructed 1918 influenza virus	Peste des petits ruminants virus
South American hemorrhagic fever viruses (Flexal, Guranito, Junin, Machupo, and Sabia)	Rinderpest virus
Tick-borne encephalitis-complex viruses	Sheep pox virus
Variola major virus	Swine vesicular disease virus
Variola minor virus	Virulent Newcastle disease virus
Toxins	Vesicular stomatitis virus (exotic)
Abrin	
Botulinum neurotoxins	
Clostridium perfringens epsilon toxin	
Conotoxins	
Diacetoxyscirpenol	
Ricin	
Saxitoxin	
Shiga-like ribosome inactivating proteins	
Shiga toxin	
Staphylococcal enterotoxins	
Tetrodotoxin	

Table 1B. Regulated select agents and toxins. Adapted from Kastenmayer and coworkers [7].

Regulated by USDA (plant pathogens)	Overlap agents
Bacteria	***Bacteria***
Ralstonia solanacearum race 3, biovar 2	*Bacillus anthracis*
Rathayibacter toxicus	*Brucella abortus*
Xanthomonas oryzae	*Brucella melitensis*
Xylella fastidiosa (citrus variegated chlorosis strain)	*Brucella suis*
Fungí	*Burkholderia mallei*
Peronosclerospora philippinensis	*Burkholderia pseudomallei*
Phoma glycinicola	***Viruses***
Sclerophthora rayssiae var zeae	Hendra virus
Synchytrium endobioticum	Nipah virus
	Rift Valley fever virus
	Venezuelan equine encephalitis virus

BIOLOGICAL BIOTERRORIST AGENTS

These agents have been reported to present multiple effects on different organs and systems among them the thyroid system. Anthrax was reported to induce hypertrophy of the left lobe of the thyroid gland [18]. Moreover, ricin, which is a highly toxic plant-stable toxin that affects different organs like the liver, kidneys, lungs, pancreas, intestine and the thyroid, depending on the route of entry into the body, has been reported to disrupt the thyroid system. Its toxic mechanism is based on the induction of oxidative stress in the affected cells, resulting in destruction of thyroid follicles with consequent reduction of circulating hormones [14], but it has been suggested that other mechanisms could be implicated in these effects [19].

Furthermore, *Clostridium botulinum* neurotoxin A (Btx) has been reported to alter thyrotropin stimulating hormone (TSH) levels. This effect has been suggested to be due to a possible pathogenetic link between Btx and autoimmune thyroid diseases, because Btx and thyroid autoantigens share a homologous amino acid sequence; some of these homologous domains contain epitopes of both Btx and thyroid autoantigens and some of such domains contain HLA-DR3 and/or HLA-DR7 binding motifs, which prevail over other HLA-DRs and could led to autoimmune thyroid disease [15, 20]. *Clostridium perfringens* beta-toxin has been described to induce a moderate degree of thyroid hyperplasia in Appaloosa foals [21]. In addition, Staphylococcus enterotoxin B (SEB) has been shown to reduce iodine thyroid uptake that could be explained through a trapping mechanism of iodine by SEB [14] which could lead to hypothyroidism.

Microorganism infections can also induce thyroid disruption. In this regard, severe cases of hemorrhagic fever with renal syndrome (HFRS) induced by hantavirus infections have been reported to cause severe hormonal disorders [22]. Similarly, milder cases of epidemic nephropathy (NE) also show long-term alterations of thyroid hormones, developing primary hypothyroidism, but not serving as a predictor of the severity of disease caused by infection with Puumala hantavirus [22]. Moreover, pathogens could colonized the thyroid gland and induce thyroiditis. In this sense, Brucella, particularly *B. melitensis* may secondarily colonize the thyroid gland and cause acute thyroiditis [23, 24].

BIOREGULATORS

Bioregulators, a class of agents between chemical and biological warfare agents, are endogenous proteic or lipid substances produced by the human organism that have regulatory physiological activities on biological processes [25]. This group includes substance P, neuropeptide Y, adrenaline and serotonin, non-volatile amines (histamine, cadaverine, putrescine, spermine, among others), angiotensin, enkephalins, endorphins, endothelins, somatostatin and TSH among others [10, 26-29].

Progress in biotechnology have created the potential for the misuse of bioregulators in assault biological weapons programs. Synthetic derivatives or faintly modified forms of these substances can have drastic toxic results. They are a new type of weapon that can impair the nervous system, disrupt mood, trigger psychological changes, and kill. Several of these substances may be potent enough to be many hundreds of times more powerful than the conventional chemical warfare agents. The potential military or terrorist utilization of bioregulators is similar to that of toxins [13].

Some of the important characteristics that would provide notable military advantages are novel mechanisms of toxic action; quick and precise effects; penetration of protective filters and equipment and militarily efficient physical incapacitation. Furthermore, bioregulators are very important regulatory molecules of many physiological functions. In this regard, their range of action covers the whole living system, from mental processes (*e.g.* endorphins) to many features of health like control of mood, consciousness, temperature control, heart rate, immune responses, sleep, and emotions, exerting regulatory effects on the body. As such, they are produced in very small quantities that are indispensable for the body's regular homeostatic functions [30]. Because they occur naturally in the organism they could be used on specific targets without such use being discovered.

Some of these compounds have been reported to be able to disrupt the thyroid system. Endothelins (ET) or endothelium-derived contracting factors (EDCFs) have been described to be able to disrupt thyroid hormones. They constitute a family of four peptide isoforms of 21 amino acids with two disulfide bridges that are encoded by four different genes. These isoforms are endothelin-1 (ET-1), endothelin-2 (ET-2), endothelin-3 (ET-3) and vasoactive intestinal contractor (VIC). The physiological action of endothelin is related to a powerful contraction of the vessels and smooth muscles (uterus, bladder and intestine) they induce; in fact the ET-1 is the most potent vasoconstrictor peptide discovered. Endothelins and their receptors have been described to be present in endocrine glands and to be able to modulate the release of prolactin, gonadotropins, growth hormone, as well as TSH [30-33].

Another bioregulator that could disrupt the thyroid system is somatostatin (somatotropin release inhibiting hormone - SRIF) that is synthesized as part of a larger precursor, prepro-SRIF, consisting of a signal peptide and a pro-region of 80-90 amino acids. In mammals the prepro-SRIF molecule undergoes tissue-specific processing to generate the mature hormone, which exists as two different bioactive species. Somatostatin is found in the hypothalamus and in the Peripheral and Central Nervous System as well as in the gastrointestinal tract. Its main biological effect is inhibition of hormone release, such as growth hormone and TSH, among others [30].

The factor that these substances have in common is that they cause direct or indirect effects on the thyroid, with or without altering production and release of thyroid hormones. With the development of biomedical sciences and the interest of the pharmaceutical industry these substances can be obtained in sufficient quantity for them in short time to be disseminated for military and terrorist aims [25-29]. Thus, an in-depth study of these compounds is needed to elucidate their possible effects on thyroid system and to counteract the possible harm they could cause.

IMMUNIZATION AGAINST BIOTERRORIST AGENTS

Due to the potential military or terrorist use of *B. anthracis*, the United States (US) authorities as well as the British and Canadians among others, initiated an immunization program against this deadly agent [34]. The program is implemented in the case of pre- or post-exposure with chemoprophylaxis using ciprofloxacin or doxycycline in order to reduce the consequences of the spread of the agent. Other countries like Spain chose not to implement immunization, although they established a reserve of these vaccines for possible use in case of intentional dissemination.

The implementation of the program of vaccination against anthrax in the early '90s, among other immunization programs, generated a strong opposition from the military, due to the fact that they related the vaccine to serious side effects, even associating it with Gulf War Syndrome, which caused greater fear of the vaccine than of the disease [35, 36].

The decision to vaccinate in the US was adopted, taking into account the risk-benefit balance that any vaccine has, and since the first Gulf War, a program of vaccination against anthrax was implemented. Veterans' associations, due to the appearance of so-called Gulf War Syndrome, informed the authorities that the vaccine could cause moderate or serious local reactions at the point of inoculation, with or without fever, chills and nausea that resolved without permanent damage. However, veterans reported that some of those immunized had developed permanent immune disorders and chronic fatigue syndrome, persistent headaches, severe joint pain and arthritis, numbness and muscle weakness, severe memory loss, paralysis, convulsions and death. Between 20 and 48 percent of all vaccine recipients developed some sort of reaction to the vaccine against Anthrax.

Given the certainty that the vaccine had adverse effects it was included in the Vaccine Adverse Event Reporting System (VAERS), communicated both individually and through the doctors, in order to establish the actual record of adverse reactions to the vaccine [37].

To date, a statistically significant relationship between the adverse effects on the thyroid and the vaccine against anthrax was not observed in any of the studies performed. A statistically significant relationship between vaccination and thyroid disorder has not found in military personnel deployed in Southwest Asia [38]. The troops deployed in South Korea were immunized since 1998 against anthrax, and the ratios of hospitalization that might be associated with vaccination against anthrax, as well as vaccination against hepatitis A have been analyzed. These data showed that hospitalization ratios had remained stable since the '90s, and no relationship between the vaccine against anthrax or against hepatitis A with a higher rate of adverse events was found [39].

However, in a comparison made of the occurrence of thyroid disorders in military personnel vaccinated against anthrax from 1998 to 2000, recording the hospitalization rate before and after receiving one vaccine dose, it was reported that after vaccination 334 individuals (ratio of 9.9 per 100,000) were hospitalized with thyroid disorders in compassion to 48 unvaccinated individuals (ratio of 6.5

per 100,000) [37]. Thus, there are conflicting data, and more studies are needed to elucidate the safety of immunization on the thyroid system.

THYROIDITIS

Pathogenic infestation by BSATs may cause an inflammation of the thyroid gland (thyroiditis) that could lead to a disruption of the thyroid system. The American Thyroid Association defines thyroiditis as a disease caused by injury to the gland causing inflammation and damage to thyroid cells. Thyroiditis is a heterogeneous group of thyroid diseases, etiologically and clinically different, that have in common the existence of infiltration of the gland by inflammatory cells [40-42].

From the seven main types of thyroiditis only two have an infectious origin; subacute thyroiditis (Quervain's thyroiditis) that has a possible viral origin, and acute thyroiditis, also called suppurative thyroiditis or thyroid abscess, where the most common origin is bacterial. Chronic thyroiditis could be cause by microorganism infection or through other causes. In addition, thyroiditis may also be produced in the treatment of infectious diseases with drugs such as interferons or cytokines, and even some vaccines used in the biodefense context (Table **2A** and **2B**) [41].

Table 2A. Types and causes of infectious thyroiditis. Adapted from Lucas Martin and Puig Domingo [41, 42].

Type	Names		Cause	
Acute	Suppurative Acute thyroiditis	Acute thyroiditis or Thyroid abscess or Infectious thyroiditis	Bacterial infection	*Staphylococcus, Streptococcus, Enterobacter* and others
			Fungal infection	*Aspergillus, Candida, Coccidioides, Histoplasma and Pneumocystis*
Subacute	Thyroiditis subacute, Granulomatous thyroiditis De Quervain's Thyroiditis Subacute	Viral thyroiditis	Mumps virus, Echovirus, Coxsackie virus, Epstein-Barr virus, Influenza and Adenovirus	
	Subacute lymphocytic thyroiditis, silent or painless			

Table 2B. Types and causes of infectious thyroiditis. Adapted from Lucas Martin and Puig Domingo [41, 42].

<table>
<tr><td rowspan="6">Chronic</td><td>Chronic autoimmune thyroiditis</td><td colspan="3">Atrophic thyroiditis, focal lymphocytic thyroiditis, Hashimoto's thyroiditis</td></tr>
<tr><td rowspan="5">Chronic non autoimmune thyroiditis</td><td>Riedel's thyroiditis</td><td colspan="2"></td></tr>
<tr><td rowspan="3">Chronic suppurative thyroiditis</td><td>Bacterial</td><td>Mycobacterium, Treponema pallidum</td></tr>
<tr><td>Fungal</td><td>Aspergillus, Candida, Coccidioides, Histoplasma and Pneumocystis</td></tr>
<tr><td>Parasitic</td><td>Echinococcus, Strongylus, Cysticercus</td></tr>
<tr><td colspan="3">Chronic non suppurative thyroiditis</td></tr>
<tr><td rowspan="3">Others</td><td>Radiation</td><td colspan="3">Radioactive Thyroiditis (Follows treatment with radioactive iodine for hyperthyroidism or external beam radiation therapy for certain cancers. OR Nuclear accident OR Radiological Terrorism incident with radioactive iodine)</td></tr>
<tr><td>Traumatic</td><td colspan="3"></td></tr>
<tr><td>Drugs</td><td colspan="3">Interferon-a
Interleukin-2
Amiodarone and Lithium
Sunitinib and other inhibitors of tyrosine kinases</td></tr>
</table>

Acute Thyroiditis

Acute thyroiditis is a rare condition (0.1 to 1% of thyroid disorders), due to a primary infection or secondary to a variety of infectious diseases. This low frequency of acute thyroiditis seems to be due to the rich blood supply of the gland, its large lymphatic drainage, its high content of iodine and the existence of a protective capsule [42]. There is a greater predisposition to thyroiditis in individuals with previous thyroid disease, a history of immunosuppression or who have fistulas in the thyroid gland [41, 42].

Aerobic bacteria typically isolated in the infections are *Staphylococcus aureus*, *Streptococcus pyogenes*, *Streptococcus epidermidis*, and *Streptococcus pneumoniae*. The most common anaerobic bacteria are Gram negative bacilli and *Peptostreptococcus spp*. Other rarely isolated microorganisms include *Klebsiella spp.*, *Haemophilus influenzae*, *Streptococcus viridans*, *Salmonella spp.*,

Enterobacteriaceae (*Escherichia coli*), and even *Treponema pallidum* [17, 43, 44]. Fungal species of *Aspergillus*, *Candida*, *Coccidioides*, *Histoplasma* or *Pneumocystis* could also induce this effect. In these cases the infection often becomes chronic and affects mainly immunocompromised patients [45]. Fig. (**1**) shows the infectious etiologies that cause thyroiditis [46].

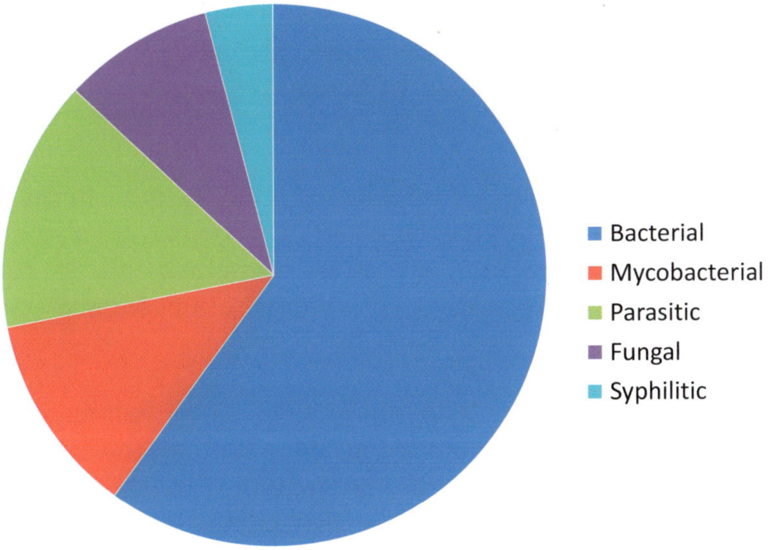

Figure 1: Infectious etiology of thyroiditis.

The most important infection routes are hematogenous (most common), lymphatic, by direct contact, by trauma, due to a persistent thyroglossal duct (presence of a vestigial pyriform sinus of the fourth gill pouch that connects the oropharynx and thyroid) [47] or due to the existence of a fistula between the left piriform sinus and the left lobe of the thyroid [44]. The latter is the second most ordinary cause of this disorder mainly in children and young adults (between 20 and 40 years old). While in the elderly, it is associated with prolonged goiter and degeneration of malignant neoplasm of the thyroid gland, usually associated with pre-existing consistent nodules with areas of involution that favor the settlement and development of germs in the thyroid gland [48, 49].

Patients, usually women since they present a greater predisposition, referred localized flare-up of pain in the throat that radiated to the ear, jaw or occipital region, which was relieved by bending the neck and increase in swallowing or neck movements. It often presented fever, dysphagia and erythema in the area, and was accompanied by fatigue and loss of appetite and even with dyspnea, cough and hoarseness [45]. On examination, signs of diffuse or localized thyroid inflammation with intense pain at palpation were observed. If there was suppuration, the skin was thickened and fluctuation could be observed in the area. Laboratory data showed marked leukocytosis with increased sedimentation rate (ESR ↑↑↑), but usually thyroid function was normal, except in chronified forms where there could be hypothyroidism. The scan image showed a cold nodule and ultrasonography showed a liquid or mixed picture [41]. In non suppurative thyroiditis, puncture allows isolation of the causal agent. If it is suppurative the germ isolation can be performed directly.

The differential diagnosis must be established with thyroid cancer, with cellulite and cervical adenitis, as well as bleeding and intranodular perichondritis and with subacute thyroiditis. For this aim, ultrasound sometimes allows the differential diagnosis between acute thyroiditis, if abscesses are formed, with subacute thyroiditis [45].

Initial treatment is performed with analgesics, anti-inflammatory and broad-spectrum antibiotics as long as there are no microbiology results. When the germ inductor of this process is isolated, the treatment is modified according to antibiotic sensitivity. Non suppurative thyroiditis improves with antibiotic treatment without sequelae in 10-14 days. Conversely, suppurative forms can produce a fistula, draining outward or inward, affecting the trachea, the esophagus or mediastinum (proving to be useful radiographic controls for controlling the fistulous ducts). Usually they resolve without sequelae with antibiotic treatment, except in extensive thyroiditis. Sometimes it may be necessary to perform surgical cleaning of the abscess [41]. Acute thyroiditis may complicate, because of antibiotic failure, with tracheal obstruction, sepsis, retropharyngeal abscess, mediastinitis and jugular vein thrombosis [45].

Subacute Thyroiditis

De Quervain's thyroiditis, also known as granulomatous, viral, simple acute, giant cell or pseudotuberculous thyroiditis, is a potentially self-limited, of viral origin, painful disorder of the thyroid gland that is preceded by an upper respiratory tract infection caused by mumps or measles virus, echovirus or Coxsackie virus [17]. A genetic predisposition cannot be ruled out since over 70% of patients with this disease have the HLA-B35 gene [41, 42]. It has to be taken into account that the viral etiology is determined by seasonal clustering of cases in summer and autumn, as well as a common environmental cluster. However, no antiviral antibodies appear and there is no laboratory evidence to confirm that etiology [42]. Women are three to six times more likely to develop this condition than men. The most frequent age of presentation is between 30 and 50 years. It also has a seasonal basis, mainly during the summer or in the fall [48].

Subacute granulomatous thyroiditis presents clinically as an acute pain in the region of the thyroid that increases when turning the head or swallowing and that radiates to the jaw, the ears or chest, usually preceded by a prodromal period of viral infection with involvement of the upper respiratory tract, fever, fatigue and malaise [40, 41]. The diagnosis of subacute thyroiditis goes unnoticed at times as it is confused with a sore throat. On exploration the gland has a firm and nodular touch. Subacute granulomatous thyroiditis clinically involves four distinct phases over time that usually develops within four to six months. It starts with an acute phase that lasts between three and six weeks, where the main symptom is pain along with thyrotoxicosis. This is followed by a phase where hormone levels tend to normalize. It continues with symptoms of hypothyroidism that may last weeks or months, or may even be permanent (up to 5 percent of patients). The final stage is a recovery interval during which the thyroid function tests are normalized.

The white blood cell count (WBC) is normal or feebly elevated, sedimentation rate is high. 50% of patients have signs of thyrotoxicosis in the acute phase of the disease, T4 values are very high compared to T3. Serum TSH levels are low, while the thyroglobulin levels are high. Thyroid hormone levels vary depending on the stage of the disease; initially there is a thyrotoxic phase (T3 and T4 high), in a second stage hypothyroidism and in a third phase recovery is observed [45]. However, sometimes it can evolve into permanent hypothyroidism when the parenchyma of the gland has been destroyed [41].

Physical examination, increased erythrocyte sedimentation rate, increased thyroglobulin levels and low radioactive iodine uptake (RAIU) confirm the diagnosis.

On examination, the gland appears enlarged, with more consistency. The initial pathological lesions are follicles infiltrated by mononuclear cells, with breaks of the epithelium, basement membrane fragmentation and loss of colloid that evolves into granulomatous lesions with a central core surrounded by colloid multinucleated giant cells.

Differential diagnosis must be established with infections of throat or upper respiratory tract, as well as thyroid disease that occur with hyperthyroidism with low uptake or hypothyroidism [41].

Anti-inflammatory therapy is based on the use of acetylsalicylic acid at high doses (1,5 - 2 g/day) or nonsteroidal anti-inflammatory drugs (NSAIDs). Glucocorticoids could be added, if the clinical situation demands it, as well as prednisone in doses of 40-60 mg/day in decreasing pattern during 4-8 weeks. Throughout the entire clinical course, levothyroxine administration at low doses may be necessary when the hypothyroid phase occurs [41, 45].

Chronic Thyroiditis

Chronic suppurative thyroiditis is associated with primary or secondary invasion of the gland by microorganisms such as mycobacteria like *Mycobacterium tuberculosis* and other atypical mycobacteria, which could complicate other forms of thyroiditis [17, 41, 50-52]. Other causes that can induce chronic thyroiditis may be fungal infections in immunocompromised patients. *Aspergillus species* of the genus (*Aspergillus spp*.) are the fungi most frequently isolated, although other fungi of the genera *Candida spp*, *Coccidioides immitis*, *Histoplasma* and *Pneumonia* cannot be ruled out [17, 53]. Clinical presentation is similar to other thyroiditis disorders, developing fever, inflammation of the gland that can eventually lead to dysphagia and dysphonia; although the outlook is less favorable than in other infectious thyroiditis disorders due to delayed diagnosis and treatment [54, 55].

Clinical symptoms are gradual emergence of a painless mass in the region of the thyroid that typically retains normal thyroid function.

Another form of chronic thyroiditis is caused by parasites that colonize the thyroid indirectly through the hematogenous route such as *Echinococcus spp*, *Strongylus spp*, or *Cisticercus spp*. [17, 56, 57].

The diagnosis is confirmed by aspiration cytology of the gland, accompanied by microbiological culture, in the case of bacteria or fungi that demonstrates the causative agent [41].

CONCLUDING REMARKS

BSATs represent a hazard for the human population producing potentially catastrophic impact on plants or animals. For this reason, there is a increasing concern that these agents may be used for intentional damage or to produce public panic. For example in the 2001 anthrax assaults, beside of murdering five people and infecting 22, these attacks had an impressive effect on population and were estimated to have had a direct economic effect of more than $1 billion. Therefore it is important that a variety of vaccines, antibiotics, and other drugs are developed against these agents to limit their possible adverse effects especially on the health of the human population, but also in animals and plants, and to prevent their use as terror weapons.

Otherwise, there is little information about the effect of these agents on thyroid systems. Thyroid hormones are important for many physiological functions and their disruption has been associated with many pathological effects, among them cognitive dysfunctions. They are necessary during critical period of time in the development of organisms especially of the central nervous system. For this reason, it is necessary to perform a complete study of the BSATs known to alter the thyroid system and to screen the remainder of agents for their possible involvement in thyroid disruption and the mechanisms through which they may induce these effects.

CONFLICT OF INTEREST

The author confirms that author has no conflict of interest to declare for this publication.

ACKNOWLEDGEMENTS

Declared None.

REFERENCES

[1] Opresko DM, Young RA, Faust RA, *et al.* Chemical warfare agents: estimating oral reference doses. Rev Environ Contam Toxicol 1998; 156:1-183.

[2] Romano JA, Luckey BJ, Salem H. Chemical Warfare Agents. Chemistry, Pharmacology, Toxicology, and Therapeutics. CRC Press, 2nd Edition. 2008.

[3] Page WF. Long-term healtg effects of exposure to sarin and Other anticholinestase chemical warfare agents. Mil Med 2003; 168(3): 239-245.

[4] Directorate General of Civil Defense and Emergencies. Notebooks Civil Protection Legislation. Notebook VIII. Basic Nuclear Emergency Plan. Madrid, Spain: Spanish Interior Ministry. 2004.

[5] Becker D, Demidchik EP, Nagataki S, Pinchera A, Williams ED. Post-Chernobyl scientific perspectives: Thyroid effects. IAEA Bulletin 1996; 38(3): 31-32.

[6] Pesatori AC, Consonni D, Bachetti S, *et al.* Short- and Long-term morbidity and mortality in the population exposed to dioxin after the "Seveso acident" Ind Health 2003; 41(3): 127-138.

[7] Kastenmayer RJ, Moore RM, Bright AL, Torres-Cruz R, Elkins WR. Select agent and toxin regulations: beyond the eighth edition of the Guide for the Care and Use of Laboratory Animals. J Am Assoc Lab Anim Sci 2012; 51: 333-338.

[8] Steele KE. Guest editorial: special focus on the pathology of biological select agents and toxins in animals and research challenges in biological defense. Vet Pathol 2010; 4: 772-773.

[9] Christopher GW, Cieslak TJ, Pavlin JA, Eitzen EM. Biological warfare. A historical perspective. JAMA 1997; 278 (5): 412-417.

[10] Wheelis M. Biological warfare before 1914. In: Moon JE van Courtland, Ed. Biological and toxin weapons: Research, development, and use from the middle ages to 1945. Vol. 1. Stockholm, Sweden: Stockholm International Peace Research Institute; 1991; pp. 8-34.

[11] Centers for Disease Control and Prevention (CDC). Bioterrorism Overview. Atlanta, USA: CDC, 2006. Available at: http://www.bt.cdc.gov/bioterrorism/overview.asp

[12] Centers for Disease Control and Prevention (CDC). Bioterrorism Agents. Emergency Preparedness and Response. Atlanta, USA: CDC. Available at: http://www.bt.cdc.gov/bioterrorism/index.asp

[13] Bokan S, Orahovec Z. An Evaluation of Bioregulators/Modulators as Terrorism and Warfare Agents. In: Stopa P, Orahovec Z, Eds. Technology for Combating WMD Terrorism. Springer Netherlands, 2004; pp. 29-40.

[14] Kumar O, Sugendran K, Vijayaraghavan R. Oxidative stress associated hepatic and renal toxicity induced by ricin in mice. Toxicon 2003; 41(3): 333-338.

[15] Atassi MZ, Deitiker PR. Does Clostridium botulinum neurotoxin A exhibit molecular mimicry with thyroid autoantigens and cause thyroid complications in predisposed persons? Endocrine 2011; 40: 140-141.

[16] Rapoport MI, Hodoval LF, Grogan EW, McGann V, Beisel WR. The influence of specific antibody on the disappearance of staphylococcal enterotoxin B from blood. J Clin Invest 1966; 45: 1365-1372.

[17] Brook I. Microbiology and management of acute suppurative thyroiditis in children. Int J Pediatr Otorhinolaryngol 2003; 67(5): 447-51.

[18] Plotkin SA, Brachman PS, Utell M, Bunford FH, Atchison MM. An epidemic of inhalation anthrax, the first in the twentieth century. I Clinical features. Am J Med 1960:992-1001.

[19] Sadani GR, Soman CS, Deodhar KK, Nadkarni GD. Reactive oxygen species involvement in ricin-induced thyroid toxicity in rat. Hum Exp Toxicol 1997; 16: 254-256.

[20] Gregoric E, Gregoric JA, Guarneri F, Benvenga S. Injections of *Clostridium botulinum* neurotoxin A may cause thyroid complications in predisposed persons based on molecular mimicry with thyroid autoantigens. Endocrine 2011; 39: 41-47.

[21] Niilo L, Chalmers GA. Hemorrhagic Enterotoxemia Caused by *Clostridium perfringens* Type C in a Foal. Can Vet J 1982; 23: 299-301.

[22] Mäkelä S, Jaatinen P, Miettinen M, *et al.* Deficiencias hormonales durante y después de la infección por hantavirus Puumala. Eur J Clin Microbiol Infect Dis 2010; 29(6): 705-713.

[23] Vermiglio F, Stassi G, Finocchiano MD, Trimarchi F. Thyroiditis due to Brucella melitensis. J Endocrinol Invest 1995; 18(4): 308-310.

[24] Azizi F, Katchoui A. Brucella infection of the thyroid gland. Thyroid 1996; 6(5): 461-463.

[25] Organization for the Prohibition of Chemical Weapons. Convergence of Chemistry and Biology. Report of the Scientific Advisory Board's Temporary Working Group Organization for the Prohibition of Chemical Weapons. The Netherlands 2014.

[26] Bajgar J, Kassa J, Fusek J, Kuca K, Jun D. Other toxic chemicals as potential chemical warfare agents. In: Gupta RC, Eds. Handbook of toxicology of chemical warfare agents. 1st Ed., Academic Press, 2009; pp. 342-343.

[27] Guillermet-Guibert J, Lahlou H, Cordelier P, Bousquet C, Pyronnet S, Susini C. Physiology of somatostatin receptors. J Endocrinol Invest 2005; 28(11 Suppl International): 5-9.

[28] Immer HU, Sestanj K, Nelson VR, Götz M. Synthesis of Somatostatin. Preliminary communication. Helv Chim Acta 1974; 57(3): 730-734.

[29] Mattern R, Moore SB, Tran TA, Rueter JK, Goodman M. Synthesis, biological activities and conformational studies of somatostatin analogs. Tetrahedron 2000; 56: 9819-9831.

[30] Bokan S. The toxicology of bioregulators as potential agents of bioterrorism. Arh Hig Rada Toksikol 2005; 56: 205-211.

[31] Colin IM, Selvais PL, Rebai T, *et al.* Expression of the endothelin-1 gene in the rat thyroid gland and changes in its peptide and mRNA levels in goiter formation and iodide-induced involution. J Endocrinol 1994; 143: 65-74.

[32] Chu CH, Lee JK, Keng HM, *et al.* Hyperthyroidism is associated with higher plasma endothelin-1 concentrations. Exp Biol Med 2006; 231: 1040-1043.

[33] Virgilio F, Sciarrillo R, Laforgia V, Varano L. Response of the thyroid gland of the lizard Podarcis sicula to endothelin-1. J Exp Zool A Comp Exp Biol 2003; 296: 137-142.

[34] Grabenstein JD, Pittman PR, Greenwood JT, Engler RJ. Immunization to protect the US Armed Forces: heritage, current practice, and prospects. Epidemiol Rev 2006; 28: 3-26.

[35] Steele L. Prevalence and patterns of Gulf War illness in Kansas veterans: association of symptoms with characteristics of person, place, and time of military service. Am J Epidemiol 2000; 152: 992-1002.

[36] Unwin C, Blatchley N, Coker W, *et al*. Health of UK servicemen who served in Persian Gulf War. Lancet 1999; 353. 169-178.

[37] Joellenbeck LM, Zwanziger LL, Durch JS, Strom BL. The anthrax vaccine: is it safe? Does it work? Committee to assess the safety and efficacy of the anthrax vaccine, medical follow-up agency. Institute of Medicine. National Academic Press. Washington D.C. 2002.

[38] Rehme PA, Williams R, Grabenstein JD. Ambulatory medical visits among anthrax-vaccinated and unvaccinated personnel after return from southwest Asia. Mil Med 2002; 167: 205-210.

[39] Lange JL, Lesikar SE, Rubertone MV, Brundage JF. Comprehensive systematic surveillance for adverse effects of anthrax vaccine adsorbed, US Armed Forces, 1998-2000. Vaccine 2003; 21(15):1620-1628.

[40] Lucas Martín AM, Puig Domingo M. Tiroiditis. In: Farreras, Rozman, Eds. Medicina Interna Vol II. XVII Edición. Elsevier 2012; pp. 1890-1893.

[41] Hurst, J.W. Medicine for the Practicing Physician, McGraw-Hill Professional Publishing 1996.

[42] Bahn RS, Burch HB, Cooper DS, *et al*. Hyperthyroidism and other causes of thyrotoxicosis: management guidelines of the american thyroid association and american association of clinical endocrinologists thyroid. Endocr Pract 2011; 21(6): 593-646.

[43] Saksouk D, Salti Ibrahim S. Acute supurtative thyroiditis caused by Escherichia coli. Br Med J 1977; 2(6078): 23-24.

[44] Ghaemi N, Sayedi J, Bagheri S. Acute suppurative thyroiditis with thyroid abscess: A case report and review of the literature. Iran J Otorhinolaryngol 2014; 26(74): 51-55

[45] Jameson JL, Weetman AP. Trastornos de la glándula tiroides. In: Kasper DL, Braunwald E, Fauci AS, *et al*, Eds. Harrison. Principios de medina interna. Vol 2. 16a ed. México: McGraw-Hill; 2005; pp. 2325-2330.

[46] Farwell A, Braverman LE. Inflammatory thyroid disorders. Otolaryngol Clin North Am 1996; 29: 541-53

[47] Cases JA, Wenig BM, Silver CE, Surks MI. Recurrent acute suppurative thyroiditis in an adult due to a fourth branchial pouch fistula. J Clin Endocrinol Metab 2000; 85(3): 953-956.

[48] Slatosky J, Shipton B, Wahba H. Thyroiditis: differential diagnosis and management. Am Fam Physician 2000; 61(4): 1047-1052.

[49] Falk, S.A. Thyroid Disease: Endocrinology, Surgery, Nuclear Medicine, and Radiotherapy, Lippincott-Raven. 1997.

[50] Cuesta Hernández M, Gómez Hoyos E, Agrela Rojas E, Téllez Molina MJ, Díaz Pérez JA. Tuberculosis tiroidea: causa excepcional de bocio compresivo. Endocrinol Nutr 2013; 60(8): 11-13.

[51] Sisto M, Cucci L, D'Amore M, Dow TC, Mitolo V, Lisi S. Proposing a relationship between Mycobacterium avium subspecies paratuberculosis infection and Hashimoto's thyroiditis. Scand J Infect Dis 2010; 42(10): 787-790.

[52] Robillon JF, Sadoul JL, Gucrin P, *et al*. *Mycobacterium avium* intracellulare suppurative thyroiditis in a patient with Hashimoto's thyroiditis. J Endocrinol Invest 1994; 17(2): 133-134.

[53] Avram AM, Sturm CA, Michael CW, Sisson JC, Jaffe CA. Cryptococcal Thyroiditis and Hyperthyroidism. Thyroid 2004; 14(6): 471-475.

[54] Goldani LZ, Zavascki AP, Maia AL. Fungal thyroiditis: an overview. Mycopathologia 2006; 161(3): 129-139.

[55] Marui S, de Lima Pereira AC, de Araújo Maia RM, Borba EF. Suppurative thyroiditis due to aspergillosis: a case report. J Med Case Rep 2014, 8:379

[56] De Oliveira Filho JR, de Nadai TR. Parasitic thyroid nodules in patient with nontoxic multinodular goiter: a case report. J Med Case Rep 2014, 8:66

[57] Gupta S, Sodhani P. Clinically unsuspected thyroid involvement in cysticercosis: a case report. Acta Cytol 2010; 54(5 Suppl): 853-856.

CHAPTER 5

Thyroid Toxicity

Immacolata Cristina Nettore and Paolo Emidio Macchia*

Department of Molecular and Clinical Endocrinology and Oncology, University of Naples Federico II, Naples, Italy

Abstract: Thyroxine is one of the most widely used drugs all over the world. Normally thyroid hormones are used in the treatment of hypothyroidism or goiter, but cases of drug overdose have been frequently reported (thyrotoxicosis factitia). This chapter will focus on the prevalence, consequences and the treatment of the thyrotoxicosis factitia, as a complication of inappropriate L- thyroxine treatment for obesity, following the ingestion of beef contaminated with thyroid gland and after accidental thyroid hormone ingestion.

Keywords: Intoxication, overdose ingestion, thyroid hormones, thyrotoxicosis factitia, treatment.

INTRODUCTION

Thyroid hormones (TH) are considered one of the most important regulators in cellular metabolism in both animals and humans.

The hypothalamic-pituitary-thyroid axis regulates serum TH levels. The hypothalamus releases thyroid releasing hormone that stimulates the pituitary to produce thyroid-stimulating hormone (TSH). Mature TSH reaches the thyroid and induces thyroid hormone synthesis and secretion. The thyroid produces two types of hormones, thyroxine (T4) and the triiodothyronine (T3). Serum THs inhibit TRH and TSH production and secretion with a negative feedback mechanism [1].

The thyroid produces predominantly T4 rather than T3 (~ 80 µg T4 per day, *versus* ~ 4 µg/day of T3). The latter is the more active form of TH, and is locally synthetized in the peripheral organs by deiodinases. Most of the THs are bound to plasma protein and are principally metabolized by the liver [1]. The half-life of T4 is 5-7 days, while T3 half-life is only 1 day [2].

Levothyroxine (L-T4) is one of the more commonly prescribed drugs around the world [3, 4]. L-T4 is used in hormone replacement therapy to treat hormone

*Corresponding author Paolo Emidio Macchia: Department of Molecular and Clinical Endocrinology and Oncology, University of Naples Federico II, Naples, Italy; E-mail pmacchia@unina.it.

deficiencies in hypothyroidism, and to reduce circulating TSH (suppressive therapy) in order to inhibit the growth of thyroid nodules and goiter [5].

In the past, replacement and suppressive therapies were preferentially performed using preparations containing both T3 and T4 obtained from lyophilization of animal thyroid tissue. Use of such "natural" drugs was associated with a high risk of thyrotoxicosis, because of the elevated T3 content and the high variability in the preparations. Then synthetic levothyroxine (L-T4) preparations became available for both oral and intravenous administration. Nowadays, L-T4 is the most common form of thyroid preparation involved in both unintentional and intentional over exposure, especially in children [6]. Indeed, in the USA the L-T4 tablets are prepared in different colors in order to avoid dosage errors, however their very colored appearance makes them particularly attractive to young children.

Since T3 is the more active form of the thyroid hormones, T3-containing preparations (liothyronine) can generate thyrotoxicosis, but T3 preparations are less frequently used in the clinical practice.

Elevated circulating thyroid hormone levels are defined as thyrotoxicosis. With the exception of thyrotoxicosis associated with thyroid hormone resistance or pituitary TSH secreting adenomas, elevated T3 and T4 serum levels are associated with a decrease in circulating TSH. In a very large study evaluating thyroid hormone concentrations in almost 26000 subjects during the Colorado 9th Health Fair, a decreased TSH level was found in 2.2% of the studied population [7]. Thyrotoxicosis can be caused by overproduction of thyroid hormone from the thyroid gland (hyperthyroidism) or can result from other causes, including destruction of thyroid tissue as a consequence of inflammatory processes (thyroiditis) and release of pre-synthetized hormones; intentionally, unintentionally, or accidentally poisoning by short- or long- term assimilation of excess thyroid hormone ("thyrotoxicosis factitia"); as well as by over-dosage of TH-containing drugs.

This report will focus on the prevalence, consequences and treatment of thyrotoxicosis factitia.

EPIDEMIOLOGICAL DATA

The first relevant outbreak of TH intoxication was reported between April 1984 and August 1985 among residents of southwestern Minnesota and adjacent areas of South Dakota and Iowa [8]. During the outbreak, one hundred and twenty-one individuals had symptoms of thyrotoxicosis associated with consumption of ground beef prepared from neck trimmings and processed by a single slaughtering plant. The association between thyrotoxicosis and ground beef consumption was confirmed by the findings of high concentrations of thyroid hormone in the samples of ground beef [8].

According to the Annual Report of the American Association of Poison Control Center's National Poison Data System, 13,005 cases of thyroid hormone poisoning were identified in 2008. Overall, 9,006 were from a exposure to a single dose [9], and the division by age for single dose was the following:

- 5,026 children younger than 6 years;
- 554 people aged 6-19 years;
- 2,957 people older than 19 years.

Among these, only 3 cases of major harm were described, but fortunately no deaths were reported. No association between toxic thyroid hormone ingestion and race and/or sex distribution was found [9].

A recent study on TH poisoning reviewed all requests to the Danish Poison Information Centre (DPIC) between March 2007 and September 2012. As a result, 181 patients were evaluated (112 children), taking a record of the following parameters: multiple drug intake and symptoms, time from ingestion, age and dose. Ingested L-T4 doses ranged from 10 to 9000 µg. Initially asymptomatic subjects were subsequently contacted by DPIC to verify the occurrence of delayed events. In this report, the most frequent cause of L-T4 ingestion was accidental assimilation discovered in children younger than 6 years of age (53.9%). The other events (24.7%) were reported in adolescents or adults (≥14 years), as suicide attempts.

To better analyze the risk regarding L-T4 assimilation in 47 subjects younger than 14 years, a review of the GlaxoSmithKline safety database (GSK safety database) between November 2002 and February 2012 was performed. Cases were found in Argentina, Brazil, India, Israel, Germany, United Kingdom, United States, Switzerland, Spain and Canada. The exposure range was 100–9,900 µg in 10 symptomatic children *versus* 25–9,600 µg in asymptomatic children [10].

Thyroid hormones and synthetic derivatives of T4 and T3 (Tetraidothyroacetic acid, TETRAC and Triiodothyroacetic acid, TRIAC) have also been used in weight-loss therapy. Despite the very high risks of thyrotoxicosis and a larger effect of these hormones on the lean mass rather than on the fat mass metabolism, such treatment are common because of the rapid weight loss [11]. Several cases of long- or short-term abuse of thyroid supplements have been reported in patients taking a massive amounts of thyroid hormones or TRIAC- or TETRAC-containing pills as a method of weight control [12].

Finally, almost 20 years ago an outbreak of thyrotoxicosis was reported in Spain in patients receiving substitutive therapy for hypothyroidism, as a consequence of errors in the preparation of the pharmaceutical agents [13]. Similarly, three cases were observed in women in the Paris area, where the thyroid hormones were prescribed not for hypothyroidism treatment but as “dietary pills”. The pills were labeled “phytotherapy-homeopathy” and usually contained aminophylline, metformin, carrageenan, sibutramine, thyroid compounds, caffeine, diazepam, and infra-therapeutic doses of L-thyroxine (25 μg), but in these cases the pills accidentally contained 30 mg of thyroxine. In addition to these patients, of 34 more women who took those pills 15 were admitted to hospital and nine to the intensive care unit [14].

BIOCHEMICAL MECHANISMS

Levothyroxine overdose has clinical manifestations on cardiovascular, gastrointestinal, and neurologic systems through a presumed activation of the adrenergic system.

The metabolic effects of THs are regulated by DNA transcription and protein synthesis. At a cellular level, T3 and T4 control development, growth and metabolism; promote gluconeogenesis, glycogen store mobilization and usage, and increase protein synthesis and basal metabolic rate.

Thyroxine toxicity is probably modulated *via* biochemical mechanisms: there is evidence suggesting that, in response to large L-T4 doses, the body increases production of reverse triiodothyronine (rT3), an inactive molecule that acts as competitive inhibitor at receptor site, preserving a relative euthyroid state and inhibiting L-T4 poisoning [15-17].

In addition, in the bloodstream, T4 is tightly bound to thyroxine binding globulin (TGB), transthyretin (TTR) and albumin [18], plasma proteins that may act as a buffering system and contribute to preventing toxicity from TH abuse [19].

SYMPTOMS

Symptoms associated with thyroid hormone ingestion are very variable. The toxic effects of L-T4 can appear from 6 hours to 11 days after the ingestion. This delay can be determined by the slow conversion of T4 into T3 and by the diffusion of T3 into peripheral tissues.

In case of ingestion of T3-containing preparations, clinical manifestations can appear more rapidly, beginning within the first 24 hours after ingestion.

The taking of mixtures containing T4 and T3 can have both instantaneous and retarded clinical effects.

Thyroid Hormone Toxicity in Children

Generally, L-T4 exposure in children follows a benign course. Indeed, during childhood (with the exception of the neonatal period) the liver has an increased metabolic capacity and babies tolerate more L-T4 than adults.

Children may be completely asymptomatic or have mild clinical manifestations. Several studies confirmed that there is no association between the quantity of adsorbed L-T4, onset and severity of manifestations, and serum concentrations of either T3 or T4 [3].

Golightly and coworkers-evaluated 41 children (1-5 years) and described minimal manifestations such as fever, tachycardia and hyperactivity. In one child, the ingestion of 13 mg of L-T4 produced no clinical complications [20].

In another study, only four of 78 children (<12 years) [19] had symptoms after the ingestion of L-T4. These included fever (peak recorded temperature: 38.3°C), supraventricular tachycardia of <175 bpm, lethargy, irritability, and mild gastrointestinal distress [16].

Tenenbein and Dean [15] reported a group of 69 pediatric subjects exposed to L-T4 doses ranging from 1.8 to 30 mg. None of the subjects developed clinical signs of thyrotoxicosis. Kulig and coworkers [21] described a 30-month-old boy who developed seizures, tremors, irritability, tachycardia, diaphoresis, and watery diarrhea but not fever after ingestion of a possible total dose of 18 mg of L-T4.

None of the subjects reported in these studies needed any anti-thyroid preparations.

In the GSK's safety database, 10 childhood cases were reported to have symptoms that included tachycardia, agitation, hyperhidrosis, anxiety, vomiting, dizziness, insomnia, tremor, pyrexia, hyperactivity, diarrhea, irritability, decreased appetite, and flushing. A few subjects had also skin manifestations including oral mucosal discolorations, cutaneous lichenoid eruptions, skin exfoliations and alopecia [10].

At the time of inquiry, 85% (153 of 181) patients of the DPIC report presented no clinical manifestations of intoxication. Within 24 hours, 9 subjects (≤15 years) reported tremors, diaphoresis, hyperactivity, insomnia, tachycardia, fever and headache. The L-T4 assimilated doses ranged from 0.3 to 15 mg.

Thyroid Hormone Toxicity in Adults

After overdose of LT4, adults have major clinical manifestations compared to those observed in children. These may include cardiac arrhythmias, coma, and malignant hyperthermia. Severe arrhythmias and loss of consciousness are very likely to occur after L-T4 overdose ingestion in adults with chronic renal disease and heart pathologies.

In the DPIC report a total of 23 adult patients were symptomatic at the time of enquiry, but no statistical difference was demonstrated between asymptomatic and symptomatic subjects. In the total group of patients (>20 years), 45 ingested one or more drugs in addition to L-T4. Of note, in these patients clinical manifestations of T4 intoxication were more frequent and significant [10].

During the outbreak in the Paris area [14], three women were admitted to the intensive care unit for thyrotoxicosis after the ingestion of dietary pills containing high levels of thyroxine. One patient developed febrile confusion and died from malignant hyperthermia. The second had progressive confusion requiring mechanical plasma exchange therapy with a favorable outcome, while the third one had very moderate symptoms.

Thyroid hormone intoxication was described in an 18-year-old female who spontaneously ingested L-T4 for six months to reduce her weight. She was brought to the hospital with thyroid storm clinical manifestation, systolic hypertension (180/74 mm Hg), tachycardia (125 beats per minute), a stuporous mental state and acute respiratory failure [22].

The differences in clinical manifestations between children and adults after poisoning doses of L-T4 make it difficult to prepare general guidelines on management of TH intoxication. In general, adults are more predisposed to develop symptoms. Often, underlying comorbidity (renal, hepatic or cardiac disorder) may activate unfavorable responses and can be associated with more frequent ingestion of other drug(s) together with L-T4.

DIAGNOSIS AND TREATMENT

Most asymptomatic patients do not require specific diagnostic tests, in particular immediately after the drug exposure. In the evaluation of patients after poisoning with L-T4, the following examinations can be considered:

- FT3 and FT4 serum levels can be sent to the lab within 2-6 hours after ingestion. It should however be considered that serum free thyroid hormones are not useful during the acute phase of clinical management and do not help in prognosis;
- Complete blood count;
- Electrolytes (*e.g.*, calcium, magnesium, phosphorous);
- Urinalysis;
- Serum acetaminophen level (in patients with intentional exposures and suicidal ideations);
- Arterial blood gas (ABG);
- ECG is indicated to evaluate symptomatic patients for myocardial ischemia, myocardial infarction and cardiac dysrhythmias (*e.g.*, atrial fibrillation);
- Lumbar puncture (LP) should be considered in patients with hyperthermia and change of mental status for the differential diagnosis with CNS infection.

The initial lack of symptoms and the variable individual responses make the medical treatment of patients with acute levothyroxine exposure controversial.

In most symptomatic pediatric patients, gastrointestinal decontamination (GID) alone is the standard treatment, however some clinicians suggest different treatments according to the degree of L-T4 overdose. In children who ingest <0.5

mg, no gastrointestinal decontamination is required. For those with exposures of between 0.5 and 3.0 mg, ipecac-induced emesis at home is suggested. Finally, all children with ingestions of >3.0 mg must receive ipecac-induced emesis followed by a dose of activated charcoal [16, 20].

In adults, to neutralize the dangerous consequences of thyroid hormone excess, the administration of β-blocking agents, barbiturates, digoxin, hydrocortisone, and cooling blankets has been suggested. Hospitalization is not considered initially necessary, but all patients required supportive care and strict clinical observation [15].

Sodium-ipodate (Oragrafin), a well-tolerated agent used for oral cholecystography, can be useful for the control of T4 thyrotoxicosis factitia, because it is a potent inhibitor of type I iodothyronine 5'-monodeiodinase (5'-MDI), the enzyme that catalyzes the conversion of T4 to T3 [23]. Oral administration of sodium-ipodate (0.5 g/day) until the normalization of serum T4 and T3 levels reduces tissue uptake of thyroid hormones and inhibits the nuclear binding of T3 [24].

Plasmapheresis or therapeutic plasma exchange (TPE) may be proposed only for life-threatening conditions [25, 26], since both of these methods can remove only 25-30% of the total absorbed L-T4 amount, and can be responsible for several complications [25].

CONFLICT OF INTEREST

The author confirms that author has no conflict of interest to declare for this publication.

ACKNOWLEDGEMENTS

Declared None.

REFERENCES

[1] http://www.thyroidmanager.org. South Dartmouth, MA: ENDOCRINE EDUCATION Inc; 2015.
[2] http://emedicine.medscape.com/article/819692-overview: Emedicine; 2010 Apr 23.
[3] Jagadishkumar K, Manjunath VG, Rashmi N, Mamatha S. Accidental levothyroxine ingestion in a child. Iran J Pediatr 2013; 23(6): 711-2.
[4] Prescribed drug spending in Canada, 2012. Healthc Q 2014; 17(1): 66.
[5] Baumgartner C, Blum MR, Rodondi N. Subclinical hypothyroidism: summary of evidence in 2014. Swiss Med Wkly 2014; 144: w14058.
[6] Majlesi N, Greller HA, McGuigan MA, Caraccio T, Su MK, Chan GM. Thyroid storm after pediatric levothyroxine ingestion. Pediatrics 2010; 126(2): e470-3.

[7] Canaris GJ, Manowitz NR, Mayor G, Ridgway EC. The Colorado thyroid disease prevalence study. Arch Intern Med 2000; 160(4): 526-34.
[8] Hedberg CW, Fishbein DB, Janssen RS, *et al.* An outbreak of thyrotoxicosis caused by the consumption of bovine thyroid gland in ground beef. N Engl J Med 1987; 316(16): 993-8.
[9] Bronstein AC, Spyker DA, Cantilena LR, Jr., Green JL, Rumack BH, Giffin SL. 2008 Annual Report of the American Association of Poison Control Centers' National Poison Data System (NPDS): 26th Annual Report. Clin Toxicol 2009; 47(10): 911-1084.
[10] Nygaard B, Saedder EA, Dalhoff K, Wikkelsoe M, Jurgens G. Levothyroxine poisoning - symptoms and clinical outcome. Basic Clin Pharmacol Toxicol. 2015; 117(4): 280-5.
[11] Poon WT, Ng SW, Lai CK, Chan YW, Mak WL. Factitious thyrotoxicosis and herbal dietary supplement for weight reduction. Clin Toxicol 2008; 46(4): 290-2.
[12] Chan WB, Chow CC, Cockram CS. A patient with low free T4 and low thyroid-stimulating hormone without hypopituitarism. Int J Clin Pract 2004; 58(10): 983-4.
[13] Binimelis J, Bassas L, Marruecos L, *et al.* Massive thyroxine intoxication: evaluation of plasma extraction. Intensive Care Med 1987; 13(1): 33-8.
[14] Ioos V, Das V, Maury E, *et al.* A thyrotoxicosis outbreak due to dietary pills in Paris. Ther Clin Risk Manag 2008; 4(6): 1375-9.
[15] Tenenbein M, Dean HJ. Benign course after massive levothyroxine ingestion. Pediatr Emerg Care 1986; 2(1): 15-7.
[16] Litovitz TL, White JD. Levothyroxine ingestions in children: an analysis of 78 cases. Am J Emerg Med 1985; 3(4): 297-300.
[17] Matthews SJ. Acute thyroxine overdosage: two cases of parasuicide. Ulster Med J 1993; 62(2): 170-3.
[18] Oppenheimer JH. Role of plasma proteins in the binding, distribution and metabolism of the thyroid hormones. N Engl J Med 1968; 278(21): 1153-62.
[19] Lehrner LM, Weir MR. Acute ingestions of thyroid hormones. Pediatrics 1984; 73(3): 313-7.
[20] Golightly LK, Smolinske SC, Kulig KW, *et al.* Clinical effects of accidental levothyroxine ingestion in children. Am J Dis Child 1987; 141(9): 1025-7.
[21] Kulig K, Golightly LK, Rumack BH. Levothyroxine overdose associated with seizures in a young child. JAMA 1985; 254(15): 2109-10.
[22] Yoon SJ, Kim DM, Kim JU, *et al.* A case of thyroid storm due to thyrotoxicosis factitia. Yonsei Med J 2003; 44(2): 351-4.
[23] Berkner PD, Starkman H, Person N. Acute L-thyroxine overdose; therapy with sodium ipodate: evaluation of clinical and physiologic parameters. J Emerg Med 1991; 9(3): 129-31.
[24] DeGroot LJ, Rue PA. Roentgenographic contrast agents inhibit triiodothyronine binding to nuclear receptors *in vitro*. J Clin Endocrinol Metab 1979; 49(4): 538-42.
[25] May ME, Mintz PD, Lowry P, Geller R, Curnow RT. Plasmapheresis in thyroxine overdose: a case report. Journal of toxicology Clin Toxicol 1983; 20(5): 517-20.
[26] Muller C, Perrin P, Faller B, Richter S, Chantrel F. Role of plasma exchange in the thyroid storm. Ther Apher Dial 2011; 15(6): 522-31.

CHAPTER 6

Drug-Induced Thyroid Toxicity

Giuseppe Barbesino*

Thyroid Unit, Massachusetts General Hospital, Harvard Medical School, Boston, Masachusettso 2114, USA

Abstract: The thyroid is a highly specialized endocrine organ devoted to the production of thyroid hormone, *via* organification of inorganic iodine. To accomplish this task, the thyroid follicular cell employs a rather complex of unique enzymes, transporters and regulatory factors. Both a classical endocrine feedback mechanism and less understood intracellular mechanisms maintain a constant output of thyroid hormone in normal physiology. Such a complex system can be altered by a number of pharmacological interferences. These interferences can be grouped under two broad categories: direct toxic effects on the thyroid gland, and immune mediated effects precipitated by immune modulators. Drug effects on the thyroid have been studied for several decades thanks to the availability of accurate methods for assessing thyroid physiology. The effects of some of these drugs, such as amiodarone and lithium have been known for many years, but novel antineoplastic agents introduced more recently have been the focus of intense attention over the past few years. This chapter concisely summarizes our current knowledge on drugs capable of altering thyroid function or structure, with attention to underlying mechanisms.

Keywords: Alemtuzumab, amiodarone, endocrine disruption, drugs, interferon-α, interferon-β, interlekin-2, lithium, thyroid gland, toxicity, tyrosine kinase inhibitors.

INTRODUCTION

The thyroid gland is an extremely specialized endocrine organ, whose only purpose is the manufacturing of the thyroid hormones, tetraiodothyronine (thyroxine-T4), and triiodothyronine (T3). The thyroid is unique in that it is the only gland using a micronutrient (iodine) to manufacture its hormones. There are several important consequences to this feature:

1) The enzymatic reactions necessary for the organification of atomic iodine into thyroid hormones require a complex array of transporters and enzymes, uniquely expressed within the follicular cell and therefore subject to specific pharmacologic influences (see [1] for an extensive review of the follicular cell molecular biology).

***Corresponding author Giuseppe Barbesino:** Thyroid Unit, Massachusetts General Hospital, Harvard Medical School, Boston, Masachusettso 2114, USA; E-mail: gbarbesino@mgh.harvard.edu

Javier Del Pino, Maria Jesus Diaz and Maria Teresa Frejo (Eds)

2) The high concentration of iodine in the thyroid gland is thought to be associated with an elevated immunogenicity of several key proteins, most importantly, thyroglobulin (Tg) [2]. This results in a high incidence of immune-mediated thyroid dysfunction.

3) Likely due to the general scarcity of iodine in the environment, the evolution of the thyroid gland has developed a mechanism for storing large amounts of iodinated hormones in the colloid, capable of providing several weeks or months' worth of the daily thyroid hormone needs.

As a consequence of such complexity, several therapeutic substances can result in thyroid toxicity. Two main pathways are typically recognized: direct toxicity, and immune-mediated toxicity. Interestingly, some of the drugs can act through either pathway, such as amiodarone, lithium and, probably, interferon-α. It is also important to recognize that the clinical manifestations of a toxic event are also variable, with some compounds resulting in hypothyroidism, while others, usually more acute in effect, resulting in rapid discharge of pre-formed thyroid hormone in the circulation, resulting in thyrotoxicosis. This latter phenomenon, termed "destructive thyrotoxicosis" (DT) is seen in clearly autoimmune processes (such as, for example, the early phase of Hashimoto's thyroiditis) but also in processes that are deemed to be inflammatory, such as some forms of amiodarone-induced thyrotoxicosis (AIT) and of interferon-α induced thyroiditis (IIT). DT is characterized by mild or moderate thyrotoxicosis, with low radioiodine neck uptake, negative TSH receptor antibody (TRAb). In DT, an early phase of thyrotoxicosis lasting a few weeks is followed by transient or permanent hypothyroidism. In all forms of DT so far studied, vascular flow to the thyroid is reduced by Color Doppler ultrasound analysis. Finally, some immune modulators can precipitate Graves' disease (GD), with manifestations that are indistinguishable from the spontaneous variety of the condition. This chapter aims to provide a comprehensive review of important pharmacologic influences on the thyroid gland, but will dedicate special space to most recently introduced drugs.

INTERFERON-α

Interferon-α is one of the earliest isolated and synthesized cytokines. While a recapitulation of the multiple properties of this central mediator of the immune response is beyond the scope of this chapter, interferon-α enhances several aspects of the immune response by activating natural killer cells, increasing the expression of MHC antigens, inducing resistance to viral infections [3]. As a consequence, interferon-α has been studied in clinical trials for many conditions, such as leukemia, malignant melanoma, Kaposi's sarcoma and other malignant and infectious conditions, most importantly, hepatitis B and C. Hepatitis C remains the most common indication to interferon-α therapy and most of the data derives from series of such patients. Interferon-α therapy has been associated with a significant increase in the incidence of thyroid dysfunction in many studies [4] and therefore has prompted several clinical and basic investigations. The induction of thyroid autoantibodies (most often thyroid peroxidase antibody–TPO-Ab) is the most commonly observed event, in 10-40% of patients. This phenomenon, likely caused by the proliferation of autoreactive lymphocytes has no clinical consequences in most cases. However, in many such cases a thyroid ultrasonographic pattern reminiscent of classical Hashimoto's thyroiditis has been recognized, even in the absence of thyroid dysfunction, suggesting lymphocytic infiltration of the gland [5]. Once acquired, TPO-Ab are persistent in the majority of cases, but up to one third of patient will become seronegative after cessation of interferon-α therapy [6]. Similarly to what seen in the clinical spectrum of spontaneous autoimmune thyroid disease, a fraction of patients with positive TPO-Ab develop hypothyroidism, and this is more likely to happen in patients who have positive TPO-Ab before the initiation of interferon-α therapy [7].

Thyrotoxicosis can also be seen during interferon-α therapy. In a minority of cases this is due to classical Graves' disease, with positive TRAb, and ongoing even after interferon-α therapy [8]. However the majority of thyrotoxicosis patients presents with the clinical features of DT. Interestingly most of these patients have negative TPO-Ab, suggesting a non-autoimmune, albeit probably inflammatory, etiology [4]. The clinical course of DT in such cases is similar to other forms of the disease, with a hypothyroid phase following the thyrotoxic phase. Return to euthyroidism is the most common outcome, but relapses have been described [9].

The pathogenesis of immune-mediated interferon-α-induced thyroid toxicity remains poorly understood. Several association studies suggest that hepatitis C infection itself predisposes to thyroid autoimmunity, but this point remains controversial [4]. As mentioned above, the presence of TPO-Ab prior to therapy has been uniformly noted as a risk factor. Genetic factors, such as some HLA haplotypes also play a role, at least in select populations [10]. Interestingly, besides the HLA, a number of other loci not previously associated with thyroid autoimmune disease has been recently identified as possibly responsible for interferon-α, immune-mediated thyroid dysfunction [11]. This suggests that the autoimmune pathways followed by this condition may be unique.

It has been postulated that DT observed during interferon-α therapy is the result of direct toxicity of the drug on thyroid follicular cells and therefore distinct from immune mediated phenomena. This is supported by studies showing several effects, including non-apoptotic cell death, induced by interferon-α on isolated thyroid cells and experimental animals [12]. The only available human pathology data, based on cytology of patients receiving both interferon-α and interleukin-2, suggests an increased expression of MHC molecules and a dense lymphocytic infiltrate, very reminiscent of classical Hashimoto's thyroiditis, therefore challenging the hypothesis of a specific pathway, not mediated by immune cellular effectors, to thyroid toxicity [13].

INTERFERON-β

Interferon-β is a cytokine belonging to the same family as interferon-α. Interferon beta and its derivatives and analogues are nowadays mostly used in the treatment of multiple sclerosis (MS). A large number of studies have analyzed the effect interferon-β on thyroid dysfunction. While some studies have suggested no effect [14], the most extensive studies suggest an increase incidence of thyroid autoimmune phenomena, such as the appearance of TPO-Ab (up to 40% of cases) and of clinical thyroid autoimmune disease (*i.e.* with measurable thyroid dysfunction-up to 15%) during treatment with interferon-β [15, 16]. Hypothyroidism is the most common form of thyroid dysfunction observed, but cases of Graves' disease requiring anti-thyroid drugs have been observed as well [17]. In most cases, the onset of thyroid autoimmunity is observed early on [16], during the first year of treatment. This suggests the existence of a pool of predisposed subjects who will experience thyroid dysfunction early on, with the remaining subjects not being susceptible to this effect even with prolonged treatment. Interestingly, glatiramer, another drug used in MS whose mechanism of action remains poorly understood, seems not to have this effect [16]. It was therefore suggested that risk factors for thyroid autoimmunity such as the presence of TPO-Ab should be included in the algorithm used to select the appropriate immune modulator for MS patients [18].

The mechanisms underlying interferon-β-induced thyroid toxicity remain unclear. Some *in vitro* studies suggest that interferon-β markedly enhances the expression of CXCL10 on thyroid follicular cells [19], a chemokine involved in the recruitment of T-cell to target tissues in autoimmunity [20]. Similarly to what observed with interferon-α, thyrocyte apoptosis also appears to be stimulated by interferon-β [21].

INTERLEUKIN-2

Treatment with interleukin-2 for malignant melanoma and renal cell carcinoma is also associated with an increased incidence of thyroid dysfunction. As with other cytokines described earlier, the presence of circulating TPO-Ab predisposes patients to development of thyroid dysfunction [22] in up to 50% of cases. Earlier suggestions of an association between the development of thyroid dysfunction and response to the therapy [22, 23] have been subsequently dismissed [24]. Hypothyroidism is most commonly observed, but cases of DT have been reported as well. Of great interest, a description of a few cases of such an occurrence also described thyroid cytology findings at the time of the thyrotoxic phase. As mentioned above, thyroid cytology from such patients, treated with both interlekin-2 and interferon-α, showed findings suggestive of Hashimoto's thyroiditis [13].

ALEMTUZUMAB AND THE IMMUNE RECONSTITUTION SYNDROME

Alemtuzumab is a humanized monoclonal antibody targeting the CD52 cell-surface antigen. Upon binding of Alemtuzumab onto its target, complement-mediated lysis of CD52 positive cells, including most lymphocytes, occurs. This quite effective and protracted anti-lymphocyte therapy has been studied in several autoimmune conditions, but found to be most effective in MS [25]. In an early pilot study, one in three patients treated with alemtuzumab developed classical Graves' disease, with unremitting hyperthyroidism, and positive TSAb [26]. Some of these patients even developed Graves' eye disease, recapitulating the whole spectrum observed in sporadic Graves' disease. Following this observation, a careful re-evaluation of thyroid dysfunction in a large trial of alemtuzumab *vs.* interferon-βin patients with MS has been presented [27]. Thyroid dysfunction was observed at some point in one third of patients on alemtuzumab, while a lower incidence (7%) was observed in interferon-β treated patients. Among the patients on alemtuzumab Graves' disease occurred in 22% of cases, hypothyroidism in 7%, DT in 4%. Of note, several of the patients with hypothyroidism had positive TSAb, an unusual feature in spontaneous autoimmune hypothyroidism. Several patients had multiple episodes of thyroid dysfunction and Graves' disease often evolved to hypothyroidism spontaneously. There was no distinctive time course to the onset of thyroid dysfunction, with new case distributed evenly along the period of observation. This extraordinary incidence of drug-induced Graves' disease is unique to immunotherapy with alemtuzumab, and appears to be limited to patients with MS. For example patients receiving the drug in the setting of B-cell leukemia do not seem to develop thyroid dysfunction at any increased rate

[28]. It seems reasonable to suppose that at least patients with MS have a genetic background predisposing them to autoimmunity and that alemtuzumab is capable to precipitate thyroid autoimmunity in this setting alone. It should be noted however that patients with MS do not seem to have a particularly high predisposition to thyroid autoimmune disease *per se* [29], so open questions remain.

Alemtuzumab is thought to cause thyroid autoimmunity indirectly. It is hypothesized that the rapid generalized lymphocyte depletion induced by the drug is followed by a phase of rapid clonal expansion, during which previously dormant autoreactive T-lymphocyte clones are expanded. It appears that in the case of alemtuzumab, a shift from Th-1 type autoimmunity (cell-mediated, typical of Hashimoto's thyroiditis) to a Th-2 type is observed, with mostly antibody-mediated autoimmune phenomena, typical of Graves' disease [30]. This is also suggested by the observation that the second most common complication of alemtuzumab treatment is another antibody-mediated condition, immune thrombocytopenic purpura.

A similar mechanism has been invoked to explain autoimmune phenomena occurring after initiation of high activity anti-retroviral therapy (HAART) in patients with the human immunodeficiency syndrome. A few studies have demonstrated a 1-2% incidence of Graves' disease in this setting [31]. While this incidence is not higher than what seen in the general population, the clustering of cases in relationship to the initiation of HAART is significant. It is also intriguing that, as seen with alemtuzumab, Graves' disease predominates, which is at odds with the spontaneous autoimmune thyroid diseases, in which hypothyroidism from Hashimoto's thyroiditis is vastly predominant.

TYROSINE KINASE INHIBITORS

Novel anti-neoplastic agents have gained tremendous interest over the past two decades, with the promise of targeting tumor-specific pathways in a selective way, therefore eliminating the widespread, dose-limiting side effects of conventional cytotoxic chemotherapy. The number of targeted molecules and pathways is ever growing, but the largest group of drugs targets tyrosine kinases, cell surface receptors involved in cell replication, tumor angiogenesis, and inhibition of apoptosis. While the original goal of tyrosine-kinase inhibitors (TKI) was targeting mutated or overexpressed oncogenes within the target cells, it has become clear that some of these molecules target other "wild type" kinases in the tumor environment, such as VEGFR, EGFR, PDGFR and others. This lack of selectivity seems to be important in several models, contributing to the overall efficacy of these drugs, by interfering with the tumor's vascular supply, modifying cell adhesion properties, and the ability to metastasize [32]. As a consequence of this incomplete selectivity, non-cancer cell types and tissues are affected by TKI treatment leading to a large array of side effects. Several of these agents have been shown to affect thyroid function and thyroid anatomy. Some of these drugs, such as imatinib, pazopanib, cabonzantinib, vandetinib and others mostly affect the levothyroxine levels in athyreotic patients, causing hypothyroidism in previously well-replaced patients [33]. These effects are clearly non-thyroidal and reflect either an increase metabolic clearance, or a reduced absorption of levothyroxine, and will not be reviewed in detail in this chapter, mostly concerned with direct thyroid toxicity.

Sunitinib, one of the earliest approved TKIs, is probably the best-studied drug in this category. Sunitinib is used in the treatment of metastatic renal cell carcinoma, gastrointestinal stromal tumor, and pancreatic neuroendocrine tumors. Sunitinib has inhibitory activity on the VEGFRs, PDGFR, RET, and KIT. Desai and colleagues reported the first series of cases of thyroid dysfunction on patients treated with sunitinib. These authors observed some degree of thyroid dysfunction in 62% of patients. Persistent or transient hypothyroidism was found in 53% of cases [34]. Interestingly, 10% of patients experienced transient, likely destructive thyrotoxicosis. In two cases described in a separate report, complete thyroid atrophy was observed by thyroid ultrasound, even in patients with pre-existing nodular goiter [35]. The incidence of hypothyroidism was positively correlated to the number of treatment courses [34]. In a following study [36], thyroid function and physiology was analyzed in more detail. The authors of this report observed worsening hypothyroidism after each sunitinib cycle. TPO-Ab tests were negative and radioiodine uptake was reduced during treatment courses. Additional information was added by the recognition that atrophic thyroid changes and hypothyroidism were associated with a decline in thyroidal blood flow by ultrasound color Doppler analysis [37]. Animal studies have indeed shown marked regression of the thyroid capillary bed during treatment with sunitinib [38].

In summary, it appears that sunitinib affects the thyroid by acutely reducing its vascular supply. The damage is cumulative, with additional damage with each cycle of treatment, leading to irreversible thyroid atrophy and hypothyroidism. In the early phases however, it can be acute enough to precipitate mild DT. Sunitinib is a TKI with inhibitory effect on several tyrosine kinases, including VEGFR1,

VEGFR2, PDGFR and others. It has been hypothesized that several targets are involved in TKI-induced thyroid damage [39]. Indeed, several other multitargeted TKI have been shown to directly affect thyroid function [33]. Although their mechanism of action has been less studied, it is likely to be similar to the effect of sunitinib.

Axitinib is another TKI, used in advanced renal cell carcinoma, which seems to share with sunitinib an intense anti-thyroid effect. Axitinib has intense inhibitory effect on the VEGFRs, but not on PDGFR, RET, or KIT. In several small studies, mostly from Japan, axitinib treatment was followed by symptomatic hypothyroidism in 80-100% of patients [40]. Subsequent larger phase III studies suggested a lower incidence of hypothyroidism, at around 20%, in European patients. It has therefore been suggested that Japanese patients might be extraordinarily susceptible to axitinib-induced thyroid toxicity [39].

Treatment with sorafenib (also used for renal cell carcinoma and hepatocellular carcinoma) is associated with hypothyroidism in 10-30% of patients [41]. Similarly to sunitinib, cases of presumed DT were observed, suggesting that sorafenib acts with a similar mechanism. The incidence of hypothyroidism seems to be twice as high in Japanese patients taking sorafenib similarly to what seen with axitinib, a phenomenon that remains unexplained [42]. While autoimmune hypothyroidism is more common in Japan as in many other iodine-replete countries [43], the incidence of autoimmune phenomena such as positive TPO-Ab seems to be low in affected patients, therefore other genetic or environmental co-factors must be at play.

Several other TKIs have been associated with hypothyroidism, although the clinical data remains limited: pazopanib, dasatinib, ilotinib and others [33].

Most TKIs capable of directly affecting thyroid function seem to act through destructive phenomena. These are all multitargeted TKIs, with affinity for at least one but more often all receptors belonging to the VEGFR family. As well demonstrated in the case of sunitinib, it is likely that all these drugs affect the microvascular supply of the thyroid gland inducing several degrees of follicular cell damage, eventually leading to irreversible primary hypothyroidism. The primary role of VEGFR inhibition in thyroid toxicity is supported by data indicating a 25% incidence of hypothyroidism in patients treated with bevacizumab, an antagonist of VEGF, the main VEGFR ligand [44]. Some of these drugs such as pazopanib [45] also reduce thyroid hormone levels in thyroidectomized patients receiving levothyroxine. This effect is possibly due to increased metabolism of the drug and therefore could also affect non-thyroidectomized patient. Data from other potent stimulators of thyroid hormone metabolism such as rifampicin, suggest that such a mechanism could cause hypothyroidism in patients whose thyroids' capacity of adapt to increased thyroid hormone demand is limited by thyroid autoimmunity [46]. It is therefore possible that TKI act through two different mechanisms, on the one hand by severely affecting the anatomic integrity of the thyroid gland, on the other hand by increasing the thyroid hormone demand on an already ailing gland.

The thyroid is an excellent model of tissue toxicity given the ease of measuring its function, and its accessibility to imaging. One wonders whether these drugs are also capable to affect other endocrine glands, less easily explored such as the adrenal and the pituitary and what role these effects might have on the safety of these drugs. This is a rapidly moving field and the years to come are sure to bring more information on these topics.

AMIODARONE

The effects of amiodarone on the thyroid have long been recognized. Amiodarone is a potent anti-arrhythmic agent with unique properties, very effective in restoring and maintaining sinus rhythm in patients with atrial fibrillation [47]. Because of its efficacy and uniqueness, the drug is widely used. Amiodarone is an amphophilic drug, with a very large volume of distribution and long half-life of about 40 days (50 days for its principal active metabolite, desethyl-amiodarone). Its benzofuran ring contains 37% iodine by weight and one 200 mg dose contains 75 mg iodine. About 10% of the iodine is released as inorganic iodine daily, providing 30-100 times the recommended daily allowance of 150 mcg (48). Amiodarone accumulates in many tissues, including the thyroid and this explains its toxicity profile, which includes the skin, the lung, the eye, the liver, and the thyroid. It is generally thought that amiodarone can affect the thyroid through its intrinsic properties, or through the inorganic iodine it constantly releases within the organism. Amiodarone accumulates in lysosomes of susceptible tissues, where it binds to intralysosomal phospholipids and interferes with their turn-over [49]. The resulting phospholipidosis is suspected to play a role in amiodarone-induced tissue toxicity, but the data is indeed limited. Other potential mechanisms also include a direct effect of high intracellular concentrations of inorganic iodine and the formation of free radicals [48]. Amiodarone also affects thyroid hormone metabolism by reducing the peripheral deiodination of T4 to triiodothyronine T3, hence causing a slight increase in T4 and a slight decrease in T3 [50].

Amiodarone Induced Hypothyroidism (AIH)

Hypothyroidism is the most common thyroidal side effect of amiodarone. Transient and mild elevations of TSH are often observed early during treatment with amiodarone [51]. The cause of these changes is unclear. It is possible that the reduced formation of triiodothyronine in the pituitary as a consequence of the known effect of amiodarone on deiodinase is responsible for increased TSH secretion. In alternative, or in addition, the Wolff-Chaikoff effect, caused by a rapid increase in the intrathyroidal level of iodine deriving from amiodarone metabolism, might cause a transient decrease in thyroid hormone secretion [52]. Overt and persistent hypothyroidism is observed in 5-12% of patients [53]. Risk factors for hypothyroidism include living in an area of iodine sufficiency, female gender, and pre-existing positive TPO-Ab [54]. Amiodarone induced hypothyroidism usually occurs within 6-18 months after initiation of amiodarone therapy.

It is generally thought that the pathogenesis of AIH involves a failure to escape from the Wolff-Chaikoff phenomenon in patients whose thyroid carries an organification defects, for example as a consequence of thyroid autoimmunity. Normal thyroid are able to escape the Wolff-Chaikoff phenomenon by down regulating the trans membrane iodine transport mechanism. Iodinated lipids that are formed during iodine organification processes are likely to mediate the down regulation of iodine transport. Thyroid autoimmunity seems to impair the organification of iodine, thus decreasing the formation of regulatory iodolipids, which in turn results in a persistence of high intracellular iodine levels and persistence of the Wolff-Chaikoff effect [55]. As a proof of concept, treatment of patients with perchlorate, a potent inhibitor of the iodine symporter, promptly resolves AIH [56]. This also suggests that this effect of amiodarone is mostly related to its iodine content, and not to the amiodarone molecule in itself.

Other *in vitro* and *vivo* studies have shown a variety of additional direct cytotoxic effects of amiodarone on the thyroid cells (reviewed in detail in [51]), but the relative importance of these effects remains unclear.

Discontinuation of amiodarone often results in restoration of euthyroidism, but treatment with levothyroxine is equally effective if amiodarone is to be continued.

Amiodarone-induced Thyrotoxicosis (AIT)

Thyrotoxicosis is a clinically very significant complication of amiodarone treatment. Patients treated with amiodarone are the most vulnerable to the complications of thyrotoxicosis as they almost universally have a mixture of cardiac arrhythmias and/or congestive heart failure likely to be significantly worsened by thyroid hormone excess. Risk factors for AIT mirror AIH: AIT is more common in men and in areas of moderate iodine deficiency [54]. Given the influence of dietary iodine, the incidence of AIT vary, but it is estimated at 15% in areas of iodine deficiency, around 10% in areas of moderate iodine replenishment and 2% in the United States [54, 57]. It has been long recognized that two distinct pathogenic mechanisms can precipitate AIT and this results in markedly different clinical features and management.

Type I AIT occurs most commonly in areas of iodine deficiency. Type I AIT appears to be caused by the effect of excessive inorganic iodine released by amiodarone on glands predisposed to the development of thyroid autonomy, such as with multinodular goiters or latent Graves' disease [51, 53]. According to this interpretation the sudden iodine load causes unremitting hyperthyroidism in such glands. The role of iodine deficiency is complex. First, autonomous nodular disease is more common in areas of iodine deficiency [58]. Second, a sudden increase in dietary iodine levels is associated with an increased risk for thyroid autoimmunity and Graves' disease [59]. Third, it appears that thyroid glands accustomed to low dietary levels of iodine have relatively inactive intracellular regulatory pathways for the handling of a sudden increase in the iodine level.

Clinically, the hyperthyroidism of type I AIT is therefore similar to the "garden variety" Graves' disease or toxic multinodular goiter, with some important differences. The high iodine content of the thyroid gland causes a high level of iodination of antithyroid drugs within the thyroid cell, resulting in inactivation of the molecule [60]. As a consequence, patients with type I AIT needs very high doses of antithyroid drugs and the response to treatment is often delayed. Because of the large amount of body iodine, treatment with radioactive iodine is usually not feasible, as the radioactive iodine uptake in the thyroid gland is usually too low to allow the delivery of an effective dose to the thyroid.

Type II AIT is believed to result from toxicity of the amiodarone molecule to the thyroid gland [48, 51]. *In vitro* studies have shown direct cytotoxic effects of amiodarone on thyroid cell lines although some of the effects appeared to be mediated by the released iodine [61], as some protection could be gained by the addition of Methimazole to the culture medium. However, in animal studies, amiodarone causes dramatic structural changes of the thyroidal endoplasmic reticulum, changes that were not seen when iodine alone was administered [62]. Similarly, amiodarone was found to cause be associated with widespread thyroid structural abnormalities in human cases of thyrotoxicosis submitted to thyroidectomy [63].

At striking difference with type I AIT, the thyrotoxicosis is self-limited and responsive to glucocorticoids.

The most important problem for the clinician confronting the problem of AIT is distinguishing between the two forms, as treatment is critically different: type I AIT is treated with high dose antithyroid drugs (perchlorate, not available in the United States, is also used in Europe) while type II AIT is treated with oral glucorticoid [64]. At difference with non-amiodarone-induced thyrotoxicosis, the radioactive iodine uptake is not very useful, as a low uptake can be seen in both forms. The differential diagnosis therefore relies on a number of indirect parameters. Typically, type II AIT presents with a moderate diffuse goiter, a poorly vascular gland on Color Doppler ultrasound studies [65], negative TSH receptor antibody tests. The time course can also be helpful, in that the median onset of type I AIT is just 3 months after initiation of therapy, while the median onset of type II is 30 months after initiation [66]. Considerable overlap exists, however. It should also be noted, that likely due to an improved iodine nutrition, type I AIT is becoming proportionally less common in developed countries [67]. However, uncertainty sometimes remain, for example a patient with AIT and a thyroid nodules does not necessarily have type I AIT, or a patient with negative TSH receptor antibodies and diffuse goiter may still have type I AIT. As a consequence patients, especially if critically ill from the cardiac condition and the thyrotoxicosis are sometimes initially treated with both modalities.

LITHIUM

Lithium is an alkaline metal, a monovalent cation, administered orally as a carbonate or citrate salt. Lithium is currently the drug of choice in the long-term management of bipolar disorders. The mechanism of action of lithium on the CNS is poorly understood. Several hypotheses have been presented, probably not mutually exclusive, recently reviewed in [68].

Lithium is completely absorbed in the gut. Being a cation, it undergoes no metabolism, its half-life is about 12 hours and the elimination is renal. The volume of distribution corresponds to the intracellular and extracellular fluid.

The effects of lithium on the thyroid gland have been long recognized. Thyroid cells concentrate lithium with an unknown mechanism [69]. The main effect of lithium on the thyroid seems to an increase in the intracellular concentrations of iodine [70]. While the iodine uptake in the thyroid gland is not affected by lithium, the release of inorganic iodine and possibly of thyroid hormone is diminished in rats [69, 71]. In spite of these effects, the serum thyroxine level is not grossly decreased [72] in humans. Clinically, the most commonly observed effect of lithium is the occurrence of a diffuse goiter [70], with a highly variable in different studies [73]. The etiology of this phenomenon remains unclear. It is possible that a subtle decrease in thyroid output of thyroid hormone results in a minimal elevation of TSH capable of causing thyroid growth over a period of years or decades. However, there are studies suggesting a direct effect of lithium on the proliferation of thyroid cells [74], an appealing explanation for the clinical presentation with goiter and no obvious thyroid dysfunction for most patients. Clinical or subclinical hypothyroidism has been reported also with highly variable incidence, from 3.8% to 62% [73], owing to differences in the populations studied with regard to duration of therapy, definition of hypothyroidism, age distribution and other factors. The presence of thyroid autoimmunity increased the risk of hypothyroidism in patients taking lithium in one study [75], with a relative risk of 8.6.

DT also appeared to be a specific complication of lithium treatment. In a population of patients with thyrotoxicosis of many causes, lithium exposure was found more often in the patients with DT than in the group of patients with other forms of thyrotoxicosis, indicating a significant association [76].

Overall, lithium effects on the thyroid gland are usually mild and relatively uncommon. However, hypothyroidism can precipitate lithium toxicity, so routinely screening thyroid function in patients on lithium seems advisable. Patients with hypothyroidism can easily be treated with levothyroxine without interruption of lithium treatment, while DT is a usually mild and transient. An interesting and unanswered is whether treatment with levothyroxine can prevent the occurrence of goiter in patients taking lithium.

The effects of lithium in increasing intrathyroidal iodine levels and therefore effectively increasing the intracellular half-life of iodine have been exploited with the goal of increasing the concentration of radioactive iodine at the time of treatment for thyroid cancer or hyperthyroidism, therefore allowing to decrease the total delivered activity. Indeed several studied have demonstrated enhanced efficacy of radioiodine treatment for hyperthyroidism [77], and thyroid cancer [78] when a short course of lithium was administered. However the benefits have not been judged significant enough to warrant routine use.

CONFLICT OF INTEREST

The author confirms that author has no conflict of interest to declare for this publication.

ACKNOWLEDGEMENTS

Declared None.

REFERENCES

[1] Kopp PA, Carrasco N. Thyroid hormone synthesis and secretion. In: Werner & Ingbar's, Eds. The Thyroid [Internet]. Lippincott Williams & Wilkins, 2005.

[2] McLachlan SM, Rapoport B. Breaking tolerance to thyroid antigens: changing concepts in thyroid autoimmunity. Endocr Rev 2014; 35(1): 59-105.

[3] Pfeffer LM, Dinarello CA, Herberman RB, *et al.* Biological properties of recombinant alpha-interferons: 40th anniversary of the discovery of interferons. Cancer Res 1998; 58(12): 2489-99.

[4] Mandac JC, Chaudhry S, Sherman KE, Tomer Y. The clinical and physiological spectrum of interferon-alpha induced thyroiditis: toward a new classification. Hepatology 2006; 43(4): 661-72.

[5] Friedrich-Rust M, Theobald J, Zeuzem S, Bojunga J. Thyroid function and changes in ultrasound morphology during antiviral therapy with pegylated interferon and ribavirin in patients with chronic hepatitis C. J Viral Hepat 2009; 16(3): 168-77.

[6] Carella C, Mazziotti G, Morisco F, *et al.* Long-term outcome of interferon-alpha-induced thyroid autoimmunity and prognostic influence of thyroid autoantibody pattern at the end of treatment. J Clin Endocrinol Metab 2001; 86(5): 1925-9.

[7] Roti E, Minelli R, Giuberti T, *et al.* Multiple changes in thyroid function in patients with chronic active HCV hepatitis treated with recombinant interferon-alpha. Am J Med 1996; 101(5): 482-7.

[8] Lisker-Melman M, Di Bisceglie AM, Usala SJ, Weintraub B, Murray LM, Hoofnagle JH. Development of thyroid disease during therapy of chronic viral hepatitis with interferon alfa. Gastroenterology 1992; 102(6): 2155-60.

[9] Parana R, Cruz M, Lyra L, Cruz T. Subacute thyroiditis during treatment with combination therapy (interferon plus ribavirin) for hepatitis C virus. J Viral Hepat 2000; 7(5): 393-5.

[10] Kakizaki S, Takagi H, Murakami M, Takayama H, Sato K, Mori M. HLA-A2 subtype in patients with interferon-alpha-induced autoimmune thyroid disorders in chronic hepatitis C. Liver 2000; 20(5): 423-4.

[11] Hasham A, Zhang W, Lotay V, *et al.* Genetic analysis of interferon induced thyroiditis (IIT): evidence for a key role for MHC and apoptosis related genes and pathways. J Autoimmun 2013; 44: 61-70.

[12] Akeno N, Smith EP, Stefan M, *et al.* IFN-alpha mediates the development of autoimmunity both by direct tissue toxicity and through immune cell recruitment mechanisms. J Immunol 2011; 186(8): 4693-706.

[13] Pichert G, Jost LM, Zobeli L, Odermatt B, Pedia G, Stahel RA. Thyroiditis after treatment with interleukin-2 and interferon alpha-2a. Br J Cancer 1990; 62(1): 100-4.

[14] Kivisakk P, Lundahl J, von Heigl Z, Fredrikson S. No evidence for increased frequency of autoantibodies during interferon-beta1b treatment of multiple sclerosis. Acta Neurol Scand 1998; 97(5): 320-3.

[15] Caraccio N, Dardano A, Manfredonia F, *et al.* Long-term follow-up of 106 multiple sclerosis patients undergoing interferon-beta 1a or 1b therapy: predictive factors of thyroid disease development and duration. J Clin Endocrinol Metab 2005; 90(7): 4133-7.

[16] Frisullo G, Calabrese M, Tortorella C, *et al.* Thyroid autoimmunity and dysfunction in multiple sclerosis patients during long-term treatment with interferon beta or glatiramer acetate: an Italian multicenter study. Mult Scler 2014; 20(9): 1265-8.

[17] Kreisler A, de Seze J, Stojkovic T, *et al.* Multiple sclerosis, interferon beta and clinical thyroid dysfunction. Acta Neurol Scand 2003; 107(2): 154-7.
[18] Rotondi M, Bergamaschi R, Chiovato L. Disease modifying therapies in multiple sclerosis: could a baseline thyroid check-up drive the therapeutic choice between interferon-beta and glatiramer acetate? Mult Scler 2014; 20(14): 1918-9.
[19] Rotondi M, Stufano F, Lagonigro MS, *et al.* Interferon-beta but not Glatiramer acetate stimulates CXCL10 secretion in primary cultures of thyrocytes: a clue for understanding the different risks of thyroid dysfunctions in patients with multiple sclerosis treated with either of the two drugs. J Neuroimmunol 2011; 234(1-2): 161-4.
[20] Rotondi M, Chiovato L, Romagnani S, Serio M, Romagnani P. Role of chemokines in endocrine autoimmune diseases. Endocr Rev 2007; 28(5): 492-520.
[21] Caraccio N, Cuccato S, Pratesi F, *et al.* Effect of type I interferon(s) on cell viability and apoptosis in primary human thyrocyte cultures. Thyroid 2009; 19(2): 149-55.
[22] Weijl NI, Van der Harst D, Brand A, *et al.* Hypothyroidism during immunotherapy with interleukin-2 is associated with antithyroid antibodies and response to treatment. J Clin Oncol 1993; 11(7): 1376-83.
[23] Atkins MB, Mier JW, Parkinson DR, Gould JA, Berkman EM, Kaplan MM. Hypothyroidism after treatment with interleukin-2 and lymphokine-activated killer cells. N Engl J Med 1988; 318(24): 1557-63.
[24] Phan GQ, Attia P, Steinberg SM, White DE, Rosenberg SA. Factors associated with response to high-dose interleukin-2 in patients with metastatic melanoma. J Clin Oncol 2001; 19(15): 3477-82.
[25] Coles AJ, Compston DA, Selmaj KW, *et al.* Alemtuzumab *vs.* interferon beta-1a in early multiple sclerosis. N Engl J Med 2008; 359(17): 1786-801.
[26] Coles AJ, Wing M, Smith S, *et al.* Pulsed monoclonal antibody treatment and autoimmune thyroid disease in multiple sclerosis. Lancet 1999; 354(9191): 1691-5.
[27] Daniels GH, Vladic A, Brinar V, *et al.* Alemtuzumab-related thyroid dysfunction in a phase 2 trial of patients with relapsing-remitting multiple sclerosis. J Clin Endocrinol Metab 2014; 99(1): 80-9.
[28] Demko S, Summers J, Keegan P, Pazdur R. FDA drug approval summary: alemtuzumab as single-agent treatment for B-cell chronic lymphocytic leukemia. Oncologist 2008; 13(2): 167-74.
[29] Marrie RA, Yu BN, Leung S, *et al.* The incidence and prevalence of thyroid disease do not differ in the multiple sclerosis and general populations: a validation study using administrative data. Neuroepidemiology 2012; 39(2): 135-42.
[30] Weetman A. Immune reconstitution syndrome and the thyroid. Best Pract Res Clin Endocrinol Metab 2009; 23(6): 693-702.
[31] Weetman AP. Thyroid abnormalities. Endocrinol Metab Clin North Am 2014; 43(3): 781-90.
[32] Zhang J, Yang PL, Gray NS. Targeting cancer with small molecule kinase inhibitors. Nat Rev Cancer. 2009; 9(1): 28-39.
[33] Illouz F, Laboureau-Soares S, Dubois S, Rohmer V, Rodien P. Tyrosine kinase inhibitors and modifications of thyroid function tests: a review. Eur J Endocrinol 2009; 160(3): 331-6.
[34] Desai J, Yassa L, Marqusee E, *et al.* Hypothyroidism after sunitinib treatment for patients with gastrointestinal stromal tumors. Ann Intern Med 2006; 145(9): 660-4.
[35] Rogiers A, Wolter P, Op de Beeck K, Thijs M, Decallonne B, Schoffski P. Shrinkage of thyroid volume in sunitinib-treated patients with renal-cell carcinoma: a potential marker of irreversible thyroid dysfunction? Thyroid 2010; 20(3): 317-22.
[36] Mannavola D, Coco P, Vannucchi G, *et al.* A novel tyrosine-kinase selective inhibitor, sunitinib, induces transient hypothyroidism by blocking iodine uptake. J Clin Endocrinol Metab 2007; 92(9): 3531-4.
[37] Makita N, Miyakawa M, Fujita T, Iiri T. Sunitinib induces hypothyroidism with a markedly reduced vascularity. Thyroid 2010; 20(3): 323-6.
[38] Kappers MH, van Esch JH, Smedts FM, *et al.* Sunitinib-induced hypothyroidism is due to induction of type 3 deiodinase activity and thyroidal capillary regression. J Clin Endocrinol Metab 2011; 96(10): 3087-94.
[39] Makita N, Iiri T. Tyrosine kinase inhibitor-induced thyroid disorders: a review and hypothesis. Thyroid 2013; 23(2): 151-9.

[40] Daimon M, Kato T, Kaino W, *et al.* Thyroid dysfunction in patients treated with tyrosine kinase inhibitors, sunitinib, sorafenib and axitinib, for metastatic renal cell carcinoma. Jpn J Clin Oncol 2012; 42(8): 742-7.

[41] Tamaskar I, Bukowski R, Elson P, *et al.* Thyroid function test abnormalities in patients with metastatic renal cell carcinoma treated with sorafenib. Ann Oncol 2008; 19(2): 265-8.

[42] Miyake H, Kurahashi T, Yamanaka K, *et al.* Abnormalities of thyroid function in Japanese patients with metastatic renal cell carcinoma treated with sorafenib: A prospective evaluation. Urol Oncol 2010; 28(5): 515-9.

[43] McLeod DS, Cooper DS. The incidence and prevalence of thyroid autoimmunity. Endocrine 2012; 42(2): 252-65.

[44] Reismuller B, Azizi AA, Peyrl A, *et al.* Feasibility and tolerability of bevacizumab in children with primary CNS tumors. Pediatr Blood Cancer 2010; 54(5): 681-6.

[45] Bible KC, Suman VJ, Molina JR, *et al.* Efficacy of pazopanib in progressive, radioiodine-refractory, metastatic differentiated thyroid cancers: results of a phase 2 consortium study. Lancet Oncol 2010; 11(10): 962-72.

[46] Curran PG, DeGroot LJ. The effect of hepatic enzyme-inducing drugs on thyroid hormones and the thyroid gland. Endocr Rev 1991; 12(2): 135-50.

[47] Singh BN. Amiodarone: a multifaceted antiarrhythmic drug. Curr Cardiol Rep 2006; 8(5): 349-55.

[48] Eskes SA, Wiersinga WM. Amiodarone and thyroid. Best Pract Res Clin Endocrinol Metab 2009; 23(6): 735-51.

[49] Rabkin SW. Effect of amiodarone on phospholipid content and composition in heart, lung, kidney and skeletal muscle: relationship to alteration of thyroid function. Pharmacology 2006; 76(3): 129-35.

[50] Burger A, Dinichert D, Nicod P, Jenny M, Lemarchand-Beraud T, Vallotton MB. Effect of amiodarone on serum triiodothyronine, reverse triiodothyronine, thyroxin, and thyrotropin. A drug influencing peripheral metabolism of thyroid hormones. J Clin Invest 1976; 58(2): 255-9.

[51] Martino E, Bartalena L, Bogazzi F, Braverman LE. The effects of amiodarone on the thyroid. Endocr Rev 2001; 22(2): 240-54.

[52] Wolff J, Chaikoff IL. The inhibitory action of excessive iodide upon the synthesis of diiodotyrosine and of thyroxine in the thyroid gland of the normal rat. Endocrinology 1948; 43(3): 174-9.

[53] Wiersinga WM. Amiodarone and the thyroid. In: Weetman AP, Grossman A, Eds. Pharmacotherapeutics of the thyroid gland. Berlin: Springer; 1997; p. 225-87.

[54] Trip MD, Wiersinga W, Plomp TA. Incidence, predictability, and pathogenesis of amiodarone-induced thyrotoxicosis and hypothyroidism. Am J Med 1991; 91(5): 507-11.

[55] Wiersinga WM, Touber JL, Trip MD, van Royen EA. Uninhibited thyroidal uptake of radioiodine despite iodine excess in amiodarone-induced hypothyroidism. J Clin Endocrinol Metab 1986; 63(2): 485-91.

[56] Martino E, Mariotti S, Aghini-Lombardi F, *et al.* Short term administration of potassium perchlorate restores euthyroidism in amiodarone iodine-induced hypothyroidism. J Clin Endocrinol Metab 1986; 63(5): 1233-6.

[57] Martino E, Aghini-Lombardi F, Bartalena L, *et al.* Enhanced susceptibility to amiodarone-induced hypothyroidism in patients with thyroid autoimmune disease. Arch Intern Med 1994; 154(23): 2722-6.

[58] Laurberg P, Pedersen KM, Vestergaard H, Sigurdsson G. High incidence of multinodular toxic goitre in the elderly population in a low iodine intake area *vs.* high incidence of Graves' disease in the young in a high iodine intake area: comparative surveys of thyrotoxicosis epidemiology in East-Jutland Denmark and Iceland. J Intern Med 1991; 229(5): 415-20.

[59] Burgi H, Kohler M, Morselli B. Thyrotoxicosis incidence in Switzerland and benefit of improved iodine supply. Lancet 1998; 352(9133): 1034.

[60] Davidson B, Soodak M, Neary JT, *et al.* The irreversible inactivation of thyroid peroxidase by methylmercaptoimidazole, thiouracil, and propylthiouracil *in vitro* and its relationship to *in vivo* findings. Endocrinology 1978; 103(3): 871-82.

[61] Chiovato L, Martino E, Tonacchera M, *et al.* Studies on the *in vitro* cytotoxic effect of amiodarone. Endocrinology 1994; 134(5): 2277-82.

[62] Pitsiavas V, Smerdely P, Li M, Boyages SC. Amiodarone induces a different pattern of ultrastructural change in the thyroid to iodine excess alone in both the BB/W rat and the Wistar rat. Eur J Endocrinol 1997; 137(1): 89-98.

[63] Smyrk TC, Goellner JR, Brennan MD, Carney JA. Pathology of the thyroid in amiodarone-associated thyrotoxicosis. Am J Surg Pathol 1987; 11(3): 197-204.

[64] Bogazzi F, Bartalena L, Tomisti L, *et al.* Glucocorticoid response in amiodarone-induced thyrotoxicosis resulting from destructive thyroiditis is predicted by thyroid volume and serum free thyroid hormone concentrations. J Clin Endocrinol Metab 2007; 92(2): 556-62.

[65] Bogazzi F, Bartalena L, Brogioni S, *et al.* Color flow Doppler sonography rapidly differentiates type I and type II amiodarone-induced thyrotoxicosis. Thyroid 1997; 7(4): 541-5.

[66] Tomisti L, Rossi G, Bartalena L, Martino E, Bogazzi F. The onset time of amiodarone-induced thyrotoxicosis (AIT) depends on AIT type. Eur J Endocrinol 2014; 171(3): 363-8.

[67] Bogazzi F, Bartalena L, Dell'Unto E, *et al.* Proportion of type 1 and type 2 amiodarone-induced thyrotoxicosis has changed over a 27-year period in Italy. Clin Endocrinol (Oxf) 2007; 67(4): 533-7.

[68] Oruch R, Elderbi MA, Khattab HA, Pryme IF, Lund A. Lithium: a review of pharmacology, clinical uses, and toxicity. Eur J Pharmacol. 2014; 740: 464-73.

[69] Berens SC, Wolff J, Murphy DL. Lithium concentration by the thyroid. Endocrinology 1970; 87(5): 1085-7.

[70] Barbesino G. Drugs affecting thyroid function. Thyroid. 2010; 20(7): 763-70.

[71] Spaulding SW, Burrow GN, Bermudez F, Himmelhoch JM. The inhibitory effect of lithium on thyroid hormone release in both euthyroid and thyrotoxic patients. J Clin Endocrinol Metab 1972; 35(6): 905-11.

[72] Berens SC, Bernstein RS, Robbins J, Wolff J. Antithyroid effects of lithium. J Clin Invest. 1970; 49(7): 1357-67.

[73] Lazarus JH. Lithium and thyroid. Best Pract Res Clin Endocrinol Metab 2009; 23(6): 723-33.

[74] Rao AS, Kremenevskaja N, Resch J, Brabant G. Lithium stimulates proliferation in cultured thyrocytes by activating Wnt/beta-catenin signalling. Eur J Endocrinol 2005; 153(6): 929-38.

[75] Bocchetta A, Cocco F, Velluzzi F, Del Zompo M, Mariotti S, Loviselli A. Fifteen-year follow-up of thyroid function in lithium patients. J Endocrinol Invest 2007; 30(5): 363-6.

[76] Miller KK, Daniels GH. Association between lithium use and thyrotoxicosis caused by silent thyroiditis. Clin Endocrinol (Oxf) 2001; 55(4): 501-8.

[77] Bogazzi F, Giovannetti C, Fessehatsion R, *et al.* Impact of lithium on efficacy of radioactive iodine therapy for Graves' disease: a cohort study on cure rate, time to cure, and frequency of increased serum thyroxine after antithyroid drug withdrawal. J Clin Endocrinol Metab 2010; 95(1): 201-8.

[78] Yamazaki CA, Padovani RP, Biscolla RP, *et al.* Lithium as an adjuvant in the postoperative ablation of remnant tissue in low-risk thyroid carcinoma. Thyroid 2012; 22(10): 1002-6.

CHAPTER 7

Metals and Thyroid Toxicity

María Jesús Díaz, Javier Del Pino[*] and María Teresa Frejo

Departament of Toxicology and Pharmacology, Veterinary School, Complutense University of Madrid, Madrid, Spain

Abstract: The thyroid system, due to its complex histological structure and functions, is often the target of many endocrine toxins, including metals. In this regard, metals such as Cd, Pb, Cr, Mn, Hg and Cu are known to induce thyroid toxicity in man and animals. On the other hand, other metals are essential for the proper functioning of thyroid system such as Se, Zn, Fe among others, and their deficiency has been related to thyroid disruption. Metals could alter the thyroid system at many levels. In this regard, metals could reduce iodide uptake, alter production of thyroid stimulation hormone (TSH) at the pituitary level, alter thyroid hormones (THs) synthesis and release *via* many different mechanisms at the thyroid gland level and/or could induce histopathological alterations of the thyroid. In addition, metals could alter the metabolism of THs or action on their receptors. This chapter is focused on the main metals reported to induce thyroid toxicity, and the mechanisms through which their effects occur.

Keywords: Endocrine disruption, metals, thyroid, toxicity.

INTRODUCTION

Due to its complex histological structure and functions, the thyroid gland is often the target of many endocrine toxins, including heavy metals [1, 2]. In this regard, metals, such as cadmium (Cd), lead (Pb), chromium (Cr), arsenic (As), manganese (Mn), mercury (Hg) and copper (Cu) are known to induce thyrotoxicity in man and animals [3-8]. On the other hand, other metals are essential for the normal function of thyroid system such as selenium (Se), zinc (Zn), iron (Fe) among others, and their deficiency has been related to thyroid disruption [9, 10].

Alterations in thyroxine (T4) and triiodothyronine (T3), and thyroid-stimulating hormone (TSH) serum concentration reflect changes in their glandular synthesis and/or secretion as well as disruptions in their extrathyroid peripheral metabolism, so they are often used as reliable indicators of thyroid function in people and

[*]**Corresponding author Javier Del Pino:** Department of Toxicology and Pharmacology, Complutense University of Madrid, Madrid, Spain; E-mail: jdelpino@pdi.ucm.es

Javier Del Pino, Maria Jesus Diaz and Maria Teresa Frejo (Eds)

experimental animals [11, 12]. Therefore, alteration of their serum concentrations could be used as a good biomarker of the action of metals on thyroid function.

Several elements of the thyroid system can be disrupted by metal actions. In this regard, metals can reduce the iodide uptake. Moreover, their accumulation in the thyroid gland can alter TH production and release *via* many different mechanisms and/or could induce histopathological alterations in the thyroid, whereas accumulation of metals in the pituitary gland could lead to modifications in the feedback mechanisms and signaling pathways that regulate the synthesis of THs [13].

In addition, metals can alter TH metabolism or their action on their receptors (Fig. **1**) [14]. However, research to date does not provide in many cases, an evident cause-and-effect picture of how metals may alter thyroid-system functions or TH actions.

Multiple factors can affect the thyroid toxicity effect induced by these metals such as, gender, length of exposure, route, dosage, type and age, which are important to take into account to evaluate the risk to their exposure.

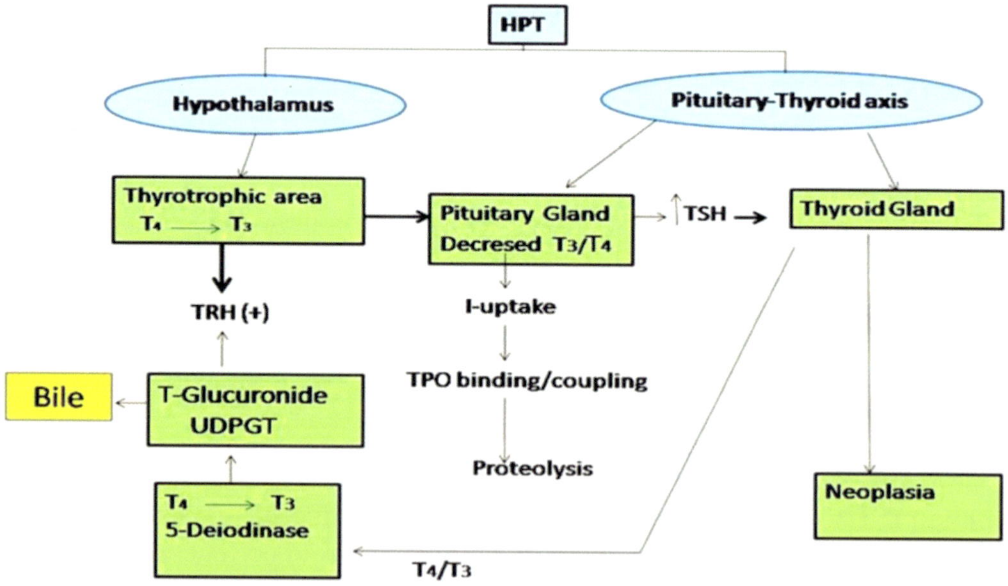

Figure 1: Multiple sites of hypothalamic-pituitary-thyroid (HPT) axis disruption by metal species. UDPGT, uridine diphosphate glucuronyltransferase; TSH, thyroid stimulating hormone; T4, thyroxine; T3, triiodothyronine; I, iodine; TPO, thyroperixidase. Adapted from Rana [14].

CADMIUM

Cadmium is an extensive industrial and environmental pollutant metal used in batteries, pigments, metal coatings, plastics and some metal alloys [15]. Conversely to other toxic heavy metals, cadmium is easily transferred from soil to plants, it is not biodegradable and can be greatly accumulated in the food chain [16], with a biological half-life of 7-30 years [17]. Contaminated food is the primary source of cadmium exposure for the population [18], and the second largest source is tobacco [19]. Cadmium is accumulated in the body and has been described to produce severe impairment to a variety of organs, including lung, liver, kidney, testis, placenta, brain and thyroid gland [20-22]. Women have been reported to present a higher level of Cd than men, which could induce higher toxic effects on them [23].

Cadmium induces its toxic effects by interfering the action of calcium, disrupting cellular energy metabolism [24]. Moreover, it generates free radicals [25] and lessens the cellular defense mechanism against oxidation, inducing oxidative stress [26], which influence plenty cellular components, such as DNA, lipids and proteins [27, 28], and subsequently may result in apoptotic cell death or induction of neoplasias [29, 30]. Cadmium is classified as a category I human carcinogen [31].

Autopsy data have shown that significantly higher concentrations of cadmium in the human thyroid gland are present only after 20 years of age [32]. It had been shown that Cd concentration in blood is positively correlated with its accumulation in the thyroid gland [33]. Different reports have indicated that Cd could induce structural and functional damage of the follicular and neuroendocrine apparatus of the thyroid gland [3, 33, 34]. Moreover, in epidemiologic studies, a positive association between T4 and T3 hormones with urinary Cd levels has been described, so an increase of Cd levels induces an increase of these hormones [35].

The damaging effects of Cd on thyroid function and morphology have been widely studied in animals. Chronic exposure to cadmium has been described to cause many histological and metabolic changes in the thyroid gland. Histopathologic changes in the thyroid are dose-dependent and are manifested by flattening of follicular cells, by their desquamation inside the follicular cells, by increasing interstitial fibrous tissue between follicular cells, and by mononuclear cellular infiltration in the stroma around the follicular cells [33]. Statistically significant lower follicular epithelium in cadmium toxicosis was also established in fish [36]. Moreover, chronic studies in rats (15 mg/kg) showed a spectrum of preneoplastic changes on thyroid follicular cells [3], and an increase in weight of the gland [9].

Cadmium thyrotoxicosis induces thyroid dysfunction, which leads to an increase in TSH concentration in rats [9], and humans [37], and decrease in T4 in serum, which was confirmed in different species [9, 38-40]. With respect to T3 hormone, the literature contains many contradictory data. Some reports show a significant decrease of T3 in serum, an increase in thyroid peroxidases (TPO) activity with a subsequent increase in T3 levels, or no effect on T3 levels [34, 41]. An increase of T3 plasma levels with a decreased serum levels of T4 was also shown in people living in areas polluted with cadmium [42]. These discrepancies could be due to the length of exposure to cadmium, route, dosage, type, age and species of experimental animals. On the other hand, it has been described that Se and Zn can have a synergistic function against Cd-induced thyroid dysfunction in rats and humans [9].

The mechanisms through which cadmium induces thyroid disruption are not completely understood. Cadmium could disrupt hypothalamic–pituitary–thyroid (HPT) axis activity by influencing the hypothalamus and also pituitary gland [43]. In this regard, it has been observed in fish that cadmium exposure induces inactivation of thyrotropin-secreting cells with an accumulation of secretory products [36]. Moreover, Yoshizuka and coworkers [22], suggested that Cd exposure induced its accumulation in mitochondria of thyroid follicular epithelial cells and disrupted oxidative phosphorylation of the organelles, leading to loss of energy supply, which likely causes inhibition of thyroid hormone synthesis and release.

It has been observed that Cd inhibits conversion of T4 to T3 in several tissues [44, 45]. This effect is mediated by inhibition of 5′-deiodinase 1 (DI1) activity [41]. The mechanism through which cadmium inhibits this enzyme is unknown, but it was suggested by Jancic and Stosic [3] that it was probably due to binding to sulfhydryl enzyme groups. In this regard, cadmium has been shown to inhibit many enzymes through binding to the sulfhydryl groups of the enzyme active sites [46], and the activity of 5′-deiodinases is highly dependent on the presence of sulfhydryl groups [47].

Finally, it was observed that cadmium exposure decreases the total level of iodine in thyroid and serum, and disrupts metabolism of THs. In this regard, as a result of iodine deficiency, a decreased production of THs, both in people and animals, has been described which leads to morphological and functional changes in the thyroid gland, as well as decreased T4 production [48].

MERCURY

Mercury display in the environment in different forms including, elemental (Hg^0), inorganic (Hg^+ and Hg^{2+}), and organic mercury possessing different physicochemical characteristics and toxicity profiles [49, 50]. Mercury is a heavy metal that may penetrate the environment through natural processes (*e.g.* volcanic activity and erosion of mineral deposits), as well as from an extensive series of anthropogenic actions like metal smelting, mining, coal production, coal-fired power stations, paper/pulp production, residential heating systems, waste disposal/incinerators and chemical synthesis/use [51, 52].

The toxicokinetics of mercury depends on the form in which it is presented. In humans, elemental mercury is easily absorbed through the respiratory tract (approximately 80%), but poorly by the gastrointestinal (GI) tract (approximately 0.01%) and only to a restricted extent *via* the skin [53]. The amount of divalent mercury absorption by inhalation or dermal routes is undetermined, but oral absorption of inorganic mercuric salts may range from 2% to 38% depending upon the form and test circumstances. However, organic forms are easily absorbed by inhalation and through the GI tract. Once absorbed, elemental mercury is extensively delivered to fat-rich tissues. Organic forms are also extensively delivered, and they cross the blood-brain and placental barriers and accumulate in the brain and fetus respectively. However, due to the fact that inorganic forms present low lipophilicity, this limits their ability to penetrate the blood-brain and placental barriers [54]. Mercury may undergo metabolic interconversion. In this regard, elemental mercury may be oxidized to Hg^{2+} by catalase and hydrogen peroxide. Methylmercury (MeHg) is also transformed to inorganic mercury through the action of microbial flora and by formation of reactive oxygen species and by interactions with sulfhydryl groups [55].

All forms of mercury are poisonous. From all forms present in the environment, organic mercury is the most toxic for humans due to its lipophilicity and its accumulation in the body [56, 57]. MeHg is the most important organic form which affects people, mainly through the consumption of contaminated fish [58].

Organic and inorganic mercurial forms react with the sulfhydryl group of biological organisms and cause toxic effects on various functions [59]. In this regard, blockade of macromolecule synthesis (DNA, RNA, and protein), microtubule disruption, increase in intracellular Ca^{2+} with disturbance of neurotransmitter action, oxidative stress, and excitotoxicity, secondary to disturbed glutamate homeostasis and activation of N-methyl D-aspartate (NMDA) receptors have been observed [60].

There is some proof that thyroid gland may concentrate mercury under situations of prolonged exposure and that the thyroid enzyme systems may be disrupted [61]. The HPT axis is one of the zones where relevant accumulation of mercury occurs at concentrations that can reach the kidneys and liver. In this regard, it has been reported that retired mercury mine workers who were chronically exposed to mercury present 1,000 times higher concentrations in these endocrine organs than controls [62].

TH levels related enzyme activities have been reported to be changed in several fish and mammalian species after exposure to MeHg, $HgCl_2$, or Hg vapor. The patterns in plasma levels of TSH and protein-bound and free T3 and T4 present contradictions through literature, probably because of differences in strains, species, exposure times, doses and ages of the animals. Numerous studies described that plasma T3, T4, or both decreased following exposure to $HgCl_2$ and MeHg in fish, rats, mice and humans [63-71], and in fish exposed to Hg^0 in the field [72]. Several studies reported increased plasma T3 and T4 levels in numerous species, including fish, rats, and occupationally exposed humans [13, 72-74]. Other studies observed increases in the ratios of T4 and T3 or of other THs, such as rT3 in humans after occupational exposure to Hg vapor [13]. Nishida and coworkers [68] suggested that acute $HgCl_2$ exposure has more effect on hormonal levels than MeHg acute exposure, but after prolonged exposure MeHg presents higher effects than $HgCl_2$ long term exposure. TSH was also monitored in several studies that also produced contradictory results, which could reflect differences in mercury forms, dose and time of exposure and dosing regimen [75, 76].

Exposure to $HgCl_2$ and MeHg in fish and rats have been shown to induce hypertrophy of the thyroid epithelium or an increase in thyroid-gland weight, but MeHg was described to be more potent, inducing an alteration in the thyroid gland [75-78].

There is proof that mercury exposure result in a slight elevation in thyroid follicular-cell carcinomas in rats exposed to high concentrations of $HgCl_2$ [79], and humans with Minamata disease have been reported to have a substantial higher incidence of thyroid gland neoplasms than patients with other neurodegenerative diseases [80].

The mechanisms through which the different mercury species induce these alterations are not clear. In this regard, TPO activity was reported to be altered after mercury exposure. In rats, TPO was reported to be blocked by $HgCl_2$, but not by MeHg [76]. Nishida and coworkers [81], also described that, while $HgCl_2$ was the only mercurial species that blocked TPO-mediated oxidation of iodide, both $HgCl_2$ and MeHg-blocked the iodination of thyroglobulin. In an *ex vivo* study in mice, the authors showed that MeHg is present in the thyroid gland after oral administration, and that, therefore, the absence of susceptibility of TPO to MeHg is not due to its lack or degradation in the thyroid gland, but rather to an incapacity to block the enzyme [82].

Different studies have shown a reduction or a decreasing pattern in iodine uptake into the thyroid after organic and inorganic mercury exposure [65, 67, 68, 76], and it was suggested that this effect could be permanent [64]. The mechanism through which this effect occurred is unknown, but it was suggested that mercury forms could block iodide uptake at the NIS level by binding to it and creating a complex that can no longer pass through the NIS or by inhibition of Na^+K^+ ATPase and the Na^+ gradient needed for NIS function [65, 76].

Finally Se is an essential trace element which has been shown to protect against mercury toxicity [83]. Thus, Se deficiency may result in a higher sensitivity to mercury toxicity. Mercury has a high affinity for Se, and many of the enzymes in the thyroid are selenoproteins, which could explain why mercury is significantly accumulated in the thyroid gland [84]. In the thyroid system, the deiodinases are selenoenzymes that transform THs from one iodinated form to another, and may be targets for thyroid-system disturbances by Hg, as suggested by different studies [13] and demonstrated in pregnant dam mice exposed to MeHg [85].

The literature indicates that Hg has the capability of altering the thyroid system in multiple places as commented above, but further studies are needed for a complete understanding of mercury mechanisms that alter thyroid function.

ARSENIC

Arsenic is a potent carcinogen and one of the most toxic environmental contaminants [86-88]. Arsenic levels in the environment are increasing due to natural as well as anthropogenic actions [89]. Exposure to arsenic-contaminated water and food/feed leads to its accumulation in plants and/or animal tissues, affecting normal metabolism, particularly producing dysfunction of the liver and kidney in animals [90-92].

The intensity of arsenic toxicity depends upon many factors like its dose, valence state, and the compound of arsenic, as different arsenic compounds differ in their absorption and metabolism in the body [93, 94].

Organic compounds of arsenic are less toxic than their inorganic counterparts, mostly owing to their better absorption and difference in metabolism [94, 95]. The trivalent forms (As(III)) are more toxic than the pentavalent ones (As(V)).

Among the trivalent forms, arsenic trioxide and sodium arsenite are the most common arsenic compounds used in agriculture and many industrial formulations. As(III) is the principal form of arsenic interacting with sulfhydryl groups, producing blockade of many enzymes [96]. However, As(V) forms do not bind to the sulfhydryl group [97], but are decreased to the trivalent form during anaerobic conditions, and then could bind to sulfhydryl groups inside cells. Inorganic arsenic compounds are metabolized and transformed to monomethylarsonic acid (MMA(V)) and dimethylarsinic acid (DMA(V)) in numerous living system, including both aquatic organisms [98] and plants [99]. It is well known that methylated trivalent metabolites like monomethylarsonous acid (MMA(III)) and dimethylarsinic acid (DMA(III)) are highly reactive and responsible for arsenic intoxication. In this regard, DMA has been reported to act as a promoter of thyroid gland carcinogenesis, among other tissues in rats [100, 101].

Arsenic toxicity is imputed mainly to lipid peroxidation and oxidative stress [102]. Experimental data inferred that reactive oxygen species (ROS) are formed during arsenic metabolism [103]. Elevated ROS production has been involved in several pathologies and is considered to be crucial in inorganic arsenic induced genotoxicity and cytotoxicity [104, 105].

Trivalent and pentavalent forms of arsenic have been reported to be highly accumulated in the thyroid gland among other tissues after long term exposure [106]. Arsenic has been reported to disrupt the function of thyroid hormone nuclear receptors [107], reduce serum levels of TSH in rats [108], inhibit TPO activity *in vitro* [109], interfere with normal thyroid hormone metabolism reducing plasma levels of both T3 and T4 in guinea pigs and humans [110, 111], but induce an increase of total and free T3 levels and a decrease of hepatic 5′ deiodinase activity in rats [108], and induce goiter in humans [112].

How arsenic disrupts thyroid hormone metabolism remains unclear. Arsenic is an antagonist of selenium, and could inhibit DI1, and thus the transformation of T4 into T3, as was observed by Eybl and coworkers [108]. Moreover, arsenic can bind to protein sulfhydryl groups [113], and this could explain arsenic-induced TPO inhibition. In this regard, it has been shown that arsenic blocks TPO in a dose-dependent manner, and the minimal dose needed to inhibit this activity is between 0.1 and 1 ppm. This dose of arsenic trioxide is 100 times greater than the US Environmental Protection Agency settled maximum contaminant level of 10 ppm [109].

Otherwise, thyroid hormone/activity could influence arsenic concentration and toxicity in liver and kidney as was observed in rats [102]. THs were observed to reduce the accumulation of arsenic in these organs and decrease lipid peroxidation. Thus, hyperthyroid as well as hypothyroid conditions could restrict the accumulation of arsenic in liver and kidney.

LEAD

Lead is present in the environment both from natural sources and released by human activities. Exposure to lead and lead chemicals can take place through ingestion, inhalation or occasionally dermal contact. Occupational lead exposure remains the main source of human intoxication and occurs in lead related industries such as manufacturing industries, including mining, smelting, refining, battery manufacturing, soldering, electrical wiring and ceramic glazing [114].

In the general population, it occurs primarily through ingestion *via* lead-contaminated food or drinking water. Inhalation is the second most important pathway of exposure and may be the major contributor in occupationally lead-exposed workers. Almost all inhaled lead is absorbed into the organism, whereas 20% to 70% of ingested lead is absorbed. Workers may inhale lead dust and lead oxide fumes, as well as eat, drink, and smoke it in or near polluted areas, thereby rising their probability of lead poisoning [115].

When absorbed, lead concentrates in three compartments: blood, soft tissues and bone to exert its toxic effects. Lead toxicity is caused by its affinity to proteins and its ability to interfere with the metabolism of other biologically important metals, such as calcium, iron, and zinc, which act as cofactors in many enzymatic processes and disrupt oxidant/antioxidant balance [116]. Lead exposures also cause functional impairment of the HPT axis and disrupt thyroid hormone homeostasis [117, 118]. There is considerable evidence that lead could affect thyroid hormone homeostasis by interfering with the production, release, biological action and metabolism of THs [119].

The toxicity of lead is tightly related to age, gender, route of exposure, grade of intake, solubility, metal oxidation state, retention percentage, length of exposure, frequency of intake, absorption rate, mechanisms and efficacy of excretion. Lead can influence individuals of any age, but it has a more pronounces effect on children because their bodies absorb a larger percentage of the lead that they ingest and they exhibit lead toxicity at lower exposure levels than adults [120, 121].

Occupational exposure to inorganic lead has been associated with impaired uptake of iodine by the thyroid gland and alterations in morphology of the thyroid tissues [116, 118, 122, 123].

There are contradictory reports in the literature regarding to the effect of occupational lead exposure on thyroid functions. Diverse occupational studies have shown a pattern of low serum T4 levels in moderately to highly lead-exposed workers depending on time of exposure, suggesting that lead induces hypothyroidism [124-127]. Other studies have also related occupational lead exposure to a decrease in T3 serum levels [127]. In addition, several reports associated lead exposure with an increase of TSH [116, 128] with [127] or without [128] an effect on T4 and T3 hormones. The relevant of significant alterations in the levels of these hormones has also been reported in a few studies [117, 129-132]. The discrepancies observed in these studies could be due to the fact that results based on blood lead levels may be misleading because there are non-linear relationships between blood level and lead exposure, uptake and concentration in organs. Moreover, several factors such as gender, genetic background, nutritional status, lifestyle characteristics, diet and other environmental contaminants in the studied subjects could confuse the results. Table **1** summarizes the main epidemiology studies on lead thyroid toxicity.

Contradictory reports are also available in animals on THs levels after lead exposure. A number of studies have shown that lead administration in animals decreases serum T3 concentrations *via* reductions in hepatic DI1 [133]. Lead produces reactive oxygen species, leading to depletion of essential thiol (-SH) groups, which are involved in DI1 activity [134]. In this regard, Goldman and Dillon [135] reported that selenium supplementation of lead treated Pekin ducklings does protect against the toxic results of lead on thyroid function. Several studies also described that rat lead treatment caused a significant depression in T3 and T4 levels [118, 136]. In contrast, in cows the blood lead levels were positively correlated with T3 and T4 [137]. On the other hand, Vyskocil and coworkers [138], reported no effect on T3 and T4 in rats exposed to lead acetate.

Table 1. Epidemiological study results on effects of lead on thyroid hormones.

Study	Hormone	Age	Effect on thyroid function
Robins and coworkers. [121]	T4, T3, TSH	Adult	Reduced T4 levels without significant changes in T3 and TSH levels
Tuppurainen and coworkers [122]	T4, T3, TSH	Adult	Negative association between duration of lead exposure and both T4 and FT4
Siegel and coworkers [128]	T4	Children	No significant effect
Gustafson and coworkers. [115]	T4,T3, TSH	Adult	Higher T4 levels 10 subjects with higher levels of Pb (440 mg/dl) have significantly higher TSH levels
Schumacher and coworkers. [129]	T4, TSH	Adult	No significant effect with blood lead levels under 60 mg/dl
Lopez and coworkers [125]	T4, T3, TSH	Adult	Negative association between lead and both T4 and T3 in Pb levels greater than 50 mg/dl; positive association between lead and TSH in Pb levels lower than 50 mg/dl
Singh and coworkers [126]	T4, T3, TSH	Adult	Significantly lower T3 with the longer exposure time (17.5 years). High TSH levels which are independent of exposure time but associated with Pb levels.
Erfurth and coworkers [116]	T4, T3, TSH	Adult	No significant effect
Dundar and coworkers [124]	T4, T3, TSH	Adolescents	Reduced T4 levels without significant changes in T3 and TSH levels
Chistensen [70]	T4, T3, TSH	Adult	Decreased T4, without significant changes in T3 or TSH
Liang and coworkers[130]	T4, T3, TSH	Adult	Inhibiting deiodination of T4

Data from Duandar and coworkers [124] with modifications.

Further studies are required to clarify the contradictions observed in occupational and animal studies, and to confirm that inhibition of DI1 through a reduction of the enzyme thiol groups is among the mechanisms of action of lead, and to determine other possible mechanisms that produce this effects.

MANGANESE

Manganese is an essential trace metal in both humans and animals, which exists in a variety of oxidation states [139]. It is present in the environment as inorganic and organic species. The inorganic forms are used in the production of dry-cell batteries, in magnetic resonance imaging, glass, ceramics, dyes and pigments, and as animal feed supplements and fertilizers to alleviate nutrient deficiency. The organic forms are used as pesticides and as antiknock agents in gasoline [140].

Mn is involved in different actions such as metabolic pathways, bone mineralization, and in defense against oxidative stress as a component of the antioxidant enzymes. Mn is also a constituent of arginase and pyruvate carboxylase enzymes and acts as an activator of other enzymes [141]. Mn is not accumulated in the body and it is eliminated in a few days after exposure [142]. For the general population, the majority of Mn is obtained from the diet since Mn occurs naturally in almost all foodstuffs [143, 144].

Mn toxicity is mainly from high levels of occupational exposure [145-147]. In this regard, Mn exposure induces pulmonary toxicity in animals and humans after inhalation of particulate manganese compounds [148]. Exposure to high levels of manganese throughout fetal development can lead neurocognitive deficits, while in adults, manganese concentration in the basal ganglia can result reduced dopamine levels and cell death in a syndrome known manganism, which shares multiple characteristics with Parkinson's disease [149].

Not much is known about the interrelationships between manganese and thyroid hormones. In this regard, a substantial correlation was observed between manganese concentrations and circulating T4 concentrations [150]. Moreover, Buthieau and Autissier [151] reported that rats exposed to manganese (10 mg/kg/day as manganese sulfate [MnSO4]) for five weeks, presented high concentration of manganese in the pituitary gland, which led to a significant decrease in serum T4, T3 and in TSH concentrations. Kawada and coworkers [152] described that mice treated with excessive amount of manganese presented reduced serum levels of T4, but not T3 after seven weeks and thyroid morphology showed retention of colloid in the lumen. In an epidemiological study on welders exposed to manganese, an increase of manganese and a decrease of thyrotropin-releasing hormone (TRH) and dopamine serum levels with respect to the control group was observed [153]. The apparent contradictory results between these studies could be related to the differences between species, doses, exposure period and vehicle among other factors.

The mechanisms through which Mn could induce these alterations are not completely understood. In this regard, Buthieau and Autissier [151] suggested that Mn may interfere with thyroid hormone binding, transport, and activity at the tissue level. Soldin and Aschner [149], reported that manganese may affect thyroid hormone homeostasis because of both direct dysregulation at the level of the thyroid gland and THs, or indirectly *via* changes in dopaminergic regulation of the thyroid gland and its hormones.

Assem and coworkers [140], studied the carcinogenic effect of inorganic manganese in rats and mouse. Their results do not provide any clear evidence of carcinogenic effect on the thyroid gland (quantitative elevation in incidence of thyroid tumors in mice but not rats). Hence, they established that there is insufficient data to indicate that inorganic Mn exposure produces cancer in animals or humans.

Taken together, further studies are needed to clarify the effects of manganese on the thyroid system for correct hazard identification of this metal and the mechanisms through which it acts.

CHROMIUM

Chromium is a persistent metal which is widely present in the environment [154-156]. The three most stable forms in which chromium appear in the environment are the 0, 3^+, and 6^+ valence states. Trivalent chromium (Cr(III)) is considered an essential element both in animal feeding and human nutrition due to its influence on carbohydrate, lipid and protein metabolism through its insulin action [157]. Otherwise, hexavalent chromium (Cr(VI)), which is used in welding, plating, and chemical industries, is highly toxic and a strong oxidizing agent [158]. Most of the Cr(VI) absorbed is reduced to Cr(III) and excreted through urine in a week, but a fraction of Cr(VI) is able to cross cell membranes and can remain in the cells, tissues and organs for years, inducing its toxics effects [158].

The main transmission and exposure route for the general population is through intake of food and water with high chromium concentrations, either as Cr(III) or Cr(VI). However, another important route of transmission is by inhalation of air contaminated with chromium particles, especially in metallurgical workers and tanning industries [159].

Chromium may induce both acute and chronic toxicity. Cr(VI) has been reported to produce neurological, hepatic, renal, gastrointestinal, hematological, cardiovascular reproductive, respiratory and thyroidal toxic effects [160-164]. Moreover, several studies have associated Cr(VI) with development of pulmonary and nasal tumors [165].

The molecular mechanisms by which Cr(VI) exerts toxic effects are hypothesized to be related to its reduction to Cr(III) in cells. Throughout this process, toxic reactive chromium intermediates Cr(V) and Cr(IV), and different reactive oxygen species (ROS) are produced. In this regard, ROS as well as the Cr intermediates could directly bind to cellular constituents thereby altering them, which could explain the cytotoxicity of this metal [158, 166, 167].

Several studies have described chromium toxic effects on the thyroid gland. In this regard, Quinteros and coworkers [168] performed a study to investigate Cr(VI) (500 ppm) on the anterior pituitary gland *in vivo* (rats) and *in vitro*. Cr(VI) showed a marked elevation (4.8 fold) of Cr levels in pituitary. Cr levels in hypothalamus also increased (1.6 fold). These authors suggested that chromium accumulation in the HPT axis may have a negative effect on normal endocrine function. Mahmood and coworkers [169], studied the effect of acute Cr(VI) (30 mg/kg bw potassium dichromate) exposure on thyroid structure and function in rats. Their results showed that chromium induced thyroid hyperplasia. Follicles were disordered clustered and crumbled, while some of them were fused. Interfollicular spaces were expander. The number of follicles was increased whereas the follicular size was substantially reduced. The membrane on the apical as well as the basal lamina side was altered. Colloid retraction within the follicles was remarkable. Serum free T4 and T3 levels were decreased, while serum TSH concentration was increased. Qureshi and Mahmood [170] examined the role of ascorbic acid (120 µg/kg bw) against acute Cr(VI) (60 µg/kg bw potassium dichromate) induced damage in rat thyroid gland. Results showed that Cr(VI) induced a substantial TSH increase and a significant reduction in free T3 and T4 concentrations, but ascorbic acid reversed these alterations almost to control levels. Moreover, ascorbic acid protected against histological effects except for the follicular size that was decreased. Thus, this study suggested that Cr(VI) toxicity on the thyroid system could be produced by induction of oxidative stress, and the use of antioxidants such as ascorbic acid may have the potential to protect the thyroid gland against chromium toxicity.

Recently, Hassanin and coworkers [171] studied the effect of Cr(VI) (60 μg/kg bw) on thyroid hormones and the protective effect of Se in rats. The results showed that Cr(VI) induced hypofunction of thyroid gland and thyroid tissue damage as a result of inducing marked oxidative insult and release of reactive oxygen species. Moreover, a substantial reduction in free T3 and T4 and GSH levels was observed, which was accompanied by significant elevation in catalase, superoxide dismutase (SOD), and malondialdehyde (MDA) in the chromium-treated group compared to the control group. Se nanoparticles had a protective action on Cr(VI) induced thyroid insult as a result of the correction of the free T3 and T4 levels and reduced glutathione (GSH), catalase, SOD, and MDA compared to the Cr treated group. Histopathological studies showed alterations in the thyroid gland represented by follicular hyperplasia with large interfollicular spaces, desquamated follicles, and congested interfollicular blood vessels.

According to this data, the mechanisms through which chromium induces toxicity on the thyroid gland are mediated by increasing cellular oxidative stress and decreasing the activity of antioxidants. However, further studies are needed to confirm these data and determine the complete mechanisms that induce these effects.

MISCELLANEOUS

Besides the metals commented above, other metals have been related to thyroid disruption, but very little is known about their effects on the thyroid system. In this regard molybdenum, copper, cobalt, lithium, zinc, nickel and thallium have all been described to have certain effects on thyroid system.

Molybdenum has been reported to inhibit secretion of THs and reduce plasma T4, inducing hypothyroidism [172]. Moreover, molybdenum has been described to interact with thyroid hormone receptors, reducing T3 binding to its nuclear receptors in a 40%, but it did not show effect on T4 binding to nuclear receptors [173].

Copper is an indispensable element for humans and animals, particularly in the metabolism of the amino acid tyrosine, which is necessary for the synthesis of THs [174].Therefore, adequate levels of Cu are necessary to prevent thyroid pathologies and it can be used in the treatment of thyroid disease. Excess Cu concentration could induce hypothyroidism, goiter and other thyroid pathologies including thyroid cancer [175, 176]. Cu has been reported to present a negative effect on Fe and iodine (I) absorption and the increase of Cu in serum and urine could reduce Fe and I, which may be implicated in disturbances of thyroid metabolism [177].

Cobalt has been related to the induction of depression in iodine uptake, resulting in goiter and classic signs of hypothyroidism in patients who received 0.17–3.9 mg/kg bw/day cobalt for 6 days to 8 months showing a 20 – 90% reduction [178]. However, recently Lantina and coworkers [179] reported in an epidemiologic study that no adverse effect was observed on thyroid function after exposure to cobalt compounds in industry workers.

Lithium, a drug used for the treatment of mood disorders, has been described to induce hypothyroidism in patients treated with it [180].

Zinc has been reported to probably play a role in T3 binding to nuclear receptors as well as having a putative role in their binding to DNA [181]. A substantial reduction in the levels of serum T3 and no change in the levels of serum T4 and TSH in rats exposed to zinc have been described. The decrease in serum T3 levels may be related with disturbed thyroid conversion of T4 to T3 [182, 183]. Zinc deficiency has also been related to thyroid disease development [184].

Nickel was described to produce a decrease in T3 and T4 levels in rats, but TSH concentration was not affected. Moreover, histological alterations were also observed [185].

Finally, an epidemiological study undertaken in 2007-2008 associated elevated urinary levels of thallium and barium with a decrease in T4 (both) and T3 (barium). Moreover, cesium was associated with a decrease in TSH levels, and tungsten with an increase in their levels [71].

CONCLUDING REMARKS

Many metals have been reported to disrupt thyroid system homeostasis directly or indirectly through their deficiency, and thus, potentially impairing physiology and developmental processes. In this regard, exposure to some metals, especially during development, has been related to cognitive deficits in humans which could be induced by disruption of TH signaling. There are contradictory data on the effects of the metals on THs, which should be clarified to determine the exact effect of these metals in order to determine the risk that exposure poses to human health. Moreover, the mechanisms through which metals induce thyroid disruption are not clear, so further studies are required to elucidate them and perform an exhaustive risk assessment of these metals. It is also decisive to keep in mind that humans are constantly exposed to a numerous of pollutants, including metals, which can act together and lead to effects that are different from those of the single pollutants. A better understanding of these issues may result in changes in public policy and awareness, and make it possible to limit adverse outcomes for future generations.

CONFLICT OF INTEREST

The author confirms that author has no conflict of interest to declare for this publication.

ACKNOWLEDGEMENTS

Declared None.

REFERENCES

[1] Bekheet SH. Comparative effects of repeated administration of cadmium chloride during pregnancy and lactation and selenium protection against cadmium toxicity on some organs in immature rats' offsprings. Biol Trace Elem Res 2011; 144 (1-3): 1008-1023.

[2] Rinal PS, Meenu BN, Viral DT, Tushar DR, Pravin TR. Screening of herbal drugs for heavy metal toxicity with specific reference to arsenic and lead with its therapeutic significance. Int Bull Drug Res 2012; 1(2): 10-23.

[3] Jancic SA, Stosic BZ. Cadmium effects on the thyroid gland. Vitam Horm 2014; 94: 391-425.

[4] Singh B, Chandran V, Bandhu HK, *et al.* Impact of lead exposure on pituitarythyroid axis in humans. Biometals 2000; 13: 187-192.

[5] Mahmood T, Qureshi IZ, Iqbal MJ. Histopathological and biochemical changes in rat thyroid following acute exposure to hexavalent chromium. Histol Histopathol 2010; 25: 1355-1370.

[6] Allen T, Rana SVS. Effect of n-propylthiouracil or thyroxine on arsenic trioxide toxicity in the liver of rat. J Trace Elem Med Biol 2007; 21: 194-203.

[7] Sin YM, Teh WF. Effect of long term uptake of mercuric sulphide on thyroid hormones and glutathione in mice. Bull Environ Contam Toxicol 1992; 49: 847-854.

[8] Zhang L, Wang J, Zhu GN, Su L. Pubertal exposure to thiodiazole copper inhibits thyroid function in juvenile female rats. Exp Toxicol Pathol 2010; 62: 163-169.

[9] Hammouda F, Messaoudi I, El Hani J, Baati T, Khaled Saïd K, Kerkeni A. Reversal of cadmium-induced thyroid dysfunction by selenium, zinc, or their combination in rat. Biol Trace Elem Res 2008; 126: 194-203.

[10] Dabbaghmanesh M-H, Abdolsamad Sadegholvaad A, Ejtehadi F, Ranjbar-Omrani G. The role of iron deficiency in persistent goiter**.** Arch Iranian Med 2008; 11 (2): 157 - 161.

[11] Cormack DH. Endocrine and reproductive systems. In: Clinically integrated histology. Philadelphia, Lippincott-Raven Press, 1998; pp. 219-275.

[12] Kelly GS. Peripheral metabolism of thyroid hormones: a review. Altern Med Rev 2000; 5(4): 306-333.

[13] Ellingsen DG, Efskind J, Haug E, Thomassen Y, Martinsen I, Gaarder PI. Effects of low mercury vapour exposure on the thyroid function in chloralkali workers. J Appl Toxicol 2000; 20: 483-489.

[14] Rana SVS. Perspectives in Endocrine Toxicity of Heavy Metals—A Review. Biol Trace Elem Res 2014; 160: 1-14.

[15] Agency for Toxic Substances and Disease Registry (ATSDR). Toxicological Profile for Cadmium. Atlanta: U.S. Department of Health and Human Services 2012. Available from: http://www.atsdr.cdc.gov/toxprofiles/tp5.pdf

[16] International Programme on Chemical Safety (IPCS). Environmental Health Criteria 134. Cadmium. Geneva, Switzerland: WHO, 1992.

[17] Jin T, Lu J, Nordberg M. Toxicokinetics and biochemistry of cadmium with special emphasis on the role of metallothionein. Neurotoxicology 1998;19(4-5): 529-535.

[18] Hogervorst J, Plusquin M, Vangronsveld J, *et al.* House dust as possible route of environmental exposure to cadmium and lead in the adult general population. Environ Res 2007; 103(1): 30-37.

[19] International Agency for Research on Cancer (IARC). Cadmium and cadmium compounds. Monographs on the evaluation of carcinogenic risks to humans. Vol. 100C. Lyon, France: IARC Scientific Publications, 2012; pp. 121-145.

[20] Jahan S, Zahra A, Irum U, Iftikhar N, Ullah H. Protective effects of different antioxidants against cadmium induced oxidative damage in rat testis and prostate tissues.Syst Biol Reprod Med 2014; 60(4): 199-205.

[21] Mendez-Armenta M, Rios C. Cadmium neurotoxicity. Environ Toxicol and Pharmacol 2007; 23(3): 350-358.

[22] Yoshizuka M, Mori N, Hamasaki K, Tanaka I, Yokoyama M, Hara K. Cadmium toxicity in the thyroid gland of pregnant rats. Exp Mol Pathol 1991; 55: 97-104.

[23] Vahter M, Akesson A, Liden C, Ceccatelli S, Berglund M. Gender differences in the disposition and toxicity of metals. Environ Res 2007; 104(1): 85-95.

[24] Andersson H, Petersson-Grawé K, Lindqvist EL, Luthman J, Oskarsson A, Olson L. Low-level cadmium exposure of lactating rats causes alterations in brain serotonin levels in the Offspring. Neurotoxicol Teratol 1997; 19(2): 105-115.

[25] Shukla GS, Hussain T, Chandra SV. Possible role of regional superoxide dismutase activity and lipid peroxide levels in cadmium neurotoxicity: *in vivo* and *in vitro* studies in growing rats. Life Sci 1987; 41(19): 2215-2221.

[26] Shukla GS, Hussain T, Srivastava RS, Chandra SV. Glutathione peroxidase and catalase in liver, kidney, testis and brain regions of rats following cadmium exposure and subsequent withdrawal. Ind Health 1989; 27(2): 59-69.

[27] Figueiredo-Pereira ME, Yakushin S, Cohen G. Disruption of the intracellular sulfhydryl homeostasis by cadmium-induced oxidative stress leads to protein thiolation and ubiquitination in neuronal cells. J Biol Chem 1998; 273: 12703-12709.

[28] Rajanna B, Hobson M, Boykin M, Chetty CS. Effects of chronic treatment with cadmium on ATPases, uptake of catecholamines, and lipid peroxidation in rat brain synaptosomes. Ecotoxicol Environ Saf 1990; 20: 36-41.

[29] Yuan Y, Jiang CY, Xu H, *et al.* Cadmium-induced apoptosis in primary rat cerebral cortical neurons culture is mediated by a calcium signaling pathway. PLoS One 2013; 8(5): e64330.

[30] Huff J, Lunn RM, Waalkes MP, Tomatis L, Infante PF. Cadmium induced cancers in animals and in humans. Int J Occup Environ Health 2007; 13: 202-212.

[31] National Toxicology Program (NTP). 12th Report on carcinogens. Research Triangle Park, NC: National Institution of Environmental Health Sciences, U.S. Department of Health and Human Services, Public Health Service 2011; pp: 80-82.

[32] Tiran B, Karpf E, Tiran A. Age dependency of selenium and cadmium content in human liver, kidney, and thyroid. Arch Environ Health 1995; 50(3): 242-246.

[33] Pilat-Marcinkiewicz B, Brzoska MM, Sawicki B, Moniuszko-Jakoniuk J. Structure and function of thyroid follicular cells in female rats chronically exposed to cadmium. Bull Vet Inst Pulawy 2003; 47: 157-163.

[34] Pilat-Marcinkiewicz B, Sawicki B, Brzoska MM, Jakoniuk JM. Effect of chronic administration of cadmium on the rat thyroid: Radioimmunological and immunohistochemical studies. Folia Histochem Cytobiol 2002; 40: 189-190.

[35] Luo J, Hendryx M. Relationship between blood cadmium, lead, and serum thyroid measures in US adults - the National Health and Nutrition Examination Survey (NHANES) 2007-2010. Int J Environ Health Res 2014; 24(2): 125-136.

[36] Jadhao AG, Paul PL, Rao PD. Effect of cadmium chloride on the pituitary, thyroid and gonads in the catfish, Clarias batrachus (Linn.). Funct Dev Morphol 1994; 4(1): 39-44.
[37] Iijima K, Otake T, Yoshinaga J, *et al.* Cadmium, lead, and selenium in cord blood and thyroid hormone status of newborns. Biol Trace Elem Res 2007; 119: 10-18.
[38] Badiei K, Nikghadam P, Mostaghni K. Effect of cadmium on thyroid function in sheep. Comp Clinical Pathol 2009; 18: 255-259.
[39] Ghosh N, Bhattachary AS. Thyrotoxicity of the chlorides of cadmium and Mercury in rabbit. Biomed Environ Sci 1992; 5: 236A-240A.
[40] Hontela A, Daniel C, Ricard AC. Effects of acute and subacute exposures to cadmium on the interrenal and thyroid function in rainbow trout, Oncorhynchus mykiss. Aquat Toxicol 1996; 35: 171-182.
[41] Gupta P, Kar A. Cadmium induced thyroid dysfunction in chicken: Hepatic type I iodothyronine 5′-monodeiodinase activity and role of lipid peroxidation. Comp Biochem Physiol 1999; 123: 39-44.
[42] Nishijo M, Nakagawa H, Morikawa Y, *et al.* A study of thyroid hormone levels of inhabitants of the cadmium-polluted Kakehashi River basin. Nippon Eiseigaku Zasshi 1994; 49: 598-605.
[43] Pillai A, Priya L, Gupta S. Effects of combined exposure to lead and cadmium on the hypothalamic-pituitary axis function in proestrous rats. Food Chem Toxicol 2003; 41: 379-384.
[44] Paier B, Hagmuller K, Noli MI, Gonzalez PM, Stiegler C, Zaninovich AA. Changes induced by cadmium administration on thyroxine deiodination and sulfhydryl groups in rat liver. J Endocrinol 1993; 138: 219-224.
[45] Pavia MA, Paier B, Noli MI, Hagmuller K, Zaninovich AA. Evidence suggesting that cadmium induces a nonthyroidal illness syndrome in the rat. J Endocrinol 1997; 154: 113-117.
[46] Vallee BL, Ullmer DD. Biochemical effects of mercury, cadmium and lead. Annu Rev Biochem 1972; 41: 91-128.
[47] Chopra IJ. Sulfhydryl groups and the monodeiodination of thyroxine to triiodothyronine. Science 1978; 199: 904-906.
[48] International Council for Control of Iodine Deficiency Disorders (ICCIDD), United Nations Children's Fund (UNICEF) and WHO (World Health Organization). Assessment of iodine deficiency disorders and monitoring their elimination (2nd ed.). Geneva, Switzerland: WHO Publication 2001.
[49] Clarkson TW. The toxicology of mercury. Crit Rev Clin Lab Sci 1997; 34: 369-403.
[50] Goldman LR, Shannon MW. The Committee on Environmental Health. Technical Report: mercury in the environment: implications for pediatricians. Pediatrics 2001; 108: 197-205.
[51] Holmes P, James KA, Levy LS. Is low-level environmental mercury exposure of concern to human health? Sci. Total Environ 2009; 408:171-182.
[52] Tan SW, Meillerb JC, Mahaffeyb KR. The endocrine effects of mercury in humans and wildlife. Crit Rev Toxicol 2009; 39(3): 228-269.
[53] Health Protection Scotland (HPS). Elemental mercury Guidance Note 2. Edinburg Scodland: HPS Publications 2007. Available from: http://www.documents.hps.scot.nhs.uk/environmental/guidance-notes/elemental-mercury.pdf
[54] Agency for Toxic Substances and Disease Registry (ATSDR). Toxicological profile for mercury. Atlanta: U.S. Department of Health and Human Services 1999. Available from: http://www.atsdr.cdc.gov/toxprofiles/tp46.pdf
[55] Yasutake A, Nakano A, Miyamoto K, Eto K. Chronic effects of methylmercury in rats. I. Biochemical aspects. Tohoku J Exp Med 1997; 182: 185-196.
[56] World Health Organization (WHO). Methylmercury. Environmental health criteria (ECH) 101. Geneva, Switzerland: WHO 1990.
[57] World Health Organization (WHO). Inorganic mercury. Environmental health criteria (ECH) 118. Geneva, Switzerland: WHO 1991.
[58] Galal-Gorchev H. Dietary intake, levels in food and estimated intake of lead, cadmium, and mercury. Food Addit Contam 1993; 10: 115-128.
[59] Vallee BL, Ulmer DD. Biochemical effects of mercury, cadmium and lead. Ann. Rev. Biochem 1972; 41: 91-128.
[60] Soldin OP, O'Mara DM, Aschner M. Thyroid hormones and methylmercury toxicity. Biol Trace Elem Res 2008; 126 (1-3): 1-12.

[61] Barregård L, Lindstedt G, Schütz A, Sällsten G. Endocrine function in mercury exponed chloralkali workers. Occup Environ Med 1994; 51: 536-540.
[62] Kosta L, Byrne AR, Zelenko V. Correlation between selenium and mercury in man following exposure to inorganic mercury. Nature 1975; 254 (5497): 238-239.
[63] Bhattacharya T, Bhattacharya S, Ray AK, Dey S. Influence of industrial pollutants on thyroid function in Channa puntatus (Bloch). Indian J Exp Biol 1989; 27: 65-68.
[64] Goldman M, Blackburn P. The effect of mercuric chloride and thyroid function in the rat. Toxicol Appl Pharamacol 1979; 48: 49-55.
[65] Kawada J, Nishida M, Yoshimura Y, Mitani K. Effects of organic and inorganic mercurials on thyroidal functions. J Pharmacobiodyn 1980; 3(3): 149-159.
[66] Kirubagaran R, Joy KP. Changes in brain monoamine levels and monoamine oxidase activity in the catfish, Clarias batrachus, during chronic treatments with mercurials. Bull Environ Contamin Toxicol 1990; 45: 88-91.
[67] Mochizuki Y, Asahara H. Effect of mercuric chloride on the thyroid function in rats. Kawasaki Med J 1978; 4(2): 113-119.
[68] Nishida M, Yamamoto T, Yoshimura Y, Kawada J. Subacute toxicity of methylmercuric chloride and mercuric chloride on mouse thyroid. J Pharmacobiodyn 1986; 9(4): 331-338.
[69] Sin YM, Teh WF, Wong MK, Reddy PK. Effect of mercury on glutathione and thyroid hormones. Bull Environ Contam Toxicol 1990; 44(4): 616-622.
[70] SinYM, Teh WF. Effect of long-term uptake of mercuric sulphide on thyroid hormones and glutathione in mice. Bull Environ Contam Toxicol 1992; 49(6): 847-854.
[71] Christensen KLY. Metals in blood and urine, and thyroid function among adults in the United States 2007-2008. Int J Hyg Environ Health 2013; 216: 624- 632.
[72] Hontela A, Dumont P, Duclos D, Fortin R. Endocrine and metabolic dysfunction in yellow perch, Perca flavescens, exposed to organic contaminants and heavy metals in the St. Lawrence River. Environ Toxicol Chem 1995; 14(4): 725-731.
[73] Bleau H, Daniel C, Chevalier G, Van Tra H, Hontela A. Effects of acute exposure to mercury chloride and methylmercury on plasma cortisol, T3, T4, glucose and liver glycogen in rainbow trout (Oncorhynchus mykiss). Aquat Toxicol 1996; 34: 221-235.
[74] Kabuto M. Chronic effects of methylmercury on the urinary excretion of catecholamines and their responses to hypoglycemic stress. Arch Toxicol 1991; 65(2): 164-167.
[75] Kabuto M. Acute endocrine effects of a single administration of methylmercury chloride (MMC) in rats. Endocrinol Jpn 1986; 33(5): 683-690.
[76] Nishida M, Muraoka K, Nishikawa K, Takagi T, Kawada J. Differential effects of methylmercuric chloride and mercuric chloride on the histochemistry of rat thyroid peroxidase and the thyroid peroxidase activity of isolated pig thyroid cells. J Histochem Cytochem 1989; 37(5): 723-727.
[77] Kirubagaran R, Joy KP. Toxic effects of mercurials on thyroid function of the catfish, Clarias batrachus (L.). Ecotoxicol Environ Saf 1989; 17(3): 265-271.
[78] Ram RN, Sathyanesan AG. Effect of mercuric chloride on thyroid function in the teleost fish Channa punctatus (Bloch). Matsya 1984; 9-10: 194-196.
[79] National Toxicology Program (NTP). Toxicology and carcinogenesis studies of mercuric chloride (CAS no. 7487-94-7) in F344/N rats and B6C3F1 mice (gavage studies). Technical Report Series No. 408. Atlanta: U.S. Department of Health and Human Services, Public Health Service, National Institutes of Health, Research Triangle Park, NC 1993.
[80] Eto K, Tokunaga Y, Nagashima K, Takeuchi T. An autopsy case of Minamata disease (Methylmercury poisoning)-Pathological viewpoints of peripheral nerves. Toxicol Pathol. 2002; 30(6): 714-722.
[81] Nishida M, Sato K, Kawada J. Differential effects of methylmercuric chloride and mercuric chloride on oxidation and iodination reactions catalyzed by thyroid peroxidase. Biochem Int 1990a; 22 (2): 369-378.
[82] Nishida M, Matsumoto H, Asano A, Umazume K, Yoshimura Y, Kawada J. Direct evidence for the presence of methylmercury bound in the thyroid and other organs obtained from mice given methylmercury; differentiation of free and bound methylmercuries in biological materials determined by volatility of methylmercury. Chem Pharm Bull (Tokyo) 1990b; 38(5): 1412-1413.

[83] Nishikido N, Furuyashiki K, Naganuma A, Suzuki T, Imura N. Maternal selenium deficiency enhances the fetolethal toxicity of methyl mercury. Toxicol Appl Pharmacol 1987; 88(3): 322-328.

[84] Falnoga I, Tusek-Znidaric M, Horvat M, Stegnar P. Mercury, selenium, and cadmium in human autopsy samples from Idrija residents and mercury mine workers. Environ Res 2000; 84(3): 211-218.

[85] Watanabe C, Yoshida K, Kasanuma Y, Kun Y, Satoh H. *In utero* methylmercury exposure differentially affects the activities of selenoenzymes in the fetal mouse brain. Environ Res 1999; 80(3): 208-214.

[86] Bundschuh J, Litter MI, Parvez F, *et al.* One century of arsenic exposure in Latin America: a review of history and occurrence from 14 countries. Sci Total Environ 2012; 429: 2-35.

[87] International Agency for Research on Cancer (IARC). Arsenic in drinking water, vol. 84. Lyon, France: IARC Scientific Publications 2004; Available from: http:// monographs.iarc.fr/ENG/Monographs/vol84/mono84-6.pdf

[88] Agency for Toxic Substances and Disease Registry (ATSDR).Toxicological profile for arsenic. Draft for Public Comment. Atlanta: US Department of Health and Human Services 2007. Available at URL: http://www.atsdr.cdc.gov/toxprofiles/tp2.html.

[89] Sharma AK, Tjell JC, Sloth JJ, Holm PE. Review of arsenic contamination, exposure through water and food and low cost mitigation options for rural areas. Appl Geochem 2014; 41: 11-33.

[90] Bergqvist C, Greger. Arsenic accumulation and speciation in plants from different habitats. Appl Geochem 2012; 27: 615-622.

[91] Naujokas MF, Anderson B, Ahsan H, *et al.* The broad scope of health effects from chronic arsenic exposure: update on a worldwide public health problem. Environ Health Perspect 2013; 121: 295-302.

[92] Ghosh A, Majumder S, Awal MA, Rao DR. Arsenic exposure to dairy cows in Bangladesh. Arch Environ Contam Toxicol 2013; 64: 151-159.

[93] Mohanta RK, Garg AK, Sahoo B. Status of arsenic in certain feeds, water and animals in Bareilly and Mukteswar region. Indian J Anim Nutr 2013; 30: 428-430.

[94] Goyer RA, Clarkson TW. Toxic effects of metals. In: Casarett LJ, Klaassen CD, and Doull J. Eds. Toxicology: the basic science of poisons, 7th edn. McGraw Hill, USA 2008; pp: 931-980.

[95] Watanabe T, Hirano S. Metabolism of arsenic and its toxicological relevance. Arch Toxicol 2013; 87: 969-979.

[96] Lin S, Cullen WR, Thomas DJ. Methylarsenicals and arsinothiols are potent inhibitors of mouse liver thioredoxin reductase. Chem Res Toxicol 1999; 12: 924-930.

[97] Mizumura A, Watanabe T, Kobayashi Y, Hirano S. Identification of arsenite-and arsenic diglutathione-binding proteins in human hepatocarcinoma cells. Toxicol Appl Pharmacol 2010; 242 (2): 119-125.

[98] Phillips DJH. Arsenic in aquatic organisms—a review, emphasizing chemical speciation. Aquat Toxicol 1990; 16(3): 151-186.

[99] Dhankher OP. Arsenic metabolism in plants: an inside story. New Phytol 2005; 168(3): 503-505.

[100] Marshall G, Ferreccio C, Yuan Y, *et al.* Fifty-year study of lung and bladder cancer mortality in Chile related to arsenic in drinking water. J Natl Cancer Inst 2007; 99(12): 920-928.

[101] Wei M, Wanibuchi H, Yamamoto S, Li W, Fukushima S. Urinary bladder carcinogenicity of dimethylarsinic acid in male F344 rats. Carcinogenesis 1999; 20(9): 1873-1876.

[102] Allen T, Rana SVS. Oxidative stress by inorganic arsenic: modulation by thyroid hormones in rat. Comp Biochem Physiol C Toxicol Pharmacol 2003; 135(2): 157-162.

[103] Ito H, Okamoto K, Kato K. Enhancement of expression of stress proteins by agents that lower the levels of glutathione in cells. Biochim Biophys Acta 1998; 1397: 223-230.

[104] Liu J, Chen H, Miller DS, *et al.* Overexpression of glutathione S-transferase II and multidrug resistance transport proteins is associated with acquired tolerance to inorganic arsenic. Mol Pharmacol 2001a; 60(2): 302-309.

[105] Liu J, Kadiiska MB, Liu Y, Lu T, Qu W, Waalkes MP. Stress related gene expression in mice treated with inorganic arsenicals. Toxicol Sci 2001; 61(2): 314-320.

[106] Kotyzova D, Eybl V, Mihaljevic M, Glattre. Effect of long-term administration of arsenic (III) and bromine with and without selenium and iodine supplementation on the element level in the thyroid of rat. Biomed Pap Med Fac Univ Palaky Olomouc Czech Repub 2005; 149: 329-333.

[107] Takagi S, Hummel BC, Walfish. Thioamides and arsenite inhibit specific T3 binding to the hepatic nuclear receptor. Biochem Cell Biol 1990; 68: 616-621.
[108] Eybl V, Topolcan O, Brtko J, Caisova D, Kotyzova D, Koutensky J. The influence of long-term administration of arsenic (III), lead, and mercury on the activity of selenoenzymes and thyroid function. Biomarkers Environ 1997; 1.
[109] Palazzolo DL, Jansen KP. The minimal arsenic concentration required to inhibit the activity of thyroid peroxidase *in vitro*. Biol Trace Elem Res 2008; 126(1-3): 49-55.
[110] Meltzer HM, Maage A, Ydersbond TA, Haug E, Glattre E, Holm H. Fish arsenic may influence human blood arsenic, selenium, and T4:T3 ratio. Biol Trace Elem Res 2002; 90: 83-98.
[111] Mohanta RK, Garg AK, Dass RS, Behera SK. Blood Biochemistry, thyroid hormones, and oxidant/antioxidant status of guinea pigs challenged with sodium arsenite or arsenic trioxide. Biol Trace Elem Res 2014; 160: 238-244.
[112] Chang TC, Hong MC, Chen CJ. Higher prevalence of goiter in endemic area of blackfoot disease of Taiwan. J Formos Med Assoc 1991; 90: 941-946.
[113] Aposhian HV. Biochemical toxicology of arsenic. Rev Biochem Toxicol 1989; 10: 265-299.
[114] Veerula GR, Noah PK Clinical manifestations of childhood lead poisoning. J Trop Med Hyg. 1990; 93(3): 170-177.
[115] Doumouchtsis KK, Doumouchtsis SK, Doumouchtsis EK, Perrea DN. The effect of lead intoxication on endocrine functions. J Endocrinol Invest. 2009; 32(2): 175-83.
[116] Gustafson A, Hedner P, Schutz A, Skerfving S. Occupational lead exposure and pituitary function. Int Arch Occup Environ Health 1989; 61: 277-281.
[117] Erfurth EM, Gerhardsson L, Nilsson A, *et al*. Effects of lead on the endocrine system in lead smelter workers. Arch Environ Health 2001; 56: 449-455.
[118] Singh B, Dhawan D. Effect of lithium on thyroidal 131 iodine uptake, its clearance, and circulating levels of triiodothyronine and thyroxine in lead-treated rats. Radiat Environ Biophys 1999; 38: 261-266.
[119] Zacharewski T. Identification and assessment of endocrine disruptors: limitations of *in vivo* and *in vitro* assays. Environ Health Perspect 1998, 106: (Suppl 2): 577-582.
[120] Baht RV, Moy GG. Monitoring and assessment of dietary exposure to chemical contaminants. Geneva: WHO 1997; pp. 132-149.
[121] Abou MA. Lead Concentrations in Different Animals Muscles and Consumable Organs at Specific Localities in Cairo. Global Veterinaria 2008; 2(5): 280-284.
[122] Lasisz B, Zdrojewicz Z, Marcinkowski Z. Effect of lead on thyroid function. Wiad Lek 1992; 45: 116-119.
[123] Robins JM, Cullen MR, Connors BB, Kayne RD. Depressed thyroid indexes associated with occupational exposure to inorganic lead. Arch Intern Med 1983; 143: 220-224.
[124] Tuppurainen M, Wagar G, Kurppa K, *et al*. Thyroid function as assessed by routine laboratory tests of workers with long-term lead exposure. Scand J Work Environ Health 1988; 14: 175-180.
[125] Pearce EN, Braverman LE. Environmental pollutants and the thyroid. Best Pract Res Clin Endocrinol Metab. 2009; 23(6): 801-813.
[126] Dundar B, Oktem F, Arslan MK. The effect of long-term low dose lead exposure on thyroid function in adolescents. Environ Res 2006, 101: 140-145.
[127] Lopez CM, Pineiro AE, Nunez N, Avagnina AM, Villaamil EC, Roses OE. Thyroid hormone changes in males exposed to lead in the Buenos Aires area (Argentina). Pharmacol Res 2000, 42: 599-602.
[128] Singh B, Chandran V, Bandhu HK, *et al*. Impact of lead exposure on pituitarythyroid axis in humans. Biometals 2000; 13: 187-192.
[129] Refowitz RM. Thyroid function and lead: no clear relationship. J Occup Med 1984; 26: 579-583.
[130] Siegel M, Forsyth B, Siegel L, Cullen MR. The effect of lead on thyroid function in children. Environ Res 1989; 49: 190-196.
[131] Schumacher C, Brodkin CA, Alexander B. Thyroid function in lead smelter workers: absence of subacute or cumulative effects with moderate lead burdens. Int Arch Occup Environ Health 1998; 71: 453-458.
[132] Liang QR, Liao RQ, Su SH, Huang SH, Pan RH, Huang JL. Effects of lead on thyroid function of occupationally exposed workers. Zhonghua Lao Dong Wei Sheng Zhi Ye Bing ZA Zhi 2003; 21:111-113.

[133] Chaurasia SS, Kar A. Influence of lead on type-I iodothyronine 5'- monodeiodinase activity in male mouse. Horm Metab Res 1997; 29: 532-533.
[134] Stohs SJ, Bagchi D. Oxidative mechanisms in the toxicity of metal ions. Free Radic Biol Med 1995; 18 (2): 321-336.
[135] Goldman M, Dillon RD. Interaction of selenium and lead on several aspects of thyroid function in Pekin ducklings. Res Commun Chem Pathol Pharmacol 1982; 37(3): 487-490.
[136] Ibrahim NM, Eweis EA, El-Beltagi HS, Abdel-Mobdy YE. Effect of lead acetate toxicity on experimental male albino rat. Asian Pac J Trop Biomed 2012; 2(1): 41-46.
[137] Swarup D, Naresh R, Varshney VP, *et al.* Changes in plasma hormones profile and liver function in cows naturally exposed to lead and cadmium around different industrial areas. Res Vet Sci 2007; 82: 16-21.
[138] Vyskocil A, Fiala Z, Ettlerová E, Tenjnorová I. Influence of chronic lead exposure on hormone levels in developing rats. J Appl Toxicol 1990; 10(4): 301-302.
[139] International Programme on Chemical Safety (IPCS) Manganese and its compounds: Environmental aspects. Cicad 63. Geneva Switzerland: WHO 2004. Available at: http://www.inchem.org/documents/cicads/cicads/cicad63.htm
[140] Assem FL, Holmes P, Levy LS. The mutagenicity and carcinogenicity of inorganic manganese compounds: a synthesis of the evidence. J Toxicol Environ Health B Crit Rev 2011; 14 (8): 537-570.
[141] Agency for Toxic Substances and Disease Registry (ATSDR). Toxicological Profile for Manganese. Atlanta: U.S. Department of Health and Human Services Public Health Service 2008. Available from: http://www.atsdr.cdc.gov/toxprofiles/tp151.pdf
[142] Andersen ME, Gearhart JM, Clewel HJ. Pharmacokinetic data needs to support risk assessments for inhaled and ingested manganese. Neurotoxicology 1999; 20: 161-172.
[143] European Community, Health and Consumer Protection Directorate-General. Opinion of the Scientific Committee on Food on the tolerable upper intake level of manganese. Brussels 2000. Available from: http://ec.europa.eu/food/fs/sc/ scf/out80f_en.pdf
[144] Gerber GB, Léonard A, Hantson P. Carcinogenicity, mutagenicity and teratogenicity of manganese compounds. Crit Rev Oncol Hematol 2002; 42: 25-34.
[145] Afridi HI, Kazi TG, Kazi NG, *et al.* Evaluation of arsenic, cobalt, copper and manganese in biological samples of steel mill workers by electrothermal atomic absorption spectrometry. Toxicol Ind Health 2009; 25: 59-69.
[146] Cowan DM, Fan Q, Zou Y, *et al.* Manganese exposure among smelting workers: Blood manganese-ironratio as a novel tool for manganese exposure assessment. Biomarkers 2009; 14: 3-16
[147] World Health Organization (WHO). Manganese in drinking-water: Background document for development of WHO Guidelines for Drinking-water Quality. Geneva Switzerland: WHO 2004. Available from: http:// www.who.int/water_sanitation_health/dwq/ chemicals/manganese.pdf
[148] Roels H, Lauwerys R, Genet P, Sarhan MJ, de Fays M, Hanotiau I. Relationship between external and internal parameters of exposure to manganese in workers from a manganese oxide and salt producing plant. Am J Ind Med 1987; 11: 297-305.
[149] Soldin OP, Aschner M. Effects of manganese on thyroid hormone homeostasis: potential links.Neurotoxicology 2007; 28(5): 951- 956.
[150] Aihara K, Nishi Y, Hatano S, Kihara M, Yoshimitsu K, Takeichi N. Zinc, copper, manganese, and selenium metabolism in thyroid disease. Am J Clin Nutr 1984; 40: 26-35.
[151] Buthieau A, Autissier N. Effects of manganese ions on thyroid function in rat. Arch Toxicol 1983; 54: 243-246.
[152] Kawada J, Nishida M, Yoshimura Y, Yamashita K. Manganese ion as a goitrogen in the female mouse. Endocrinol Jpn 1985; 32: 635-643.
[153] Kim EA, Cheong H-K, Joo K-D, *et al.* Effect of manganese exposure on the neuroendocrine system in welders. NeuroToxicology 2007; 28: 263-269.
[154] Costa M. Potential hazards of hexavalent chromate in our drinking water. Toxicol Appl Pharmacol 2003; 188: 1-5.
[155] International Agency for Research on Cancer (IARC) Chromium and its Compounds. Lyon, France: IARC Scientific Publications 1990.
[156] Zayed AM, Terry N. Chromium in the environment: factors affecting biological remediation. Plant Soil 2003; 249:139-156.

[157] World Health Organization (WHO). Trace elements in human nutrition and health. Geneva Switzerland: WHO 1996; p. 155-160.
[158] O'Brien TJ, Ceryak S, Patierno SR. Complexities of chromium carcinogenesis: role of cellular response, repair and recovery mechanisms. Mutat Res 2003; 533: 3-36.
[159] Kawanishi S, Hiraku Y, Murata M, Oikawa S. The role of metals in site-specific DNA damage with reference to carcinogenesis. Free Radic. Biol. Med. 2002; 32: 822-832.
[160] Kumar S. Occupational Exposure Associated with Reproductive Dysfunction. J. Occup. Health 2004; 46: 1-19.
[161] Thompson CM, Proctor DM, Haws LC. Investigation of the mode of action underlying the tumorigenic response induced in B6C3F1 mice exposed orally to hexavalent chromium. Toxicol Sci 2011; 123(1): 58-70.
[162] Bright P, Burge PS, O'Hickey SP, Gannon PF, Robertson AS, Boran A. Occupational asthma due to chrome and nickel electroplating. Thorax 1997; 52: 28-32.
[163] Costa M. Toxicity and carcinogenicity of Cr (VI) in animal models and humans. Crit Rev Toxicol 1997; 27 :431-442.
[164] Dartsch PC, Hildenbrand S, Kimmel R, Schmahl FW. Investigations on the nephrotoxicity and hepatotoxicity of trivalent and hexavalent chromium compounds. Int Arch Occup Environ Health 1998; 71: 40-45.
[165] International Agency for Research on Cancer (IARC). Chromium and its Compounds. Lyon, France: IARC Scientific Publications 1990.
[166] Harris GK, Shi X. Signaling by carcinogenic metals and metal-induced reactive oxygen species. Mutat Res 2003; 533: 183-200.
[167] Bal W, Kasprzak KS. Induction of oxidative DNA damage by carcinogenic metals. Toxicol Lett 2002; 127: 55-62.
[168] Quinteros FA, Poliandri AHB, Machiavelli LI, Cabilla JP, Duvilanski BH. *In vivo* and *in vitro* effects of chromium VI on anterior pituitary hormone release and cell viability. Toxicol Appl Pharmacol 2007; 218: 79-87.
[169] Mahmood T, Qureshi IZ, Iqabi MJ. Histopathological and biochemical changes in rat thyroid following acute exposure to hexavalent chromium. Histol Histopathol 2010; 25(11): 1355-1370.
[170] Qureshi IZ, Mahmood T. Prospective role of ascorbic acid (vitamin C) in attenuating hexavalent chromium-induced functional and cellular damage in rat thyroid. Toxicol Ind Health 2010; 26(6): 349-359.
[171] Hassanin KMA, El-Kawi SHA, Hashem KS. The prospective protective effect of selenium nanoparticles against chromium-induced oxidative and cellular damage in rat thyroid. Int J Nanomed 2013; 8: 1713-1720
[172] Patty FA. George D. Clayton FE. Patty's Industrial Hygiene and Toxicology (Vol 2, 4rd edition). Wiley Interscience Publ 1981.
[173] Faure R, Dussault JH. Interaction of sodium molybdate with the thyroid hormone receptor. Biochem Cell Biol 1990; 68(3): 630-634.
[174] Zaichick VY, Tsyh AF, Vtyurini BM. Trace elements and thyroid cancers. Analyst 1995; 120: 817-821.
[175] Theophanides T, Anastassopoulou J. Copper and carcinogenesis. Crit Rev Oncol Hemat 2002; 42: 57-62.
[176] Aurthor KA, Kirchgessner M, Eder K. Concentrations of thyroid hormones in serum and activityof hepatic 5′-monodeiodinase in copper-deficient rats. Z Ernährungswiss 1996; 35: 288-290.
[177] Kazi TG, Kandhro GA, Afridi HI, *et al.* Interaction of copper with iron, iodine, and thyroid hormone status in goitrous patients. Biol Trace Elem Res 2010; 134: 265-279.
[178] Carson BL, Ellis HV, McCann JL. Toxicology and Biological Monitoring of Metals in Humans. Michigan, USA: Lewis Publishers Inc. 1986.
[179] Lantina AC, Mallants A, Vermeulen J, Speybroeck N, Hoet P, Lisona D. Absence of adverse effect on thyroid function and red blood cells in a population of workers exposed to cobalt compounds. Toxicol Lett 2011; 201 (1): 42-46.
[180] McKnight RF, Adida M, Budge K, Stockton S, Goodwin GM, Geddes JR. Lithium toxicity profile: a systematic review and meta-analysis. Lancet 2012; 379 (9817): 721-728.

[181] Martin I, Surks S, Irving JR, Lawrence ES, Mutukumara KS. Effect of zinc (II) and other divalent cations on binding of 3,5,3'-triiodo-L-thyronine to nuclear receptors from cultured GC cells. J Biol Chem 1989; 264 (17): 9820-9826.

[182] Moustafa SA. Effect of glutathione (GSH) depletion on the serum levels of triiodothyronine (T3), thyroxine (T4), and T3/T4 ratio in allyl alcohol-treated rats and possible protection with zinc. Int J Toxicol 2001; 20: 15-20.

[183] Chaurasia SS, Gupta P, Kar A, Maiti PK. Lead induced thyroid dysfunction and lipid peroxidation in the fish *Clarias batrachus* with special reference to hepatic type 1-5′-monodeiodinase activity. Bull Environ Contam Toxicol 1996; 56: 649-715.

[184] Nishi Y, Ryoso K, Usui T. Zinc metabolism in thyroid disease. Postgrad Med J 1980; 56: 833-837.

[185] Cheng W, Zhou Z, Yang Y, Yin C, Chai GW. Effect of nickel sulfate on the concentrations of T3, T4 and TSH in serum of rat. Wei Sheng Yan Jiu 1997; 26 (1): 53-59.

CHAPTER 8

Pesticides and Thyroid Function

Carmen Freire[1,2,3,*]

[1]*National School of Public Health, Oswaldo Cruz Foundation (FIOCRUZ), Rio de Janeiro, Brazil;* [2]*University of Granada, Granada, Spain and* [3]*Biomedical Research Centre Network for Epidemiology and Public Health (CIBERESP), Spain*

Abstract: Experimental evidence has shown the ability of multiple pesticides to affect thyroid homeostasis. The thyroid-disrupting effects of organochlorine (OC) pesticides are the most studied. OC pesticides can affect the deiodination of thyroid hormones (TH) leading to increased T3 degradation; can bind to TH-binding proteins altering circulating TH levels; may mimic TH action; and interfere with their binding to hormonal receptors, altering TH-mediated gene expression. Epidemiological studies have shown inverse relationships between exposure to OC pesticides and levels of T3 and T4, and positive associations with TSH among pregnant women, newborns and adults. Non-persistent contemporary pesticides such as organophosphates (OP), carbamate and pyrethroids may also interfere with thyroid function, as suggested by various animal studies. Evidence from human studies linking non-persistent pesticides to thyroid function is still limited and controversial. However, alterations compatible with hypothyroidism were observed in some studies, particularly in relation to OP pesticides. Overall, experimental and epidemiological studies indicate that hypothyroid effect are the general effects from pesticide exposure, supporting that pesticide exposure causes a decrease in TH, but also an increase in TSH. The varying methodological approaches used in epidemiological research particularly hamper drawing conclusions about the evidence on the topic. In addition, exposure levels, modes of action of individual substances, and genetic variability might be important sources of variation between studies. Given the important role of TH on metabolism and brain development, exposure to even low doses of thyroid-disrupting pesticides may contribute to increase the risk of thyroid disease and neurodevelopmental disorders.

Keywords: Non-persistent pesticide, organochlorine pesticides, thyroid disruption, thyroid gland, toxicity.

INTRODUCTION

Pesticides are chemicals designed to exterminate or control insects, weeds, fungi, rodents, and other unwanted organisms. Synthetic pesticides are a large and inhomogeneous group of compounds that can be widely classified as

[*]**Corresponding author Carmen Freire:** National School of Public Health, Oswaldo Cruz Foundation (FIOCRUZ), Rio de Janeiro, Brazil; E-mail: cfreire@ugr.es

Javier Del Pino, Maria Jesus Diaz and Maria Teresa Frejo (Eds)

organochlorines, organophosphates, carbamates, and pyrethroids. Organochlorine (OC) pesticides are insecticides that have the property of lipid affinity and bioaccumulation through the food chain. Due to their severe toxicity and persistence, OC pesticides have been prohibited for agricultural and domestic use since the 1970s in most industrialized countries [1]. However, due to their high environmental persistency and continuous use in some countries for pest control such as malaria [2], their presence is still detected in environmental compartments and human population [3, 4]. Actually, OC pesticides heptachlor epoxide, oxychlordane, trans-nonachlor, 1,1-dichloro-2,2-bis (p-chlorophenyl)-ethylene (p,p'-DDE), 1,1,1-trichloro-2,2-bis (4-chlorophenyl)-ethane (p,p'-DDT), dieldrin, and mirex are still found in humans [5].

Non-persistent pesticides have short biological half-lives and they became widely used after OC pesticides were banned from manufacture and use. Several different classes of pesticides make up this group, being organophosphates (OP), carbamates and synthetic pyrethroids the most common. OP are mostly insecticides, carbamates are herbicides and fungicides, and pyrethroids are insecticides. OPs are the most widely used group of insecticides in the world and they are among the most toxic of all pesticides [6]. Synthetic pyrethroid insecticides are among the most generally available to consumers today due to elevated use in recent years because of the necessity to substitute OP insecticides following use restrictions [7]. Other classes of contemporary-use non-persistent pesticides include dithiocarbamate and azole fungicides, triazine herbicides, and phenoxyacetic acids.

Over 800 active ingredients are sold worldwide in tens of thousands of pesticide products extensively utilized in agriculture, public health, domestic and urban areas. Agriculture is the main source of pesticide exposure and, thus, farmers and people living in pesticide application areas are at higher risk for exposure to these compounds. Among the general population, diet and use in homes and gardens may account for most of the exposure.

Numerous synthetic pesticides are known for their endocrine-disrupting behavior [8, 9]. The Endocrine Society defines endocrine-disrupting (ED) chemicals as "compounds natural or synthetic that through environmental or inappropriate developmental exposures alter the hormonal and homeostatic systems that enable the organism to communicate with and respond to its environment" [10]. More than 100 pesticides have been listed as confirmed or possible ED chemicals by the US Environmental Protection Agency (EPA), the International Agency for

Research on Cancer (IARC) and the European Union Community Strategy for EDs [11]. The OC pesticides p,p'-DDT, endosulphan, and aldrin; OP pesticides malathion, dimethoate, diazinon, dichlorvos, and fenitrothion; carbamates aldicarb, carbaryl, and carbofuran; and synthetic pyrethroids permethrin, cypermethrin, and deltamethrin are well known for their ED properties.

Chemicals that affect thyroid function are called "thyroid disruptors". Many animal and toxicological studies suggest that numerous pesticides may present thyroid-disrupting properties [12-14]. In humans, a number of studies have shown associations between exposure to OC pesticides and adverse effects on the thyroid function [15-22]. Regarding modern non-persistent pesticides, a growing body of epidemiological studies indicates that they may also exert thyroid dysfunction [23-28].

EXPERIMENTAL EVIDENCE

Nowadays, it is recognized that the thyroid system is a major target of ED chemicals and experimental evidence this system is vulnerable to the effects of EDs is growing [12, 13, 29]. Thyroid-disrupting chemicals may interfere with the homeostasis of the hypothalamic-pituitary-thyroid (HPT) axis by affecting either thyroid hormone (TH) synthesis in the thyroid gland, hormone transport, cellular TH uptake and availability, or TH peripheral metabolism [13, 14, 30, 31].

Numerous experimental studies have shown the ability of multiple pesticides, including herbicides, insecticides and fungicides, to affect thyroid homeostasis [12, 13, 29, 32, 33]. In particular, OC pesticides have demonstrated to influence TH and thyroid-stimulating hormone (TSH) activity and metabolism [12, 31, 34].

Organochlorine Pesticides

In general, OC compounds can affect the deiodination of TH by inducing or increasing type III deiodinase expression leading to increased T3 degradation; or can bind to TH-binding proteins (thyroid-binding globulin-TBG, transthyretin-TTR, or albumin) altering circulating T4 and T3 levels. OC pesticides may mimic TH action, and even modulate the mechanisms and interfere with their binding to hormonal receptors [31, 35, 36]. Laboratory studies have shown that OC pesticides interfere with TSH receptor function and bind to T3 and T4 receptors, altering TH-mediated gene expression [13, 37]. The thyroid-disrupting effects of DDT and hexachlorobenzene (HCB) are the most studied.

In 1968, an *in vitro* study suggested that o,p'-DDD, a metabolite of DDT, competes with T4 for TBG binding sites [38]. A study in 1974 found that biliary excretion of T4 was affected in DDT-treated rats [39]. DDD interfered with transporter TTR *in vivo* [40], while DDT interfered *in vitro* with thyroid cell function, inhibiting TSH-stimulated adenylate cyclase activity and cAMP production [41]. Expression of thyroid receptor beta (TRβ) was significantly decreased in frogs by DDE with a dose-response relationship [37]. In this study with frogs, the effect of p,p'-DDE exposure on TRβ mRNA expression was negatively correlated with tadpoles' tail length and width during the exposure period. Conversely, experiments found that the human TRβ had very low affinity for DDT and its metabolites [34].

Prenatal HCB exposure of rats increased T4-UDPGT (uridine diphosphoglucuronosyl transferase) and type II 5'deiodinase in the brain of rat pups [42], indicating an increased peripheral T4 metabolism [12]. HCB also increased hepatic metabolism of TH [43, 44] and interfered with TTR [40] in rats. Methoxychlor decreased type I 5'deiodinase activity *in vitro*, either increasing or decreasing local quantities of active TH in the liver and the kidney [45]. Insecticides lindane (also known as gamma-hexachlorocyclohexane-HCH) and endosulphan stimulated iodide-oxidizing activity of thyroid peroxidase (TPO) in experimental studies with fish [46, 47]. For its part, aldrin reduced iodine uptake by the thyroid in chicks exposed to high doses [48].

Perchlorate is an OC chemical that can be present in some fertilizers. Some animal studies have observed that perchlorate binds to the sodium-iodide symporter (NIS), disrupting the thyroid's ability to synthetize TH [49, 50]. Pentachlorophenol (PCP) has been used as an herbicide, insecticide, fungicide, algaecide, and disinfectant, and is the primary metabolite of pesticide HCB. *In vitro* studies showed TPO inhibition by chlorinated phenol compounds [51] as well as interference with thyroid binding proteins [52, 53].

In addition, several OC pesticides have estrogenic properties. Since TBG is known to increase with estrogen exposure [54], OC pesticides may mimic the estrogen-induced increase in synthesis of TBG.

Thyroid endpoints currently utilized by *in vivo* studies are mainly circulating TH levels, circulating TSH, thyroid gland weight and histopathology [31]. Numerous animal studies have shown associations between exposure to elevated concentrations of OC pesticides, including DDT, its main metabolite p,p'-DDE and HCB, with lower TH or higher TSH levels [12]. Birds exposed to DDT had reduced T4 levels

[55] and increased thyroid weight [56]. Concentration of DDT in adipose tissue of seals correlated inversely to circulating total T3 (TT3) and free T3 (FT3) [57, 58]. Total T4 (TT4) and TT3 were reduced in rodents exposed to HCB [44, 59-62]. T4 levels were decreased in ewes after PCP exposure [63, 64]. In the latter study, the OC pesticide lindane did not decrease TH levels. Animal studies have shown perchlorate to decrease circulating T4 levels in rats [65].

Non-Persistent Pesticides

For most non-persistent pesticides, mechanisms of alteration of hormonal homeostasis have not been established yet. However, reports on thyroid-disrupting effects of contemporary pesticides are emerging [13, 30, 32].

One group of thyroid-disrupting chemicals are the commonly used fungicides from the ethylene bisdithiocarbamates family, which are widely used for protection of fruits, vegetables, and field crops from fungal diseases. The main degradation product of many of the dithiocarbamates (*e.g.* maneb, mancozeb, ziram, zineb) is ethylene thiourea (ETU), which is known to interfere with iodide uptake by inhibiting TPO iodide oxidation [66]. In addition, the EPA classifies ETU as a carcinogen, based on animal data showing that it causes thyroid and other cancers in rodents [67, 68]. Due to its metabolism to ETU, mancozeb and maneb decreased thyroidal production of T3 and T4 in experimental animals [69, 70]. Increased thyroid/body weight ratio, histopathological changes, reduced serum protein-bound iodine, T4 and TPO activity have also been observed in rats treated with mancozeb [69]. In a recent study, mancozeb exposure reduced T4 levels in rat dams [71]. The metabolism of propineb and other ethylene bisdithiocarbamate fungicides proceeds mainly *via* propylenthiourea, which also inhibits TPO and deiodinase activity in peripheral tissues [72, 73].

Some fungicides from the azole family may enhance hepatic catabolism by UDPGT, increasing biliary elimination of T3 and T4 [68, 74]. The fungicide tebuconazole significantly reduced T3 in rats [75], while exposure of zebrafish larvae to both hexaconazole and tebuconazole decreased T4 and T3 levels [76]. Carbendazim, a widely used, broad-spectrum benzimidazole fungicide, caused histopathological damages in the thyroid and increased serum T3 levels in rats [77]. Animal studies have shown that aminotriazole can affect absorption of iodine by thyroid gland through inhibition of TPO [68, 78, 79], alter serum protein-bound iodide levels and induce thyroid carcinogenesis [80]. This commonly used fungicide also inhibited *in vitro* conversion of T4 to T3 through interference with 5'-deiodinase [81].

In has been suggested that more than 60% of all herbicides are endocrine disruptors [30]. Herbicides are a heterogeneous group of chemical classes mostly used in agriculture. Many modern herbicides are chlorinated compounds. Among them, acetochlor inhibited glucuronidation of TH in the liver of rodents [68]. Studies on the effects of 2,4-dichlorophenoxyacetic acid (2,4-D) in rats suggest this herbicide may interfere with iodide uptake by the thyroid gland [82] and lower plasma TH levels through interference with the T4 binding site of TTR [40]. Besides 2,4-D, a number of chlorinated and non-chlorinated herbicides, including dinitrophenols, fenoprop, linuron, bromoxynil, 2,4,5-trichlorophenoxyacetic acid, trichloroacetic acid, dichlorophenol, trichlorophenol, tetrachlorophenol and pentachlorophenol, have shown ability to lower plasma TH levels through interference with transport proteins [40].

By inhibiting brain cholinesterase activity, OP and carbamate insecticides may affect the hypothalamus and the hypophysis through muscarinic and nicotinic receptors [33], resulting in disruption of the thyroid function. The OP dimethoate inhibited extrathyroidal deiodination of T4 to T3 in mice [83]. Malathion stimulated TPO activity, increased T3 levels, reduced T4 and stimulated the extrathyroidal conversion of T4 into T3 *in vitro* [47], whereas it decreased T3 and T3/T4 ratio without altering the level of circulating T4 *in vivo* [84]. OP insecticides ethyl-parathion, malathion and ethyl-bromophos interfered with TTR *in vivo* [40]. Carbamates carbaryl and naphtol showed thyroid antagonist activity *in vitro*, acting as disruptors of the TH receptor-signaling pathway [85]. Carbaryl caused a decline in T4 level and elevation in T3 and T3/T4 ratio in fish [84].

Although they are thought to interfere with the HPT axis, thyroid disruption mechanisms of synthetic pyrethroids are still unclear. In 2010, Du and coworker. tested *in vitro* the ability of nine pyrethroid pesticides and their metabolites to interact with thyroid receptor, showing that all of tested chemicals but one triggered anti-thyroid effects. In addition, pyrethroid insecticide fenvalerate inhibited type I iodothyronine 5'-monodeiodinase activity and enhanced excessive excretion of TH in mice [83, 86]. Pyrethroid permethrin induced a decrease in levels of T4 and T3 in serum and brain of rats, whereas deltamethrin only induced decrease in the serum and brain T4 [87].

Various other contemporary pesticides can also affect thyroid function. Fipronil, which is a broad-spectrum insecticide from the new class known as phenylpyrazole, may interfere with iodine uptake and TPO activity. Dicofol, an OC acaricide still used in many countries, binds to TH transport proteins. Widely used herbicides atrazine and prometryn affect T4 to T3 conversion. Clofentenzine (insecticide), pyrimethanil (fungicide), pendimethalin and thyazopyr (herbicides) interfere with glucuronidation of TH [40, 68, 81].

Overall, experimental studies indicate that hypothyroid effect are the general effects from pesticide exposure, supporting that pesticide exposure causes a decrease in TH, but often the decrease in TT4, FT4, TT3 and FT3 is accompanied by an increase in TSH. Morphological changes and carcinogenic effects in the thyroid gland have also been observed after exposure to pesticides.

EPIDEMIOLOGICAL EVIDENCE

Organochlorine Pesticides

Human data indicate that chronic exposure to certain OC pesticides may interfere with thyroid function [19]. Several epidemiological studies conducted over the last two decades have investigated the association between OC pesticide concentrations in human tissues and circulating levels of T4, T3 and TSH in pregnant women, newborns, children, adolescents, and adults. Literature reporting on these epidemiological studies is summarized below.

Pregnant Women and Newborns

Epidemiological studies have reported different interrelations between FT4, TT4 or TT3 in birth cohorts characterized by low or moderate exposure to OC pesticides.

Among studies with pregnant women, concentrations of HCB, p,p'-DDE and cis-nonachlor in plasma of Canadian mothers were related to decrease in TT3 [22]. A divergent result was shown in a Spanish birth cohort study, which found no significant association between maternal serum p,p'-DDE and T3 [88]. Studies investigating exposure across placenta found inverse relationships between OC pesticides in placenta tissue or cord blood and TH or TBG values [20, 89, 90]. Levels of PCP in umbilical cord plasma were inversely related to cord-blood FT4, TT3 and TBG among Canadian mother-child pairs [90]. In a Belgian study, HCB cord levels were associated with lowered TT3 and FT4, while p,p'-DDE was only associated with lower FT4 [20]. Accordingly, TT4 was inversely associated with cord serum levels of DDT metabolites in a birth cohort in Thailand [89]. However, one of the Canadian studies did not find significant association between cord serum OC pesticides and TT3 or FT4 [22].

Two studies assessed exposure to OC pesticides through breast milk in relation to thyroid status of newborns [91, 92]. In the Netherlands, neonatal levels of TT4 were inversely associated with concentration of several OC pesticides in breast milk [91]. Conversely, cord-blood TH values were not associated with p,p'-DDE, HCB or trans-nonachlor levels in breast milk of Danish women [92]. The latter study also assessed the degree of cord-blood TBG saturation and found levels of p,p'-DDE and trans-nonachlor in both milk and maternal serum at 34th week of gestation to be associated with decrease in binding capacity of TBG [92].

Regarding TSH, findings in a Spanish community highly exposed to HCB showed no significant association between cord serum levels of this pesticide and TSH at birth but a close-to-significant positive association between p,p'-DDE and neonatal TSH levels above 10 mU/L was noted [21]. The earlier study also reported a positive relationship between TSH and cord serum beta-HCH. Subsequent studies in Spain found positive associations between neonatal beta-HCH, but not HCB or DDT, and infants' TSH [93, 94]. Increased serum TSH was associated with higher p,p'-DDE exposure in Spanish pregnant women [88], although TSH was not related to maternal serum levels of DDT and HCB in the US [15]. In a Spanish birth cohort, TSH values of newborns were related to placental concentrations of p,p'-DDE, endrin and endosulphan-sulfate [16]. Asawasinsopon and coworkers (2006) found no relation between cord blood TSH and maternal or cord serum levels of DDT, dieldrin, heptachlor, HCB or lindane, and there have been other reports of no association between TSH and OC pesticide concentrations [20, 22, 95].

Adults

Several studies conducted over the last decades in the area of eastern Slovakia highly polluted by a mixture of polychlorinated biphenyls, DDE and HCB have observed high prevalence of thyroid and metabolic disorders in residents of such area [19]. Among thyroid disorders, increase of thyroid volume, positive TPO antibodies in blood, increase of serum FT4 and TT3, and reduced TSH have been suggested to be related to OC exposure. Research findings also suggested that prenatal exposure to OC compounds may contribute to the increased prevalence of thyroid antibodies and increased thyroid volume in children born to highly exposed mothers [19].

For their part, Rádiková and coworkers examined the thyroid status of more than 2,000 people living in two areas in Slovakia, one of which was an area with heavy OC pollution, including pesticides DDE and HCB, and a low pollution area. They found a positive association between OC serum levels and TT3 and FT4, a weak negative association with TSH, and a positive relation with thyroid volume. In addition, authors observed autoimmunity signs, *i.e.* higher prevalence of positive TPO antibodies in people living in the high pollution area compared to the low pollution area, particularly in men [96]. Levels of TPO antibodies were also elevated in North American indigenous youth (10-16 years old) with high concentrations of p,p'-DDE, mirex, and HCB in serum [97].

Serum HCB was inversely related to T4 levels in Spanish adults [98] and indigenous adolescents [99] living in rural areas polluted with high OC compounds. In a small sample of sportsmen from New York State, TT4 and HCB serum levels were inversely associated [100]. Lowered T3 was also associated with HCB exposure in a small study among Canadian obese men [101]. p,p'-DDE serum concentration was not associated with T4 among sportsmen [100] or indigenous youth [99, 102], nor was with T3 in obese men [101] and adolescents [102]. Conversely, one study investigating more than 300 adult men recruited from an infertility clinic in the U.S. found positive association between serum p,p'-DDE, TT3 and FT4 values [36]. Conflicting results were reported in a Spanish cohort study that showed negative associations between TT3 and serum p,p'-DDT or beta-HCH, but not with p,p'-DDE or HCB among 259 children at the age of 4 years [103].

No association between HCB, DDT, p,p'-DDE and T3 or T4 values were described in adult populations elsewhere [104-106].

Regarding the effects of other OC pesticides, a recent survey was conducted in Brazil to assessed serum concentrations of 19 OC pesticides in relation to thyroid status of population residing in an area highly contaminated with OC insecticides from a manufactory plant abandoned in the 1960s [17, 18]. High prevalence of subclinical hypothyroidism and positive TPO antibodies was observed among adults (303 men and 305 women) [18]. Levels of FT4 were inversely associated with beta-HCH and p,p'-DDT in males and positively related to HCB, heptachlor, o,p'-DDT, and p,p'-DDT in females. Lowered TT3 were related to levels of endosulphan 2 in males, while they were related to p,p'-DDT, endosulphan 2, methoxychlor and alpha-chlordane in women [18]. These findings suggested that OC pesticides might affect the thyroid system through gender-specific mechanisms. In young population (<16 years old), data showed that exposure to OC pesticides produced a significant increase in serum TT3 [17].

Additional associations between OC pesticide exposure and TSH have been have been reported, *e.g.* inverse relationships with p,p'-DDE [35, 36] and HCB [35], and positive association with p,p'-DDE and beta-HCH [18, 105]. In contrast, no association between HCB or mirex and TSH were reported in Spanish adults residing near a chlor-alkali plant [98] and North American indigenous [102].

In general, epidemiological studies among pregnant women, newborns and adults have found inverse relationships with levels of T3 and T4, and some positive associations with TSH. However, epidemiological studies on the effects of OC pesticides on thyroid function cannot demonstrate consistent associations. Evidence on the effect in vulnerable groups (*e.g.* pregnant women and infants) has been particularly controversial [20, 22, 89, 93, 95]. Discrepancies in these findings might result from differences in exposure levels, sample sizes, matrices for exposure assessment (*e.g.*, maternal blood, cord blood, placenta, breast milk), specimen collection time points and mechanisms of action of individual compounds. In addition, little is known about the thyroid-disrupting potential of other OC pesticides, such as mirex, endosulphan, aldrin and methoxychlor [16, 17, 22, 89, 102].

Non-Persistent Pesticides

The effects of non-persistent pesticides on thyroid function have received little attention, and there is much controversy over their potential clinical impact, because few studies have been conducted in humans. Over the last decade, however, body of epidemiological evidence linking exposure to modern pesticides with thyroid function has grown. Few cross-sectional studies have examined exposure to OP pesticides [23, 26, 27], pyrethroids [7, 107] and dithiocarbamates [108], mostly assessed by urinary metabolites, in relation to circulating levels of T4, T3 and/or TSH. A link between agricultural working and thyroid function has been also suggested in other studies [24, 25, 28, 109, 110]. Only two cohort studies explored the association between prenatal exposure to non-persistent pesticides and TH levels [107, 111, 112].

Three studies in the U.S. investigated the association between TH concentration and biological markers of exposure to OP pesticides, carbamates or pyrethroids in non-occupationally-exposed adults [7, 23, 27]. Fortenberry and coworkers (2012) assessed the relationship between urinary levels of 5,6-trichloro-2-pyridinol (TCPY), a metabolite of the OP insecticide chlorpyrifos, and altered serum TH levels using data from 3,249 individuals 12 years and older from the U.S. National Health and Nutrition Examination Survey (NHANES). They found that increased urinary TCPY in males was associated with significant increases in serum TT4, and decreases in TSH. In women >60 years of age, exposure levels were positively associated with TSH [23]. Levels of TCPY in urine of 300 men from an infertility clinic were significantly associated with elevation in TSH levels and reduced free T4, respectively [27]. In this study, urinary 1-naphthol, metabolite of carbamate insecticide carbaryl, did not show association with hormone values. In a subsample of these men, urinary levels of the metabolite of pyrethroids cis-3-2,2-dichlorovinyl-2,2-dimethylcyclopropane carboxylic acid (cis-DCCA) were associated with lower TT3, but not FT4 or TSH [7]. However, 3-phenoxybenzoic acid (3-PBA) in urine, which has been commonly used as a generic biomarker of exposure to pyrethroid insecticides, was not related to TH.

A study among Mexican men involved in floriculture work examined TH levels in relation to urinary concentration of dialkylphosphates (DAPs), which are non-specific metabolites of the OP pesticides [26]. Levels of DAP, TSH and TT4 (but not TT3) were significantly higher in the high-exposure season compared to the low-exposure season. In addition, concentration of dimethyl metabolites (DMP) showed positive association with TSH and TT4, whereas TT3 decreased with increasing DMP.

Using data from the U.S. Agricultural Health Study, Goldner and coworkers (2010) investigated whether use of pesticides (*i.e.* herbicides, insecticides, fungicides, fumigants, OP, carbamates, and pyrethroids) increased the risk of thyroid disease among wives of pesticide applicators. They found that increased risk of hypothyroidism was associated with overall fungicide use (odds ratio [OR]= 1.4), and use of fungicide benomyl (OR= 3.1), dithiocarbamates maneb and mancozeb (OR= 2.2), and herbicide paraquat (OR= 1.8). In addition, women that reported use of maneb and mancozeb had greater risk of hyperthyroidism (OR=2.3) [25]. A study with U.S. farmworkers and a group of urban controls reported reduction in TSH and FT4 levels from summer (higher exposure) to fall (lower exposure) seasonal shifts among herbicide and fungicide applicators [24]. TSH levels in farmers who had aerial application of fungicides increased by 40% from summer to fall. Subclinical hypothyroidism in this study was noted in 5 out of 144 applicators, but not in urban control subjects [24]. A study in a group of Danish greenhouse workers exposed to more than 60 pesticides found a moderate reduction in FT4 (10-16%) among individuals working in greenhouses with a high spraying load [28]. When hormone levels between the spring (low-exposure season) and the fall (high-exposure season) were compared, it was observed 32% higher TSH level in the spring compared to the fall, and lower levels of TT3, FT3 and FT4. In Mexico, a small sample of farmers applying ethylene bisdithiocarbamates fungicides had significantly higher levels of TSH compared to non-exposed individuals. T4 levels did not differed between groups [108].

Conversely, concentration of T4 and T3 among famers from Cameroon exposed to insecticides, herbicides, nematicides, and fungicides was not significantly different from that observed in non-exposed men [110]. In Pakistan, pesticide applicators using different classes of chemicals did not show significantly lower FT4 and TSH compared to unexposed individuals [109]. A recent study among Venezuelan agricultural workers did not find correlation between blood cholinesterase activity, a biomarker of recent exposure to OP and carbamates, and serum FT4 and TSH [113].

Three studies have examined maternal-infant exposure to non-persistent pesticides in relation to TH. A Japanese mother-child cohort with 231 women without occupational exposure to pesticides assessed maternal exposure to pyrethroids by measuring its urinary 3-PBA metabolite at 10-12 gestational weeks [107, 112]. Maternal levels of FT4, TSH and TBG were not associated with urinary 3-PBA concentration [107], nor were serum FT4 and TSH of newborns [112]. A Danish cohort study with 145 mother-child pairs found lower serum TSH among 6-11 year-old children born by women working in greenhouse during pregnancy compared to children born by unexposed women [111].

Overall, epidemiological studies exploring the effects of non-persistent pesticides on thyroid function have produced quite discrepant results. Inconsistencies across studies can arise for many reasons. Exposure level and modes of action of individual substances might be important sources of variation between studies. Differences in genetic susceptibility, between both individuals and populations, may also account for the lack of clear dose-response relationships between individual compounds or compound groups and thyroid status.

Exposure to both background levels and higher doses (*e.g.* occupational) of pesticides may produce mild thyroid changes. However, for most pesticides, insufficient data are available to prove or disprove a link with an individual compound or group of compounds. It will be a challenge, thus, to identify associations with any particular substance given the large range of modern pesticides in addition to past-use OC pesticides. The key issues are to understand the mechanism by which these chemicals act and the dose at which they act. Interactions of chemical mixtures at concentrations relevant to human exposure are largely unknown and require further investigation.

RELEVANCE TO PUBLIC HEALTH

Thyroid hormones in humans are indispensable for metabolic control and for maintaining normal cardiovascular, reproductive, and nervous system functions.

Exposure to ED chemicals may potentially result in mild changes in serum TH levels, which in turn may result in significant impact on public health. Given that pesticides are used extensively today, exposure of large populations to moderate and low levels of thyroid-disrupting compounds, the effects of which can be additive, may be a major contributor to environmental burdens of clinical and subclinical thyroid disease. Although the consequences of subclinical changes in thyroid function are not well understood yet [114, 115], all factors associated with any alteration in TH levels should be investigated.

TH are of special significance in fetal development, as development of the brain is dependent on regular levels of TH [116]. Absence of TH decreases neuronal growth and differentiation in the cerebral cortex, hippocampus, and cerebellum [13]. Epidemiological studies have described that even a marginally low T4 level in a pregnant woman may give rise to reduction of cognitive functions of the offspring [117-119]. According to this, it has been speculated that some of the neurotoxic effects (*e.g.* altered psychomotor and cognitive functions) of early exposure to ED chemicals may result from disruption of the thyroid system [116]. Because even relatively minor changes in the thyroid homeostasis can result in neurodevelopmental deficiencies, early exposure to pesticides with potential to disrupt thyroid function should be a particular cause of concern.

CONFLICT OF INTEREST

The author confirms that author has no conflict of interest to declare for this publication.

ACKNOWLEDGEMENTS

Declared None.

REFERENCES

[1] United Nations Environment Programme. 2014. Stockholm Convention. http://www.unep.org/chemicalsandwaste/UNEPsWork/PersistentOrganicPollutansPOPs.

[2] Food and Agriculture Organization of the United Nations (FAO). Prevention and disposal of obsolete pesticides. 2014. Available from http://www.fao.org/agriculture/crops/obsolete-pesticides.

[3] CDC. Fourth National Report on Human Exposure to Environmental Chemicals. Atlanta: National Center for Environmental Health. 2009; pp. 520 Report N° 1. Available from http://www.cdc.gov/exposurereport/pdf/FourthReport.pdf

[4] Saoudi A, Fréry N, Zeghnoun A, *et al.* Serum levels of organochlorine pesticides in the French adult population: the French National Nutrition and Health Study (ENNS), 2006-2007. Sci Total Environ 2014; 472: 1089-99.

[5] Crinnion WJ. Chlorinated pesticides: threats to health and importance of detection. Altern Med Rev 2009; 14: 347-59.

[6] Eaton DL, Daroff RB, Autrup H, *et al.* Review of the toxicology of chlorpyrifos with an emphasis on human exposure and neurodevelopment. Crit Rev Toxicol 2008; S2: 1-125.
[7] Meeker JD, Barr DB, Hauser R. Pyrethroid insecticide metabolites are associated with serum hormone levels in adult men. Reprod Toxicol 2009; 27(2): 155-60.
[8] McKinlay R, Plant JA, Bell JNB, Voulvoulis N. Endocrine disrupting pesticides: Implications for risk assessment. Environ Int 2008; 34: 168-83.
[9] Mnif W, Hassine AI, Bouaziz A, Bartegi A, Thomas O, Roig, B. Effect of endocrine disruptor pesticides: A review. Int J Environ Res Public Health 2011; 8: 2265-303.
[10] EEC. European workshop on the impact of endocrine disrupters on human health and wildlife. Weybridge: UK 1996.
[11] PAN. List of lists: a catalogue of lists of pesticides identifying those associated with particularly harmful health or environmental impacts. Pesticide Action Network; 2005.
[12] Boas M, Feldt-Rasmussen U, Skakkebaek NE, Main KM. Environmental chemicals and thyroid function. Eur J Endocrinol Eur Fed Endocr Soc 2006; 154(5): 599-611.
[13] Boas M, Feldt-Rasmussen U, Main KM. Thyroid effects of endocrine disrupting chemicals. Mol Cell Endocrinol 2012; 355(2): 240-8.
[14] Crofton KM. Thyroid disrupting chemicals: mechanisms and mixtures. Int J Androl 2008; 31: 209-23.
[15] Chevrier J, Eskenazi B, Holland N, Bradman A, Barr DB. Effects of exposure to polychlorinated biphenyls and organochlorine pesticides on thyroid function during pregnancy. Am J Epidemiol 2008; 168: 298-310.
[16] Freire C, Lopez-Espinosa MJ, Fernández M, Molina-Molina JM, Prada R, Olea N. Prenatal exposure to organochlorine pesticides and TSH status in newborns from Southern Spain. Sci Total Environ 2011; 409(18): 3281-7.
[17] Freire C, Koifman RJ, Sarcinelli P, Rosa AC, Clapauch R, Koifman S. Long term exposure to organochlorine pesticides and thyroid function in children from Cidade dos Meninos, Rio de Janeiro, Brazil. Environ Res 2012; 117: 68-74.
[18] Freire C, Koifman RJ, Sarcinelli P, Rosa AC, Clapauch R, Koifman S. Long term exposure to organochlorine pesticides and thyroid status in adults in a heavily contaminated area in Brazil. Environ Res 2013; 127: 7-15.
[19] Langer P. The impacts of organochlorines and other persistent pollutants on thyroid and metabolic health. Front. Neuroendocrinol 2010; 31: 497-518.
[20] Maervoet J, Vermeir G, Covaci A, *et al.* Association of thyroid hormone concentrations with levels of organochlorine compounds in cord blood of neonates. Environ Health Perspect 2007; 115(12): 1780-6.
[21] Ribas-Fitó N, Sala M, Cardo E, *et al.* Organochlorine compounds and concentrations of thyroid stimulating hormone in newborns. Occup Environ Med 2003; 60: 301-3.
[22] Takser L, Mergler D, Baldwin M, Smargiassi A, Lafond J. Thyroid hormones in pregnancy in relation to environmental exposure to organochlorine compounds and mercury. Environ Health Perspect 2005; 113: 1039-45.
[23] Fortenberry GZ, Hu H, Turyk M, Barr DB, Meeker JD. Association between urinary 3, 5, 6-trichloro-2-pyridinol, a metabolite of chlorpyrifos and chlorpyrifos-methyl, and serum T4 and TSH in NHANES 1999-2002. Sci Total Environ 2012; 424: 351-5.
[24] Garry VF, Holland SE, Erickson LL, Burroughs BL. Male reproductive hormones and thyroid function in pesticide applicators in the Red River Valley of Minnesota. J Toxicol Environ Health A 2003; 66(11): 965-86.
[25] Goldner WS, Sandler DP, Yu F, Hoppin JA, Kamel F, Levan TD. Pesticide use and thyroid disease among women in the Agricultural Health Study. Am J Epidemiol 2010; 171(4): 455-64.
[26] Lacasaña M, López-Flores I, Rodríguez-Barranco M, *et al.* Association between organophosphate pesticides exposure and thyroid hormones in floriculture workers. Toxicol Appl Pharmacol 2010; 243(1): 19-26.
[27] Meeker JD, Barr DB, Hauser R. Thyroid hormones in relation to urinary metabolites of non-persistent insecticides in men of reproductive age. Reprod Toxicol 2006; 22(3): 437-42.
[28] Toft G, Flyvbjerg A, Bonde JP. Thyroidfunction in Danish Green houseworkers. Environmental Health: A Global Access Science Source 2006; 5(2): 1-8.

[29] Kandarakis ED, Bourguignon JP, Gore AC. Endocrine-disrupting chemicals: an Endocrine Society scientific statement. Endocr Rev 2009; 30(4): 293-342.

[30] Colborn T. Neurodevelopment and endocrine disruption. Environ Health Perspect 2004; 112: 944-9.

[31] Zoeller RT, Tyl RW, Tan SW. Current and potential rodent screens and tests for thyroid toxicants. Crit Rev Toxicol 2007; 37(1-2): 55-95.

[32] Howdeshell KL. A model of development of the brain as a construct of the thyroid system. Environ Health Perspect 2002; 110 (Suppl 3): 337-48.

[33] Smallridge RC, Carr FE, Fein HG. Diisopropylfluorophosphate (DFP) reduces serum prolactin, thyrotropin, luteinizing hormone, and growth hormone and increases adrenocorticotropin and corticosterone in rats: Involvement of dopaminergic and somatostatinergic as well as cholinergic pathways. Toxicol Appl Pharmacol 1991; 108(2): 284-95.

[34] Cheek AO, Kow K, Chen J, McLachlan JA. Potential mechanisms of thyroid disruption in humans: interaction of organochlorine compounds with thyroid receptor, transthyretin, and thyroid-binding globulin. Environ Health Perspect 1999; 107: 273-8.

[35] Langer P, Tajtaková M, Kocan A, *et al.* Multiple organochlorine pollution and the thyroid. Endocr Regul 2006; 40: 46-52.

[36] Meeker JD, Altshul L, Hauser R. Serum PCBs, p,p'-DDE and HCB predict thyroid hormone levels in men. Environ Res 2007; 104: 296-304.

[37] Mortensen AS, Kortner TM, Arukwe A. Thyroid hormone-dependent gene expression as a biomarker of short-term 1,1-dichloro-2,2-bis(p-chlorophenyl)ethylene (DDE) exposure in European common frog (Rana temporaria) tadpoles. Biomarkers 2006; 11(6): 524-37.

[38] Marshall JS, Tompkins LS. Effect of o,p'-DDD and similar compounds on thyroxine binding globulin. J Clin Endocrinol 1968; 28: 386-92.

[39] Bastomsky CH. Effects of a polychlorinated biphenyl mixture (Aroclor 1254) and DDT on biliary thyroxine excretion in rats. Endocrinology 1974; 95(4): 1150-5.

[40] Van den Berg KJ, van Raaij JAGM, Bragt PC, Notten WRF. Interactions of halogenated industrial chemicals with transthyretin and effects on thyroid hormone levels *in vivo*. Arch Toxicol 1991; 65(1): 15-9.

[41] Santini F, Vitti P, Ceccarini G, *et al. In vitro* assay of thyroid disruptors affecting TSH stimulated adenylate cyclase activity. J Endocrinol Invest 2003; 26: 950-5.

[42] Morse DC, Groen D, Veerman M, *et al.* Interference of polychlorinated biphenyls in hepatic and brain thyroid hormone metabolism in fetal and neonatal rats. Toxicol Appl Pharmacol 1993; 122: 27-33.

[43] Kleiman de Pisarev DL, del Carmen Rios de Molina M, San Martin de Viale LC. Thyroid function and thyroxine metabolism in hexachlorobenzene-induced porphyria. Biochem Pharmacol 1990; 35(5): 817-25.

[44] Van Raaij JAGM, Kaptein E, Visser TJ, van den Berg KJ. Increased glucuronidation of thyroid hormone in hexachlorobenzene-treated rats. Biochem Pharmacol 1993; 45(3): 627-31.

[45] Zhou LX, Dehal SS, Kupfer D, Morrell S, McKenzie BA, Eccleston ED Jr, Holtzman JL. Cytochrome P450 catalyzed covalent binding of methoxychlor to rat hepatic, microsomal iodothyronine 5'-monodeiodinase, type I: does exposure to methoxychlor disrupt thyroid hormone metabolism? Arch Biochem Biophys 1995; 322: 390-4.

[46] Sinha N, Lal B, Singh TP. Effect of endosulfan on thyroid physiology in the freshwater catfish, Clarias batrachus. Toxicology 1991; 67: 187-97.

[47] Yadav AK, Singh TP. Pesticide-induced impairment of thyroid physiology in the freshwater catfish, Heteropneustes fossilis. Environ Poll 1987; 43: 29-38.

[48] Kuzan FB, Prahlad KV. The effects of 1,2,3,4,10,10-hexachloro-1,4,4a,5,8,8a-hexahydroxy endo, exo-5,8-dimthionaphthalene (aldrin) and sodium ethylenebisdithiocarbomate (Nabam) on the chick. Poult Sci 1975; 54: 1054-64.

[49] Eskandari S, Loo DD, Dai G, Levy O, Wright EM, Carrasco N. Thyroid Na+/I- symporter. Mechanism, stoichiometry, and specificity. J Biol Chem 1997; 272(43): 27230-8.

[50] Wolff J. Perchlorate and the thyroid gland. Pharmacol Rev 1998; 50: 89-106.

[51] Schmutzler C, Hamann I, Hofmann PJ, *et al.* Endocrine active compounds affect thyrotropin and thyroid hormone levels in serum as well as endpoints of thyroid hormone action in liver, heart and kidney. Toxicology 2004; 205: 95-102.

[52] Kudo Y, Yamauchi K. *In vitro* and *in vivo* analysis of the thyroid disrupting activities of phenolic and phenol compounds in Xenopus laevis. Toxicol Sci 2005; 84: 29-37.
[53] Yamauchi K, Ishihara A, Fukazawa H, Terao Y. Competitive interactions of chlorinated phenol compounds with 3,3',5-triiodothyronine binding to transthyretin: detection of possible thyroid-disrupting chemicals in environmental waste water. Toxicol Appl Pharmacol 2003; 187: 110-7.
[54] Tahboub R, Arafah BM. Sex steroids and the thyroid. Best Pract Res Clin Endocrinol Metab 2009; 23: 769-80.
[55] Scollon EJ, Carr JA, Cobb GP. The effect of flight, fasting and p,p'-DDT on thyroid hormones and corticosterone in Gambel's white-crowned sparrow, Zonotrichia leucophrys gambelli. Comparative Biochemistry and Physiology. Toxicol Pharmacol 2004; 137: 179-89.
[56] Jefferies DJ, French MC. Avian thyroid: effect of p,p'-DDT on size and activity. Science. 1969; 166(3910): 1278-80.
[57] Chiba I, Sakakibara A, Goto Y, *et al.* Negative correlation between plasma thyroid hormone levels and chlorinated hydrocarbon levels accumulated in seals from the coast of Hokkaido, Japan. Environ Toxicol Chem 2001; 20: 1092-7.
[58] Sormo EG, Jussi I, Jussi M, Braathen M, Skaare JU, Jenssen BM. Thyroid hormone status in gray seal (Halichoerus grypus) pups from the Baltic Sea and the Atlantic Ocean in relation to organochlorine pollutants. Environ Toxicol Chem 2005; 24: 610-6.
[59] Alvarez L, Hernández S, Martinez-de-Mena R, Kolliker-Frers R, Obregón MJ, Kleiman de Pisarev DL. The role of type I and type II 5' deiodinases on hexachlorobenzene-induced alteration of the hormonal thyroid status. Toxicology 2005; 207(3): 349-62.
[60] Foster WG, Pentick JA, McMahon A, Lecavalier PR. Body distribution and endocrine toxicity of hexachlorobenzene (HCB) in the female rat. J Appl Toxicol 1993; 13(2): 79-83.
[61] Rozman K, Gorski JR, Rozman P, Parkinson A. Reduced serum thyroid hormone levels in hexachlorobenzene-induced porphyria. Toxicol Lett 1986; 30: 71-78.
[62] Smith AG, Dinsdale D, Cabral JRP, Wright AL. Goiter and wasting induced in hamsters by hexachlorobenzene. Arch Toxicol 1987; 60: 343-49.
[63] Beard AP, Bartlewski PM, Chandolia RK, Honaramooz A, Rawlings NC. Reproductive and endocrine function in rams exposed to the organochlorine pesticides lindane and pentachlorophenol from conception. J Reprod Fertil 1999; 115: 303-14.
[64] Beard AP, Rawlings NC. Thyroid function and effects on reproduction in ewes exposed to the organochlorine pesticides lindane or pentachlorophenol (PCP) from conception. J Toxicol Environ Health Part A 1999; 58: 509-30.
[65] Gilbert ME, Sui L. Developmental exposure to perchlorate alters synaptic transmission in hippocampus of the adult rat. Environ Health Perspect 2008; 116(6): 752-60.
[66] Marinovich M, Guizzetti M, Ghilardi F, Viviani B, Corsini E, Galli CL. Thyroid peroxidase as toxicity target for dithiocarbamates. Arch Toxicol 1997; 71: 508-12.
[67] Houeto P, Bindoula G, Hoffman JR. Ethylenebisdithiocarbamates and ethylenethiourea: possible human health hazards. Environ Health Perspect 1995; 103: 568-73.
[68] Hurley PM, Hill RN, Whiting RJ. Mode of carcinogenic action of pesticides inducing thyroid follicular cell tumors in rodents. Environ Health Perspect 1998; 106: 437-45.
[69] Kackar R, Srivastava MK, Raizada BR. Studies on rat thyroid after oral administration of Mancozeb: morphological and biochemical evaluations. J Appl Toxicol 1997; 17: 369-75.
[70] Trivedi N, Kackar R, Srivastava MK, Mithal A, Raizada RB. Effect of oral administration of fungicide Mancozeb on thyroid gland of rat. Ind J Exp Biol 1993; 31: 564-6.
[71] Axelstad M, Boberg J, Nellemann C, Kiersgaard M, Jacobsen PR, Christiansen S, Hougaard KS, Hass U. Exposure to the widely used fungicide mancozeb causes thyroid hormone disruption in rat dams but no behavioral effects in the offspring. Toxicol Sci 2011; 120(2): 439-46.
[72] Leonard JL, Rosenberg IN. Thyroxine 5'-deiodinase activity of rat kidney: observations on activation by thiols and inhibition by propylthiouracil. Endocrinology 1978; 103: 2137-44.
[73] Visser TJ, van Overmeeren E, Fekkes D, Docter R, Hennemann G. Inhibition of iodothyronine 5'-deiodinase by thioureylenes; structure-activity relationship. FEBS Lett 1979; 103: 314-8.
[74] Wolf DC, Allen JW, George MH, *et al.* Toxicity profiles in rats treated with tumorigenic and nontumorigenic triazole conazole fungicides: Propiconazole, triadimefon, and myclobutanil. Toxicol Pathol 2006; 34: 895-902.

[75] Taxvig C, Hass U, Axelstad M, *et al.* Endocrine-disrupting activities *in vivo* of the fungicides tebuconazole and epoxiconazole. Toxicol Sci 2007; 100: 464-73.

[76] Yu L, Chen M, Liu Y, Gui W, Zhu G. Thyroid endocrine disruption in zebrafish larvae following exposure to hexaconazole and tebuconazole. Aquat Toxicol 2013; 138-139: 35-42.

[77] Barlas N, Selmanoglu G, Kockaya A, Songur S. Effects of carbendazim on rat thyroid, parathyroid, pituitary and adrenal glands and their hormones. Hum Exp Toxicol 2002; 21: 217-21.

[78] Ealey PA, Henderson B, Loeveridge N. A quantitative study of peroxidase activity in unfixed tissue sections of the guinea-pig thyroid gland. Histochem J 1984; 16: 111-22.

[79] Mayberry WE. Antithyroid effects of 3-amino-1,2,4-trizole. Proc Soc Exp Biol Med 1968; 129(2): 551-6.

[80] Steinhoff D, Weber H, Mohr U, Boehme K. Evaluation of amitrole (aminotriazole) for potential carcinogenicity in orally dosed rats, mice, and golden hamsters. Toxicol Appl Pharmacol 1983; 69: 161-9.

[81] Ghinea E, Dumitriu L, Stefanovici G, Pop A, Oprescu, Ciocirdia C. Action of some pesticides on T4 to T3 conversion in cultured kidney and liver cells in the presence or absence of cysteine. Rev Roum Med Endocrinol 1986; 24(3): 157-66.

[82] Florsheim WH, Velcoff SM. Some effects of 2,4-dichlorophenoxyacetic acid in thyroid function in the rat: effects on iodine accumulation. Endocrinology 1962; 71(1): 1-6.

[83] Maiti PK, Kar A. Dimethoate inhibits extrathyroidal 5'-monodeiodination of thyroxine to 3,3',5-triiodothyronine in mice—the possible involvement of the lipid peroxidative process. Toxicol Lett 1997; 91(1): 1-6.

[84] Sinha N, Lal B, Singh TP. Pesticides induced changes in circulating thyroid hormones in the freshwater catfish Clarias batrachus. Comp Biochem Physiol C. 1991b; 100: 107-10.

[85] Sun H, Shen OX, Xu XL, Song L, Wang XR. Carbaryl, 1-naphthol and 2-naphthol inhibit the beta-1 thyroid hormone receptor-mediated transcription *in vitro*. Toxicology 2008; 249 (2-3): 238-42.

[86] Maiti PK, Kar A, Gupta P, Chaurasia SS. Loss of membrane integrity and inhibition of type I iodothyronine 5'-monodeiodinase activity by fenvalerate in female mouse. Biochem Biophys Res Commun 1995; 214(3): 905-9.

[87] Wang S, Shi N, Ji Z, Pinna G. Effects of pyrethroids on the concentrations of thyroid hormones in the rat serum and brain. Zhonghua Lao Dong Wei Sheng Zhi Ye Bing Za Zhi 2002; 20: 173-6.

[88] Lopez-Espinosa MJ, Vizcaino E, Murcia M, *et al.* Association between thyroid hormone levels and 4,4'-DDE concentrations in pregnant women (Valencia, Spain). Environ Res 2009; 109: 479-85.

[89] Asawasinsopon R, Prapamontol T, Prakobvitayakit O, Vaneesorn Y, Mangklabruks A, Hock B. The association between organochlorine and thyroid hormone levels in cord serum: a study from northern Thailand. Environ Int 2006; 32(4): 554-9.

[90] Sandau CD, Ayotte P, Dewailly E, Duffe J, Norstrom RJ. Pentachlorophenol and hydroxylated polychlorinated biphenyl metabolites in umbilical cord plasma of neonates from coastal populations in Québec. Environ Health Perspect 2002; 110(4): 411-7.

[91] Fiolet DCM, Cuijpers CEJ, Lebret E. Exposure to polychlorinated organic compounds and thyroid hormone plasma levels of human newborns. 1997; 34: 459-65.

[92] Julvez J, Debes F, Weihe P, Choi AL, Grandjean P. Thyroid Dysfunction as a Mediator of Organochlorine Neurotoxicity in Preschool Children. Environ Health Perspect 2011; 119: 1429-35.

[93] Alvarez-Pedrerol M, Ribas-Fitó N, Torrent M, *et al.* Thyroid disruption at birth due to prenatal exposure to beta-hexachlorocyclohexane. Environ Int 2008; 34: 737-40.

[94] Lopez-Espinosa MJ, Vizcaino E, Murcia M, *et al.* Prenatal exposure to organochlorine compounds and neonatal thyroid stimulating hormone levels. J Expo Sci Environ Epidemiol 2010; 20: 579-88.

[95] Dallaire R, Muckle G, Dewailly E, *et al.* Thyroid hormone levels of pregnant inuit women and their infants exposed to environmental contaminants. Environ Health Perspect 2009; 117(6): 1014-20.

[96] Rádiková Z, Tajtáková M, Kocan A, *et al.* Possible effects of environmental nitrates and toxic organochlorines on human thyroid in highly polluted areas in Slovakia. Thyroid 2003; 18: 353-62.

[97] Schell LM, Gallo MV, Ravenscroft J, DeCaprio AP. Persistent organic pollutants and anti-thyroid peroxidase levels in Akwesasne Mohawk young adults. Environ Res 2009; 109: 86-92.

[98] Sala M, Sunyer J, Herrero C, To-Figueras J, Grimalt J. Association between serum concentrations of hexachlorobenzene and polychlorobiphenyls with thyroid hormone and liver enzymes in a sample of the general population. Occup Environ Med 2001; 58: 172-7.

[99] Schell LM, Gallo MV, Denham M, Ravenscroft J, DeCaprio AP, Carpenter DO. Relationship of thyroid hormone levels to levels of polychlorinated biphenyls, lead, p,p'- DDE, and other toxicants in Akwesasne Mohawk youth. Environ Health Perspect 2008; 116: 806-13.

[100] Bloom MS, Weiner JM, Vena JE, Beehler GP. Exploring associations between serum levels of select organochlorines and thyroxine in a sample of New York state sportsmen: the New York State Angler Cohort Study. Environ Res 2003; 93: 52-66.

[101] Pelletier C, Doucet E, Imbeault P, Tremblay A. Associations between weight loss-induced changes in plasma organochlorine concentrations, serum T(3) concentration, and resting metabolic rate. Toxicol Sci 2002; 67: 46-51.

[102] Schell LM, Gallo MV, Decaprio AP, Hubicki L, Denham M, Ravenscroft J. The Akwesasne Task Force on the Environment, 2004. Thyroid function in relation to burden of PCBs, p,p'-DDE, HCB, mirex and lead among Akwesasne Mohawk youth: a preliminary study. Environ Toxicol Pharmacol 2004; 18: 91-9.

[103] Alvarez-Pedrerol M, Ribas-Fitó N, Torrent M, Carrizo D, Grimalt JO, Sunyer J. Effects of PCBs, p,p'-DDT, p,p'-DDE, HCB and beta-HCH on thyroid function in preschool children. Occup Environ Med 2008; 65(7): 452-7.

[104] Hagmar L, Bjork J, Sjodin A, Bergman A, Erfurth EM. Plasma levels of persistent organohalogens and hormone levels in adult male humans. Arch Environ Health 2001; 56: 138-43.

[105] Rylander L, Wallin E, Jonssson BA, Stridsberg M, Erfurth EM, Hagmar L. Associations between CB-153 and p,p'-DDE and hormone levels in serum in middle-aged and elderly men. Chemosphere 2006; 65: 375-81.

[106] Turyk ME, Anderson HA, Freels S, *et al.* Associations of organochlorines with endogenous hormones in male Great Lakes fish consumers and nonconsumers. Environ Res 2006; 102: 299-307.

[107] Zhang J, Hisada A, Yoshinaga J, *et al.* Exposure to pyrethroids insecticides and serum levels of thyroid-related measures in pregnant women. Environ Res 2013; 127: 16-21.

[108] Steenland K, Cedillo L, Tucker J, *et al.* Thyroid hormones and cytogenetic outcomes in backpack sprayers using ethylenebis(dithiocarbamate) (EBDC) fungicides in Mexico. Environ Health Perspect 1997; 105(10): 1126-30.

[109] Khan DA, Ahad K, Ansari WM, Khan H. Pesticide exposure and endocrine dysfunction in the cotton crop agricultural workers of southern Punjab, Pakistan. Asia Pac J Public Health 2013; 25(2): 181-91.

[110] Manfo FPT, Moundipa PF, Déchaud H, Tchana AN, Nantia EA, Zabot MT. Effect of Agropesticides Use on Male Reproductive Function: A Study on Farmers in Djutitsa (Cameroon). Environ Toxicol 2012; 27: 423-32.

[111] Wohlfahrt-Veje C, Main KM, Schmidt IM, *et al.* Lower birth weight and increased body fat at school age in children prenatally exposed to modern pesticides: a prospective study. Environ Health 2011; 10(79): 2-11.

[112] Zhang J, Yoshinaga J, Hisada A, *et al.* Prenatal pyrethroid insecticide exposure and thyroid hormone levels and birth sizes of neonates. Sci Total Environ 2014; 488-489: 275-9.

[113] Miranda-Contreras L, Gómes-Pérez R, Rojas G, Cruz I, *et al.* Occupational exposure to organophosphate and carbamate pesticides affects sperm chromatin integrity and reproductive hormone levels among Venezuelan farm workers. J Occup Health 2013; 55(3): 195-203.

[114] Boelaert K, Franklyn JA. Thyroid hormone in health and disease. J Endocrinol 2005; 187: 1-15.

[115] Surks MI, Ortiz E, Daniels GH, *et al.* Subclinical thyroid disease: scientific review and guidelines for diagnosis and management. JAMA 2004; 291: 228-38.

[116] Williams GR. Neurodevelopmental and neurophysiological actions of thyroid hormone. J Neuroendocrinol 2008; 20(6): 784-94.

[117] Berbel P, Mestre JL, Santamaría A, *et al.* Delayed neurobehavioral development in children born to pregnant women with mild hypothyroxinemia during the first month of gestation: the importance of early iodine supplementation. Thyroid 2009; 19(5): 511-9.

[118] Haddow JE, Palomaki GE, Allan WC, *et al.* Maternal thyroid deficiency during pregnancy and subsequent neuropsychological development of the child. N Engl J Med 1999; 341(8): 549-55.

[119] Pop VJ, Brouwers EP, Vader HL, Vulsma T, van Baar AL, de Vijlder JJ. Maternal hypothyroxinaemia during early pregnancy and subsequent child development: a 3-year follow-up study. Clin Endocrinol (Oxf) 2003; 59(3): 282-8.

CHAPTER 9

Pathologic Effects of Radiation on the Thyroid Gland

Zubair W. Baloch* **and Virginia A. LiVolsi**

Department of Pathology & Laboratory Medicine, Perelman School of Medicine, University of Pennsylvania, Philadelphia, PA, USA

Abstract: The thyroid gland is virtually unique since it can be affected by both external radiation (and thus, it shares with other organs histopathologic changes due to irradiation effects) and by the so-called "internal" radiation, wherein administration of radioactive iodide preferentially affects the thyroid gland (almost to the exclusion of all other organs). This review will focus on both types of radiation and the changes that can be seen acutely and chronically in the thyroid after it has been subjected to irradiation. In addition, the neoplastic potential of radiation exposure on thyroid follicular epithelium will be presented and illustrated.

Keywords: Radiation, carcinoma, thyroid, thyroiditis.

INTRODUCTION

"Radiation exposure causes cancer and non-cancer health effects, each of which varies greatly in the form of the dose response curve, latency, persistency, recurrence, curability, fatality and impact on the quality of life". The carcinogenic potential of ionizing radiation was shown when skin cancers developed in early X-ray workers. The first case of human dermatitis of the hand was reported in 1896 [1, 2]. Currently, it is well known that exposure to ionizing radiation is directly related to increased risk of malignancy development. The increased incidence of secondary malignant tumors in children treated by radiation for their first malignancy, and long term studies of atomic bomb survivors in Japan and known nuclear accidents/disasters throughout the world have made a major contribution to the assessment of the radiation-dose related risk of malignancy [3-7].

It is well documented that ionizing radiation affects directly or indirectly the cell genome causing instability and mutations. The genomic instability may not serve as the cause of mutations in the irradiated cells, but can lead to an increased risk

*Corresponding author Zubair W. Baloch: Department of Pathology & Laboratory Medicine, Perelman School of medicine, University of Pennsylvania, Philadelphia, PA, USA; E-mail: baloch@mail.med.upenn.edu

Javier Del Pino, Maria Jesus Diaz and Maria Teresa Frejo (Eds)

of chromosomal abnormalities and mutations in the progeny later in life. This theory has been substantiated by the "bystander effect" phenomenon; in which the genomic stability is also observed in the daughter cells derived from non-irradiated cells in close proximity to the irradiated cells. However, this bystander effect does not underscore the direct radiation induced DNA mutations; but docs provide insight into other mechanisms responsible for the consequences due to low-dose effects resulting from nuclear accident/disasters [5, 8-10].

The thyroid gland is the largest pure endocrine gland in humans and it weights approximately 20g. It comprises two lobes; right and left, which are joined by a narrow isthmus which is usually found at the level of third and fourth tracheal cartilages. Histologically, the thyroid is comprised of follicles (the functioning unit) of varying sizes, which are lined by cuboidal to attenuated epithelial cells and filled with colloid. The follicular cells actively transport iodide from the capillaries interspersed among follicles to the lumen of the follicle containing colloid. Thyroglobulin, a high molecular weight glycoprotein, is the major component of colloid and is crucial in the synthesis and formation of thyroid hormones.

The thyroid hormones, triiodothyronine-T3 and thyroxine-T4 play an important role in normal growth and development, overall energy expenditure and substrate utilization. Synthesis and release of thyroid hormones are maintained by actions of the pituitary hormone thyroid stimulating hormone (TSH). TSH exerts its effect on follicular cells *via* TSH receptor. Stimulatory effects of hypothalamic hormone, thyrotropin-releasing hormone (TRH) and the inhibitory negative feedback effects of thyroid hormones govern TSH secretion. The thyroid gland also contains neural crest derived C-cells which are not responsible for the production of T3 and T4.

The exposure of the thyroid gland to radiation can lead to a wide variety of pathophysiological changes. This was first reported in 1920s, in thyrotoxic patients receiving radiotherapy; followed by documentation of clinical use of radioactive iodine in euthyroid patients with cardiac disease to reduce basal metabolic rate [11]. The first report of hypothyroidism following radiotherapy for head and neck cancer was reported in 1960s [12].

The histologic changes in the thyroid gland following radiation exposure vary depending upon the mode (external *vs*. internal radiation) and dose of radiation; and the interval following radiation. It has been suggested that thyroid damage may be divided into acute/sub-acute and chronic/late changes. The former usually occurs within the first 3-months of exposure [5, 8, 13].

TYPES OF RADIATION INDUCED THYROID DAMAGE

There are basically two modes of radiation exposure; external and/or internal. The external exposure is dependent upon distance from radiation source (the strength of radiation falls with distance from the source of radiation) and the length of time a person remains in close vicinity to the radiation source. The internal radiation exposure occurs due to ingestion of radiation contaminated foods, inhalation of radioactive gases or aerosol particles or by surface absorption through damaged skin barrier [5, 14-18].

External Radiation

Acute effects: It is extremely rare, indeed almost impossible, to have the opportunity to examine thyroid tissue that has been subjected to external radiation acutely (within 4 weeks of exposure). Animal studies have shown that damage to the follicular epithelium, extrusion of stored colloid, and an inflammatory infiltrate, which initially is neutrophilic and then becomes mixed before becoming chronic are seen. There is stromal edema, but no significant fibrosis at this stage [14, 19].

Acute changes, as reported within 3-6 weeks of lethal atomic bomb exposures, include decrease in size and number of follicles, which are lined by low cuboidal epithelium. Thyroid glands exposed to high doses of I-131 during the course of therapy show follicular necrosis, acute vasculitis and hemorrhage followed by lymphocytic infiltration and vascular sclerosis [13, 20-22] (Figs. **1-6**).

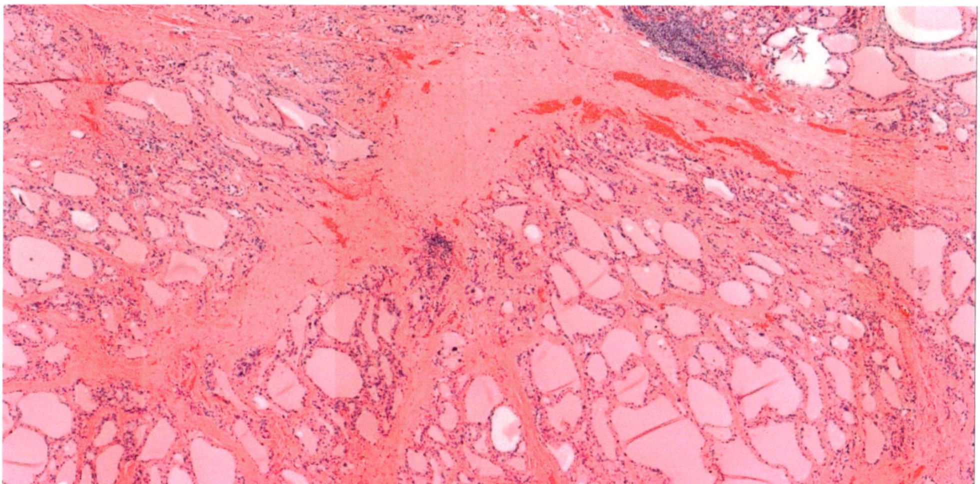

Figure 1: A case of acute radiation injury demonstrating lobules of variably sized follicles containing watery colloid and some fibrosis (Hematoxylin & Eosin stain, 10X).

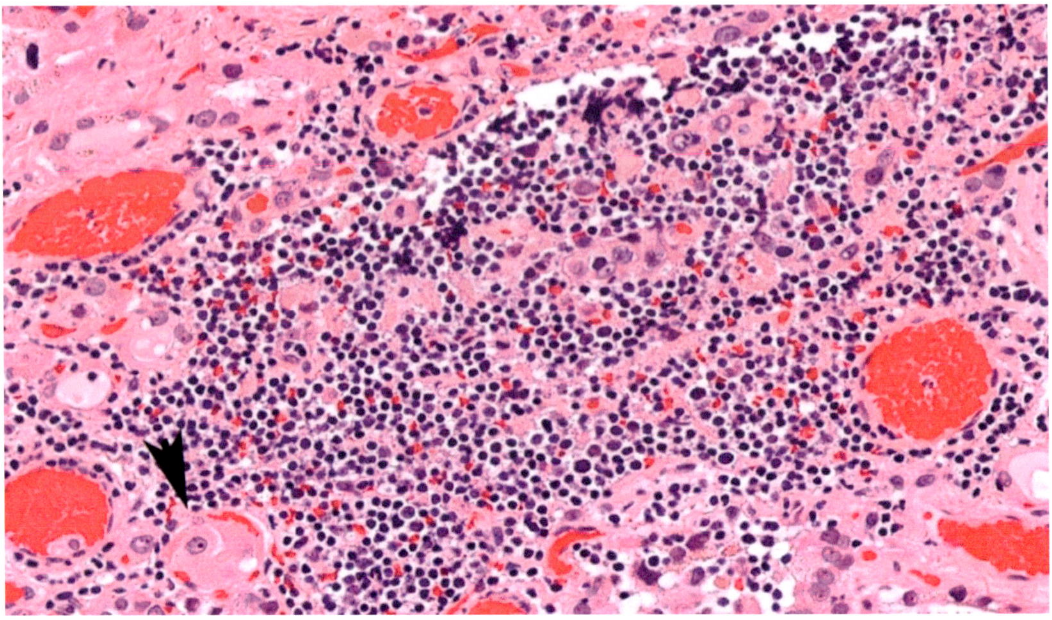

Figure 2: Acute radiation injury: Inflammatory infiltrate with follicular damage leading to oncocytic metaplasia - Arrow head (Hematoxylin & Eosin stain, 20X).

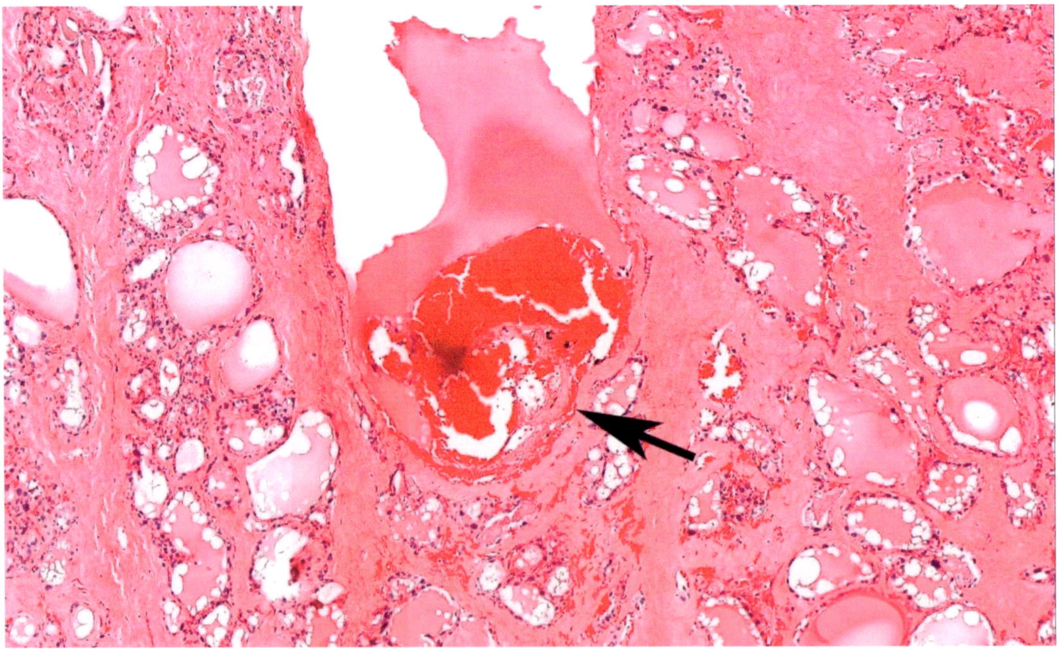

Figure 3: Acute radiation injury: Thrombosis and recanalization of an intrathyroidal vessel - Arrow (Hematoxylin & Eosin stain, 20X).

Chronic effects: The most common chronic clinical effect of external irradiation on the thyroid gland is hypothyroidism; however, hyperthyroidism can occur in a minority of patients. Hypothyroidism is usually seen in patients exposed to therapeutic doses (30-70 Gy) to the head and neck/cervical region. Subclinical hypothyroidism (elevation in TSH levels with normal serum FT4 level) is the most common finding in patients undergoing regular biochemical screening after head and neck irradiation. Overt hypothyroidism is also a frequent finding [13]. Dorp and colleagues reported 40% rate of thyroid dysfunction by analyzing 10 studies involving 4012 survivors with complications after Hodgkin's lymphoma treatment during childhood [23]. These studies also showed that in patients under the age of 17, the radiation dose has been found to be the most important risk factor for developing hypothyroidism.

On histopathologic examination, fibrosis and follicular atrophy are the main changes seen after months and/or years of exposure of the thyroid to external radiation. The fibrosis is most prominent in the inter-lobular areas although peri-follicular or trans-lobular fibrosis may also be seen. Scattered chronic inflammatory cells are noted within the areas of fibrosis; mild to moderate atypia of stromal fibroblasts and endothelial cells may accompany the fibrosis [14, 20, 21] (Figs. **7-11**).

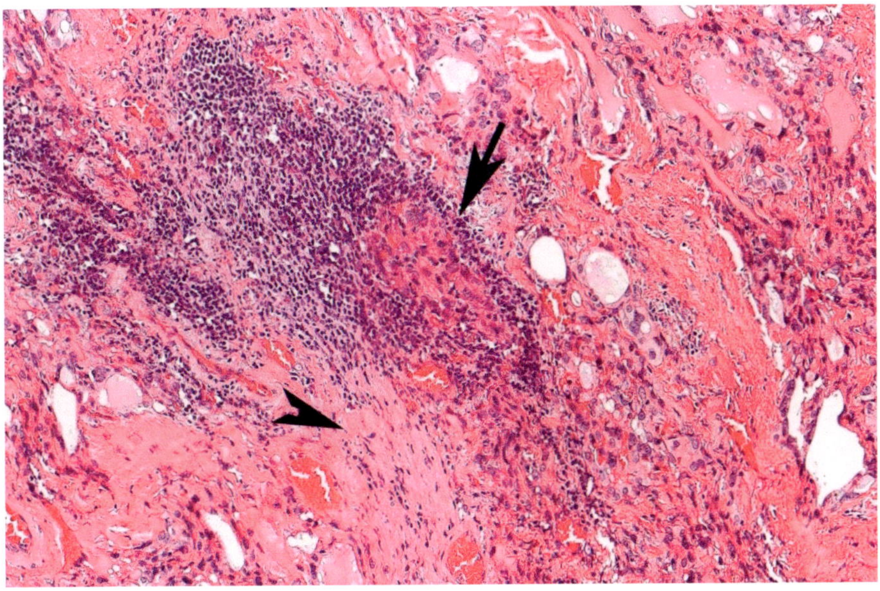

Figure 4: Acute radiation injury: Fibrosis and drop out of follicular structures (arrow head), inflammatory infiltrate and collection of histiocytes/pseudo-granuloma formation (arrow) (Hematoxylin & Eosin stain, 20X).

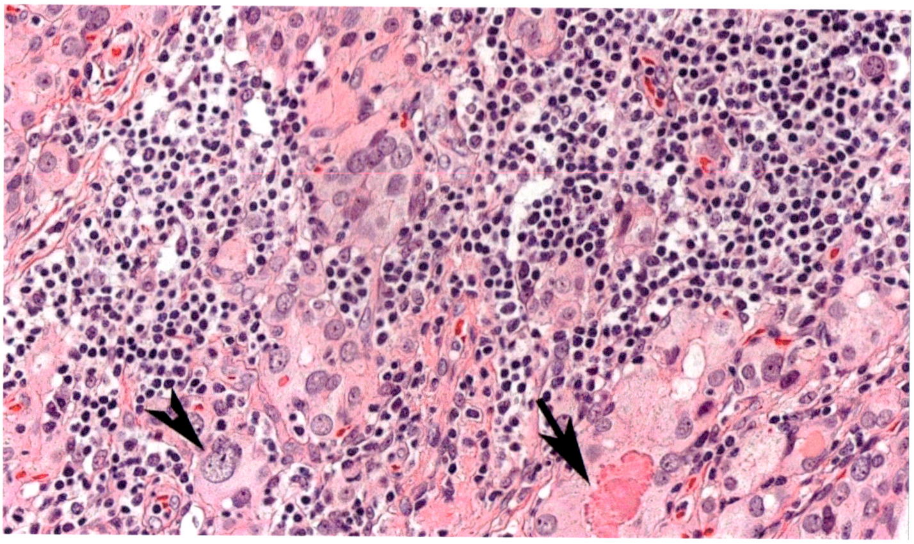

Figure 5: Acute radiation injury: Inflammatory infiltrate consisting of lymphocytes and plasma cells with follicular damage leading to oncocytic metaplasia. Notice the random nuclear enlargement (arrow head)& thick residual colloid within the follicular lumen (arrow) (Hematoxylin & Eosin stain, 40X).

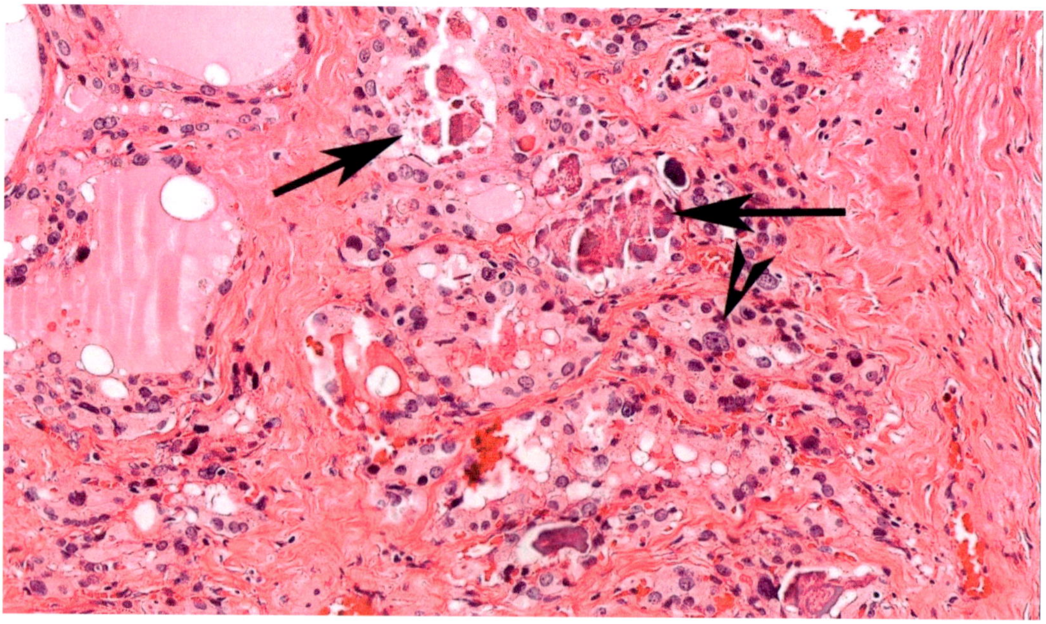

Figure 6: Acute radiation injury: Thyroid follicular structure damage leading to random nuclear enlargement/atypia (arrow head) & thick residual colloid within the follicular lumen (arrows). On the left of figure notice the residual normal follicles containing watery colloid (Hematoxylin & Eosin stain, 40X).

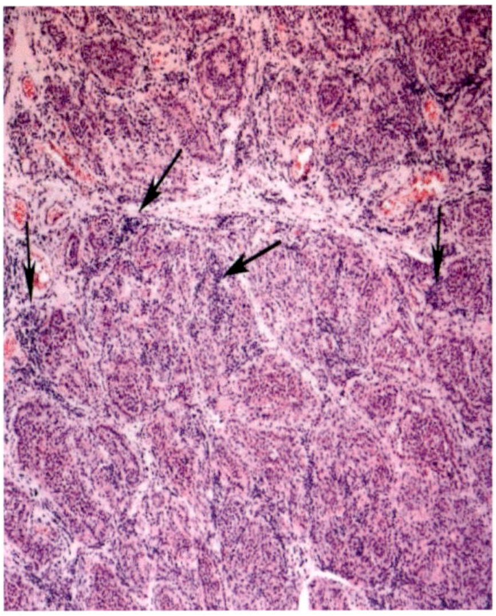

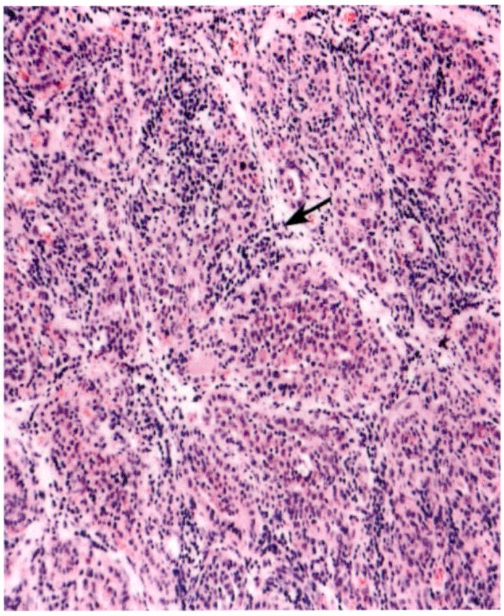

Figures 7 & 8: Chronic radiation injury: A case of Graves' disease treated with radioactive iodine demonstrating lobular architecture and inflammatory infiltrate (arrows) (Hematoxylin & Eosin stained sections, Fig. **7** 4X, Fig. **8** 10X).

The follicular epithelial cells can show a range of changes including random nuclear enlargement and hyperchromasia; metaplasia including oncocytic and squamous types; and the colloid can be shrunken and eosinophilic. In some cases, and this is probably dose dependent, the follicles themselves are small and atrophic. The other reported changes in thyroid gland after irradiation include chronic lymphocytic thyroiditis and multinodular goiter [20, 21].

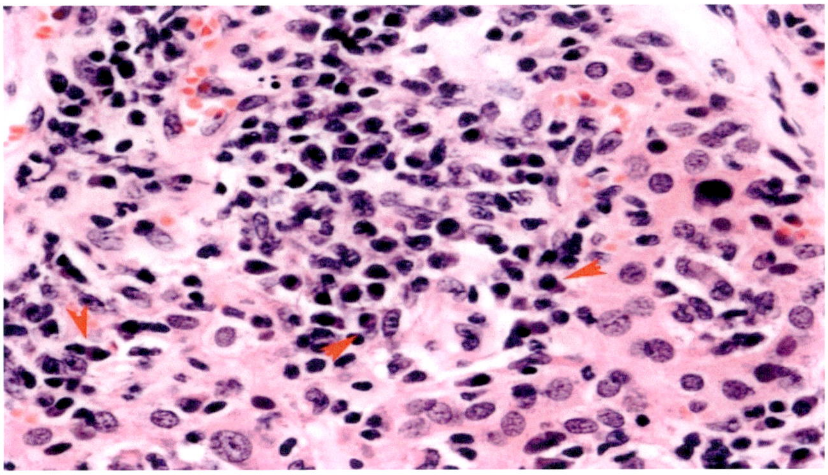

Figure 9: Chronic radiation injury. High power showing inflammatory infiltrate consisting of mostly plasma cells (red arrow head) and few lymphocytes (Hematoxylin & Eosin 40X).

Depending upon the degree of fibrosis and the extent of follicular atrophy there may be thyroid dysfunction with the development of subclinical or overt hypothyroidism. This clinical result in general is dependent upon the dose of radiation administered, the size of the gland prior to being radiated, whether or not there was nodularity to the gland before radiation, whether there was iodine deficiency in the patient and the time course over which the radiation occurred [14, 20, 21].

Internal Radiation

The effects of radioactive iodide, which is preferentially taken up by thyroid follicular epithelium, are dose dependent.

In the clinical setting, the reason for administration of radioactive iodide determines the dosage used. In the treatment of hyperthyroidism (Graves′ disease or toxic nodular goiter or toxic nodule), the radiation dose is around 30 mCi [24]. If the hyperthyroidism is caused by a diffuse hyperplasia of the gland, the distribution of the radiation dose is relatively uniform throughout the gland. The hyperplasic follicles are converted to either normal follicles or atrophic ones. Over time, the destruction of the thyroid follicles and stromal fibrosis leads to glandular shrinkage (weights of these thyroids may be 2-4 g). Histologically, in addition to fibrosis and follicular atrophy, oncocytic metaplasia and random marked nuclear pleomorphism may be identified.

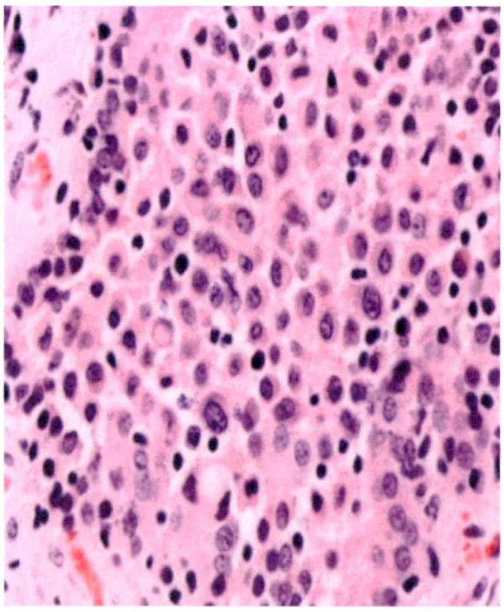

Figures 10: Chronic radiation injury. A follicular structure filled with histiocytes (Fig. **10**, Hematoxylin & Eosin 40X).

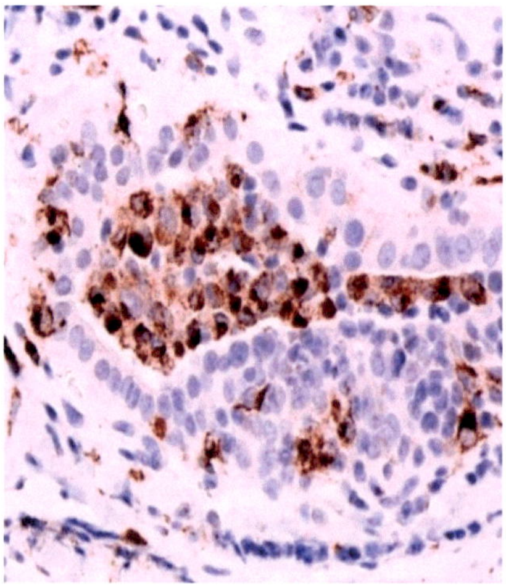

Figure 11: The histiocytic origin is confirmed by immunostains for CD68 (Fig. **11**, Immunoperoxidase stain, 20X).

If the hyperthyroidism is due to hyper functioning nodule (AKA toxic nodule) or multinodular goiter, the distribution of the iodide dose is lopsided and different areas of the thyroid may be exposed to different concentrations of iodine. Hence, as might be expected, nodular areas might be slightly less fibrotic and less affected than intervening relatively normal thyroid areas [7, 14, 20, 21] (Figs. **7-11**).

If the radioactive iodide is given for the treatment of a carcinoma of the thyroid, the doses administered are higher than 30 mCi. Hence, the degree of histologic changes would be expected to be more severe. However, most of these patients have had surgery and the iodide is given for destruction of residual normal thyroid tissue or tumor to avert local "thyroid bed" recurrence [14].

NEOPLASTIC EFFECTS OF RADIOACTIVE IODIDE AND EXTERNAL RADIATION ON THE THYROID

For many decades, it was known, anecdotally and by some epidemiological studies, that exposure of the thyroid to radiation could induce neoplastic transformation of the thyroid follicular epithelium [9, 24]. In these cases, the overall swelling type of thyroid carcinoma that developed was papillary thyroid carcinoma [23-25]. Depending on dosage, size of the gland, and thyroid function status, the effects of radiation varied.

The consequences of major nuclear fallouts/accidents have provided access to established large cohorts, known thyroid radiation doses and methods to diagnose thyroid disease(s) [5, 6, 26-29].

Atomic Bomb Survivor Data

"The Radiation Effects Research Foundation (RERF, formerly the Atomic Bomb Casualty Commission) created a longitudinal Life Span Study consisting of 120321 atomic bomb survivors in 1950 and its sub-cohort, the Adult Health Study (AHS), consisting of 19961 survivors, in 1958". In both studies, a strong correlation was found between radiation dose and development of thyroid cancer and thyroid nodules, confirmed by tumor registry and autopsy data in Hiroshima and Nagasaki.

In the atomic bomb testing experiences both in the Pacific Islands and in Western portions of the United States mainland, some of the developed tumors were histologically bizarre and some appeared to be papillary carcinomas. In the Japanese experience in World War II, the great majority of the cancers were ordinary papillary carcinomas. It must be remembered that in the latter, the diet is the world's richest in iodide [3, 7, 30, 31].

Chernobyl Nuclear Power Plant Accident

The nuclear accident at Chernobyl occurred on April 26, 1986. Large quantities of radioactive materials were released. The radioactive cloud containing large quantities of radioactive iodine reached Belarus within a few hours of the explosion, leading to concentrated exposure to thyroids of the population in the area. The acute radiation syndrome induced after radiation exposure led to fatalities in 28 people. Contamination of milk with I-131 occurred due to pasture-cow-milk pathway, resulting also in internal radiation exposure [27, 29, 32, 33].

It is widely recognized that children exposed to iodine isotope radiation due to the Chernobyl nuclear accident have suffered the most significant side-effects. This case cohort has been thoroughly investigated by teams of local and international experts to independently evaluate the clinical, morphological and epidemiological characteristics of thyroid lesions and/or carcinoma. These studies have clearly shown a substantial increase in the incidence of thyroid carcinoma as a consequence of this massive nuclear accident [6, 33].

The first clue to an increase in thyroid malignancy among those exposed to fallout was observed in 1990, *i.e.* 4 years after the accident, in Minsk and Kiev [34, 35]. The incidence of thyroid carcinoma continued to rise, and in 1995 the incidence rate of childhood thyroid carcinoma in Belarus reached 40 per million. The highest incidence was observed in the most exposed to the radiation blast in the south of Belarus, the lowest in the least exposed northern regions of the country. It is evident, from many studies of this population, that the risk for those exposed as adults is very low or absent [32].

It has been suggested that higher age-related sensitivity, seen in radiation induced thyroid carcinoma, can be explained on the basis of dose applied to child's throat, gland size, and biological factors influencing sensitivity. It is well-known that the radiation dose to the thyroid of a child during fallout is greater than that of a similarly exposed adult. However, in children, the additional exposure occurred due to the ingestion of contaminated cow's or mother milk, because of high iodine uptake and concentration by the mammary glands. The biological reason for increased sensitivity of children's thyroid to radiation is the rapid growth of thyroid cells during development, which in turn, may lead to increased susceptibility to developing mutations and rearrangements [5, 6, 18, 27, 33].

Clinical Features of Chernobyl Related Thyroid Carcinoma

According to some (but not all) published reports, the Chernobyl associated PTC's behave in an aggressive fashion with poor clinical outcomes characterized by high frequency of extra-thyroidal extension, loco-regional cervical lymph node and distant metastases. Interestingly, these aggressive features were independent of the size of the tumors [36-40].

A recent study of 1078 children and adolescents exposed to Chernobyl fallout, published by Fridman and colleagues, demonstrated lymph nodes metastases in 73.8% and distant spread in 11.1 cases at presentation. The overall survival was favorable in this cohort after total thyroidectomy and radioactive-iodine treatment [29].

Morphologic Characteristics of Chernobyl-related Thyroid Carcinoma

The earliest cases of thyroid cancers that were developed after the Chernobyl fallout were virtually all papillary carcinomas (PTCs); 98% of Belarussian and 95% of Ukranian cases; however, to date few cases of follicular and medullary carcinoma have been reported [29, 36, 37, 41-44].

The earliest publications reported that all PTCs were mostly comprised of solid growth pattern AKA solid cell type; however, later studies have found that classic variant was the most common subtype [32, 44]. A study by Fridman and colleagues studied clinical and pathological characteristics of PTCs in 1078 Belarussian children exposed to radiation during Chernobyl fallout. The histologic review was conducted in 936 of 1078 cases which showed the following distribution of various subtypes of PTC: classical variant - 38.5%, follicular variant - 31.2%, solid variant – 14.5%, diffuse sclerosing variant - 7.8%, tall cell variant - 6.9%, and oncocytic or clear cell - 1.1%, [29]. The main histologic features of classic, follicular, solid and diffuse sclerosis variant are summarized in Table **1**.

By light microscopy, the ***classic variant of PTC*** can appear as encapsulated or infiltrative tumors; the latter are commonly associated with sclerosis within or at the infiltrative edge. It is not unusual to encounter various percentages of follicle formation in close proximity or embedded within the tumor papillae. Lamellated calcification, known as psammoma bodies, can also be seen within the tumor papillae. It is not uncommon to see psammoma bodies at the infiltrative edge or away from the main tumor in the lymphatics within the normal thyroid

Table 1. Morphologic characteristics of papillary thyroid carcinoma seen in population exposed to irradiation.

Solid Variant **a.** *Low Power*: **i.** Solid and trabecular growth pattern in 50% of tumor mass **ii.** Invasion is commonly encountered **b.** *High Power*: **i.** Solid nests of tumor cells with varying amounts of surrounding by either fibrotic stroma or delicate fibrous bands
Classic Variant a. Low Power: i. Complex papillae (variably sized and inter-branching) with well-developed vascular cores b. High Power i. Cells lining the papillae show: 1. Scant cytoplasm 2. Nuclear stratification 3. Nuclear elongation 4. Irregular nuclear membrane 5. Nuclear chromatin clearing (Orphan Annie Nuclei) 6. Eccentric nucleoli 7. Intra-nuclear grooves & inclusions 8. Psammoma bodies (40-50% of cases)
Follicular Variant **a.** Low Power **i.** Encapsulated, partially encapsulated, diffuse involving both lobes **ii.** Tumor capsule invasion and/or vascular invasion of tumor capsule vessels **iii.** Growth : microfollicles, mixed macro and microfollicular, rarely pure macrofollicles (macrofollicular variant) **iv.** Dense eosinophilic luminal colloid with peripheral scalloping **b.** High power i. Cells lining the follicles show: 1. Scant to oncocytic cytoplasm 2. Nuclear features of papillary carcinoma
Diffuse Sclerosis Variant a. Low power a. Solid and papillary nests of tumor permeating the thyroid gland parenchyma b. Prominent lymphocytic infiltrate around tumor nests c. Numerous psammoma bodies d. Extrathyroidal extension is frequent b. High power a. Tumor cells i. Squamous metaplasia ii. Nuclear features of papillary carcinoma

parenchyma, which is indicative of lymphatic spread. The ultimate diagnosis of PTC lies on demonstration of typical nuclear cytology *i.e.* nuclear elongation, chromatin clearing, small eccentric nucleoli, irregular nuclear membranes, intra-nuclear grooves and inclusions [45-47] (Fig. **12**). The hallmark features of ***follicular variant of PTC*** are follicular architecture and the diagnostic PTC nuclei lining the follicles. The ***follicular variant of PTC*** can present as either completely encapsulated tumors with or without capsular and/or vascular invasion, partially encapsulated or infiltrative tumors. The tumor scan shows an admixture of large or small follicles containing thick eosinophilic colloid and variable intra-tumoral sclerosis [45, 46].

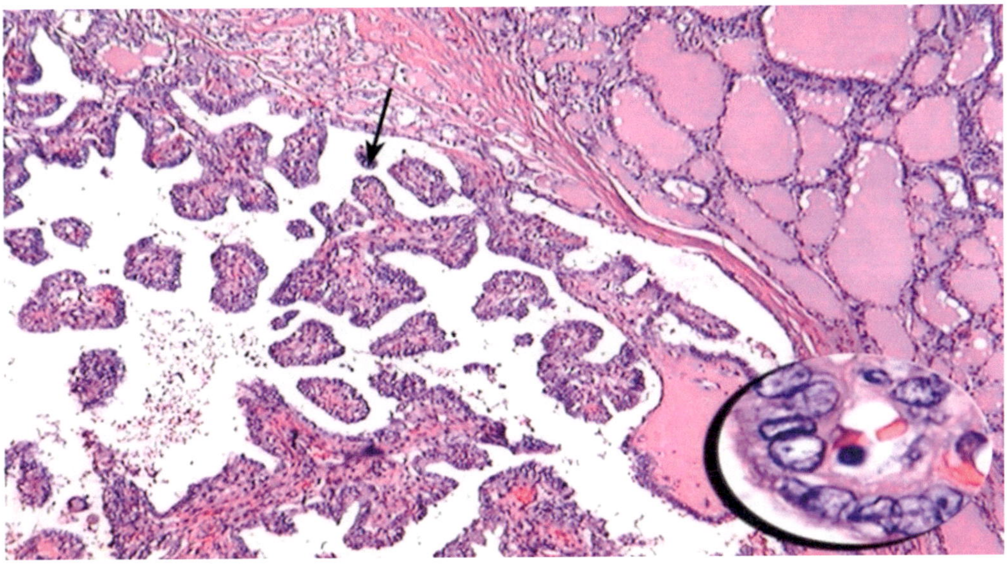

Figure 12: Classic variant of papillary thyroid carcinoma demonstrating complex papillary architecture (arrow) (Hematoxylin & Eosin stain, 10X). The inset shows diagnostic nuclear features (Hematoxylin & Eosin stain, 60X).

"A solid growth pattern is noted focally in many papillary carcinomas. When the solid growth represents >50% of the tumor mass, a diagnosis of ***solid variant of papillary carcinoma*** may be made". "It usually presents as a solid nodule with infiltration into the surrounding thyroid parenchyma. By light microscopy, the tumor shows solid nests of tumor cells with nuclear features of papillary carcinoma, separated by delicate to broad collagenous bands (Fig. **12**). Some tumors may show focal areas of follicular and papillary architecture. The nuclear features are those of papillary carcinoma, although the nuclei tend to be more rounded than oval. About 40% of these tumors show vascular invasion and extrathyroidal extension" [3, 29, 36, 41, 48, 49] (Fig. **13**).

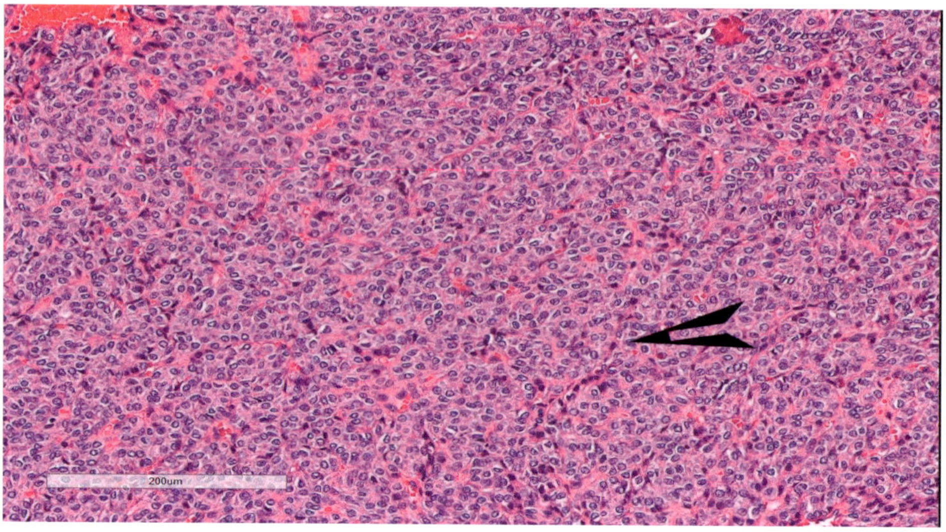

Figure 13: Solid variant of papillary thyroid carcinoma showing solid and trabecular growth pattern and thin walled vessels (arrow head)(Hematoxylin & Eosin stain 40X).

Although some studies, particularly from Japan, have considered the solid papillary carcinoma as a poorly differentiated tumor with a guarded prognosis, in North America and Europe, this has not been found. It is important to recognize these lesions as papillary carcinomas and not over-diagnose them as more aggressive tumors such as poorly differentiated (insular) carcinoma. Both papillary and non-papillary cancers of the thyroid can demonstrate areas of solid growth and/or insular growth patterns. We believe that these two should be morphologically separated; the areas of insular carcinoma usually show well-defined nests of monotonous tumor cells with round nuclei and scant cytoplasm. Loose connective tissue stroma and prominent vascularity separate the tumor nests from each other. Occasionally these areas may show foci of tumor necrosis [50].

The ***diffuse sclerosis variant (DSV)*** is a rare subtype of PTC, which was first described by Vickery and coworkers in 1985. It represents only about 1.8% of all papillary carcinomas in large series. This tumor, which most often affects children and young adults between 15 and 30 years of age is characterized by diffuse involvement of one or both lobes of the thyroid gland and may present as bilateral goiter. Grossly, the tumor is extremely hard, reflecting the extensive calcification. In addition to classic papillary nuclear features, it is histologically characterized by dense sclerosis, extensive squamous metaplasia, focal to diffuse lymphocytic infiltration, numerous psammoma bodies and small papillary to solid tumor deposits within intraglandular lymphatics [41, 51-54] (Fig. **14**). "Due to the presence of numerous psammoma bodies the ultrasound of the thyroid will show lymphatics outlined by calcium AKA "snow storm appearance". The squamous metaplasia of the tumor papillae resembles 'morular' metaplasia of the endometrium. As stated above, the lymphocytic infiltrates are found around the tumor foci; indeed, the background thyroid shows well-developed chronic lymphocytic thyroiditis. Both the histology and immunoprofile of the background thyroid are identical to Hashimoto's disease. It is unclear if the thyroiditis precedes the tumor or if it is developed as a reaction to the neoplasm. The lesions often show extra-capsular extension, distant, and nodal metastases (almost 100% will have regional node involvement at presentation) and recur in the neck. Earlier studies have shown that these tumors have a somewhat more serious prognosis than usual childhood/adolescent papillary cancer and a decreased disease-free survival when compared with the usual-type papillary carcinoma. However, the overall survival is not significantly different. The recent reports and case series have shown that the prognosis of this DSV-PTC is as good as that of classic PTC if aggressive treatment is given.

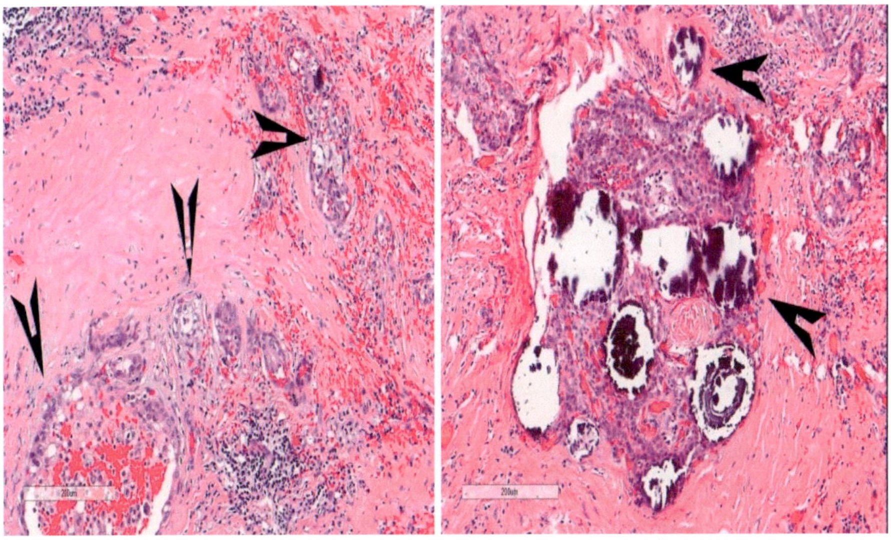

Figure 14 (a & b): Diffuse sclerosis variant of papillary thyroid carcinoma showing nests of tumor cells (arrow head) and associated sclerosis (Hematoxylin & Eosin stain 10X). High power showing characteristic lamellated clacification/psamomma bodies within the tumor nests (arrow heads) (Hematoxylin & Eosin stain 40X).

Abnormalities of E-cadherin/catenin adhesion complex have been identified in diffuse sclerosing variant and appear to be more pronounced in DSV than in classical PTC [55]. In DSV there is a pronounced reduction in its membranous expression, accompanied by a relocation to the cytoplasm compared to classic

PTC, where there is heterogeneous loss of E-cadherin expression. Inactivation of the E-cadherin/catenin complex appears to occur in DSV *via* two different pathways: [1] E-cadherin alteration either through mutation or through methylation of the E-cadherin gene promoter and [2] beta- and/or gamma-catenin alterations.

MOLECULAR BIOLOGY OF RADIATION INDUCED THYROID CARCINOMA

Rearrangements of RET gene, known as RET/PTC have been identified in papillary carcinoma of thyroid exposed to radiation [56-59]. The RET proto-oncogene is normally expressed in cells of neural crest origin and plays a role in kidney and gastrointestinal neuronal development. It is located on the long arm of chromosome 10q11.2 and codes for a cell membrane receptor tyrosine kinase. RET is relatively well conserved among species, and its homologs have been identified in several vertebrates as well as in Drosophila Melanogaster [60]. RET is encoded by 21 exons, and several RET messenger RNA (mRNA) splice variants specifying a unique protein isoform with distinct function [61].

In normal thyroid, wild type RET is only expressed in C cells and not follicular cells. RET/PTC seen in papillary carcinomas occurs due to fusion of tyrosine kinase domain of RET to the 5′ portion of various genes [56]. To date, 13 novel types of rearrangements have been described in papillary carcinoma [61, 62]. RET/PTC 1 and 3 are the most common forms that occur in sporadic papillary carcinoma. RET/PTC 1 accounts for 60% of the RET-associated PTC and is formed by fusion of RET to H4, whereas RET/PTC3 represents approximately 30% of PTCs and occurs due to fusion of RET to the ELE1 gene [63].

RET/PTC expression in thyroid follicular cells of transgenic mice leads to development of thyroid tumors with histologic features of papillary thyroid carcinoma [64]. Similarly, transfection of follicular cells in tissue culture by RET/PTC causes the cells to demonstrate nuclear features of papillary carcinoma [65]. The prevalence of RET/PTC in papillary carcinoma varies significantly among various geographic regions [66, 67]; in the United States it ranges from 11% to 43% [68]. In sporadic tumors RET/PTC1 is the most common form of rearrangement (60% to 70%) followed by RET/PTC3 (20% to 30%) [68]. The other rare forms of RET/PTC rearrangements have been mainly found in radiation induced papillary carcinomas [69].

Several studies have shown a strong association between radiation induced papillary carcinoma and expression of RET/PTC. Up to 72% of surgically resected tumors showed RET/PTC fusions as compared to 20% of non-irradiated populations [62, 68-70]. This finding is not surprising because ionizing radiation leads to double-stranded breaks in DNA; and the formation of aberrant chromosomal translocations, including those that lead to RET/PTC fusion genes are dependent on this type of DNA damage [62, 71, 72]. It has been shown that RET gene carries a particular predisposition to radiation induced fragmentation leading to RET/PTC fusions in both cultured cells and in mouse xenografts [72]. In addition, RET/PTC1 and 3 fusion are seen with high frequency in radiation-associated PTCs because of the physical proximity between RET gene on long arm of chromosome 10 and the donor genes (H4/CCD6 and RET activating gene ELE1/androgen receptor-associated protein). It has been shown RET and H4/CCD6 are directly juxtaposed in 30% of thyroid follicular cells during interphase [73].

It is interesting to note that overtime the proportion of post Chernobyl PTCs demonstrating RET/PTC have declined, but in the RET/PTC positive tumors, the proportion of RET-PTC1 has increased as compared to RET/PTC3 (opposite to that seen in early reports of Chernobyl induced PTCs)[74].

It is important to note that even though the oncogenic role of RET/PTC is specific to thyroid, studies have shown that RET/PTC expression can also occur in some benign lesions. These include hyalinizing trabecular adenoma, Hashimoto thyroiditis, and hyperplastic nodules and follicular adenoma [75-77].

Several authors have suggested an association between Hashimoto thyroiditis and papillary carcinoma [75, 76]; however, others have suggested that this association is most likely incidental since both are common [78]. Two independent studies have shown high prevalence of RET/PTC in histologically benign thyroid tissue affected by Hashimoto thyroiditis; these studies concluded that thyroiditic glands harbor multiple foci of papillary carcinoma which are not identified by histologic examination only [75, 79]. However, a study by Nikiforov and colleagues have disputed these findings and failed to reproduce these results [78].

Activation of the RAS oncogene is considered to be an important mechanism by which human cancer develops. RAS has been shown to regulate several pathways that contribute to cellular transformation including the Raf/MEK/ERK pathways [59]. Numerous studies confirm that the Raf/MEK/ERK pathway is a significant contributor to the malignant phenotype associated with deregulated RAS signaling [80, 81].

An activating mutation in BRAF has been described in 29%-69% of human papillary thyroid cancers. BRAF activating mutations in thyroid cancer are almost exclusively the BRAF V600E mutation, and have been found in 29-69% of papillary thyroid cancers, 13% of poorly differentiated cancers, and 10% of anaplastic cancers [82-84]. The role of BRAF as an oncogenic-initiating event in thyroid follicular cells has been confirmed in mouse models [84]. There is practically no concordance between papillary carcinoma with RET/PTC, BRAF or RAS mutations. The lack of this overlap provides strong evidence of this signaling pathway for thyroid follicular cells to develop into papillary carcinoma [85].

The BRAF-mutations are uncommon in post-Chernobyl related PTCs. Nikiforova and colleagues in a study of 55-post Chernobyl PTCs found BRAF point mutations in only 4% of cases as compared to 58% of cases showing RET/PTC rearrangements [86]. A study by Tronko and colleagues analyzed 35 cases, and found BRAF point mutations in 24% and RET-PTC rearrangements in 34.3% cases [36]. These differences may be either indicative of a true shift in molecular paradigm of radiation induced tumors or a result of increased screening due to Chernobyl fallout leading to increased diagnosis of non-radiation induced PTCs.

In a study of the genetic alterations in DSV, no BRAF (V600) mutations were found, but all the cases showed RET proto-oncogene (RET)/PTC rearrangements [87]. Another study supporting the above findings identified that the profile of genomic mutations detected in PTC-DSV is different from that in classic PTC [88]. None of genomic mutations of BRAF, 1p36, 3p12, 7p31, and 10q23 was detected in DSV, but a higher frequency of LOHs of 3p24, 9p21, 17q21, 21q22, and 22q13 was noted. It has been suggested that these mutations may play an important role in the different morphologic appearance and prognosis of DSV.

By molecular analysis cases of solid variant-PTC arising in association with radiation exposure has shown RET/PTC rearrangement. The RET/PTC3 rearrangement has been more frequently associated with SV-PTC [49, 77, 89], the most prevalent variant among the irradiated tumors. With the increase in latency period, both the solid variant and the RET/PTC rearrangements prevalence have declined, suggesting a strong relationship between radiation exposure, solid variant and RET/PTC3 [49]. Interestingly, a triplet deletion of the BRAF gene leading to the replacement of a valine and a lysine by a glutamate (BRAF V600E

+ K601), was first reported only in the solid variant of PTC by Trovisco and colleagues [90]; which has been confirmed by other investigators [91].

CONFLICT OF INTEREST

The author confirms that author has no conflict of interest to declare for this publication.

ACKNOWLEDGEMENTS

Declared None.

REFERENCES

[1] Grubbe EH. X-ray treatment; its introduction to medicine. J Am Inst Homeopath 1946; 39(12): 419-22.

[2] Grubbe EH. The origin and birth of x-ray therapy. Urol Cutaneous Rev 1947; 51(7): 375-9.

[3] Preston DL, Ron E, Tokuoka S, *et al.* Solid cancer incidence in atomic bomb survivors: 1958-1998. Radiat Res 2007; 168(1): 1-64.

[4] Murakami M, Oki T. Estimation of thyroid doses and health risks resulting from the intake of radioactive iodine in foods and drinking water by the citizens of Tokyo after the Fukushima nuclear accident. Chemosphere 2012; 87(11): 1355-60.

[5] Williams D. Radiation carcinogenesis: lessons from Chernobyl. Oncogene 2008; 27 Suppl 2: S9-18.

[6] Jargin SV. Chernobyl-Related Cancer and Precancerous Lesions: Incidence Increase *vs.* Late Diagnostics. Dose-response 2014; 12(3): 404-14.

[7] Imaizumi M, Usa T, Tominaga T, *et al.* Radiation dose-response relationships for thyroid nodules and autoimmune thyroid diseases in Hiroshima and Nagasaki atomic bomb survivors 55-58 years after radiation exposure. JAMA 2006; 295(9): 1011-22.

[8] Hamada N, Fujimichi Y. Classification of radiation effects for dose limitation purposes: history, current situation and future prospects. J Radiat Res 2014; 55(4): 629-40.

[9] Seo D, Han S, Kim KH, *et al.* Evaluation based on Monte Carlo simulation of lifetime attributable risk of cancer after neck X-ray radiography. Radiol Med 2015. [Epub ahead of print]

[10] Sjoblom T, Jones S, Wood LD, *et al.* The consensus coding sequences of human breast and colorectal cancers. Science 2006; 314(5797): 268-74.

[11] Blumgart HL, Freedberg AS, Kurland GS. Treatment of incapacitated euthyroid cardiac patients with radioactive iodine: summary of results in treatment of 1,070 patients with angina pectoris or congestive failure. J Am Med Assoc 1955; 157(1): 1-4.

[12] Einhorn J, Wilkholm G. Hypothyroidism after external irradiation to the thyroid region. Radiology 1967; 88(2): 326-8.

[13] Hancock SL, McDougall IR, Constine LS. Thyroid abnormalities after therapeutic external radiation. Int J Radiat Oncol Biol Phys 1995; 31(5): 1165-70.

[14] Carr RF, LiVolsi VA. Morphologic changes in the thyroid after irradiation for Hodgkin's and non-Hodgkin's lymphoma. Cancer 1989; 64(4): 825-9.

[15] Sarne D, Schneider AB. External radiation and thyroid neoplasia. Endocrinol Metab Clin North Am 1996; 25(1): 181-95.

[16] Aizawa T, Watanabe T, Suzuki N, *et al.* Radiation-induced painless thyrotoxic thyroiditis followed by hypothyroidism: a case report and literature review. Thyroid 1998; 8(3): 273-5.

[17] Nikiforov YE, Gnepp DR. Pathomorphology of thyroid gland lesions associated with radiation exposure: the Chernobyl experience and review of the literature. Adv Anat Pathol 1999; 6(2): 78-91.

[18] Fushiki S. Radiation hazards in children - lessons from Chernobyl, Three Mile Island and Fukushima. Brain Dev 2013; 35(3): 220-7.

[19] Nishiyama K, Kozuka T, Higashihara T, Miyauchi K, Okagawa K. Acute radiation thyroiditis. Int J Radiat Oncol Biol Phys 1996; 36(5): 1221-4.

[20] Fajardo LF. Basic mechanisms and general morphology of radiation injury. Semin Roentgenol 1993; 28(4): 297-302.

[21] Fajardo LF. The pathology of ionizing radiation as defined by morphologic patterns. Acta Oncol 2005; 44(1): 13-22.

[22] Fajardo LF, Berthrong M. Radiation injury in surgical pathology. Part I. Am J Surg Pathol 1978; 2(2): 159-99.

[23] van Dorp W, van Beek RD, Laven JS, Pieters R, de Muinck Keizer-Schrama SM, van den Heuvel-Eibrink MM. Long-term endocrine side effects of childhood Hodgkin's lymphoma treatment: a review. Hum Reprod Update 2012; 18(1): 12-28.

[24] Jereczek-Fossa BA, Alterio D, Jassem J, Gibelli B, Tradati N, Orecchia R. Radiotherapy-induced thyroid disorders. Cancer Treat Rev 2004; 30(4): 369-84.

[25] Sigurdson AJ, Bhatti P, Doody MM, *et al.* Polymorphisms in apoptosis- and proliferation-related genes, ionizing radiation exposure, and risk of breast cancer among U.S. Radiologic Technologists. Cancer Epidemiol Biomarkers Prev 2007; 16(10): 2000-7.

[26] Williams ED. Radiation-induced thyroid cancer. Histopathology 1993; 23(4): 387-9.

[27] Williams ED. Chernobyl and thyroid cancer. J Surg Oncol 2006; 94(8): 670-7.

[28] Dinets A, Hulchiy M, Sofiadis A, *et al.* Clinical, genetic, and immunohistochemical characterization of 70 Ukrainian adult cases with post-Chornobyl papillary thyroid carcinoma. Eur J Endocrinol 2012; 166(6): 1049-60.

[29] Fridman M, Savva N, Krasko O, *et al.* Initial presentation and late results of treatment of post-Chernobyl papillary thyroid carcinoma in children and adolescents of Belarus. J Clin Endocrinol Metab 2014; 99(8): 2932-41.

[30] Sampson RJ, Key CR, Buncher CR, Iijima S. Thyroid carcinoma in Hiroshima and Nagasaki. I. Prevalence of thyroid carcinoma at autopsy. JAMA 1969; 209 (1): 65-70.

[31] Sampson RJ, Key CR, Buncher CR, Oka H, Iijima S. Papillary carcinoma of the thyroid gland. Sizes of 525 tumors found at autopsy in Hiroshima and Nagasaki. Cancer 1970; 25(6): 1391-3.

[32] Williams ED, Pacini F, Pinchera A. Thyroid cancer following Chernobyl. J Endocrinol Invest. 1995; 18(2): 144-6.

[33] Thomas GA, Tronko MD, Tsyb AF, Tuttle RM. What have we learnt from Chernobyl? What have we still to learn? Clin Oncol (R Coll Radiol) 2011; 23(4): 229-33.

[34] Avetisian IL, Gulchiy NV, Demidiuk AP, Stashuk AV. Thyroid pathology in residents of the Kiev region, Ukraine, during pre- and post-Chernobyl periods. J Environ Pathol Toxicol Oncol 1996; 15(2-4): 233-7.

[35] Petrova GV, Tereshchenko VP, Avetis'ian IL. [The dynamics of thyroid diseases in the inhabitants of Kiev and Kiev Province after the accident at the Chernobyl Atomic Electric Power Station]. Lik Sprava 1996; 5-6: 67-70.

[36] Tronko MD, Bogdanova TI, Komissarenko IV, *et al.* Thyroid carcinoma in children and adolescents in Ukraine after the Chernobyl nuclear accident: statistical data and clinicomorphologic characteristics. Cancer 1999; 86(1): 149-56.

[37] Pacini F, Vorontsova T, Molinaro E, *et al.* Thyroid consequences of the Chernobyl nuclear accident. Acta Paediatr Suppl 1999; 88(433): 23-7.

[38] Cetta F, Montalto G, Petracci M, Fusco A. Thyroid cancer and the Chernobyl accident. Are long-term and long distance side effects of fall-out radiation greater than estimated? J Clin Endocrinol Metab 1997; 82(6): 2015-7.

[39] Nikiforov Y, Gnepp DR, Fagin JA. Thyroid lesions in children and adolescents after the Chernobyl disaster: implications for the study of radiation tumorigenesis. J Clin Endocrinol Metab 1996; 81(1): 9-14.

[40] Tuttle RM, Vaisman F, Tronko MD. Clinical presentation and clinical outcomes in Chernobyl-related paediatric thyroid cancers: what do we know now? What can we expect in the future? Clin Oncol (R Coll Radiol) 2011; 23(4): 268-75.

[41] LiVolsi VA, Abrosimov AA, Bogdanova T, *et al.* The Chernobyl thyroid cancer experience: pathology. Clin Oncol (R Coll Radiol) 2011; 23(4): 261-7.

[42] Thomas GA, Williams ED. International cooperation post-Chernobyl. Scientific project panel of the international cooperation to establish post chernobyl thyroid tissue, nucleic acid and databanks. Int J Radiat Biol 2001; 77(2): 254.
[43] Nikiforov YE, Heffess CS, Korzenko AV, Fagin JA, Gnepp DR. Characteristics of follicular tumors and nonneoplastic thyroid lesions in children and adolescents exposed to radiation as a result of the Chernobyl disaster. Cancer 1995; 76(5): 900-9.
[44] Nikiforov Y, Gnepp DR. Pediatric thyroid cancer after the Chernobyl disaster. Pathomorphologic study of 84 cases (1991-1992) from the Republic of Belarus. Cancer 1994; 74(2): 748-66.
[45] Baloch Z, LiVolsi VA. Pathology of the Thyroid Gland. Livolsi VA, Asa S, editors. Philadelphia, PA: Churchill Livingston; 2002; 61-88 p.
[46] LiVolsi VA. Well differentiated thyroid carcinoma. Clin Oncol (R Coll Radiol). 1996; 8(5): 281-8.
[47] LiVolsi VA. Surgical Pathology of The Thyroid. Philadelphia, PA: WB. Saunders; 1990.
[48] Krestinina LY, Davis F, Ostroumova E, *et al.* Solid cancer incidence and low-dose-rate radiation exposures in the Techa River cohort: 1956 2002. Int J Epidemiol 2007 36(5): 1038-46.
[49] Nikiforov YE, Erickson LA, Nikiforova MN, Caudill CM, Lloyd RV. Solid variant of papillary thyroid carcinoma: incidence, clinical- pathologic characteristics, molecular analysis, and biologic behavior. Am J Surg Pathol 2001; 25(12): 1478-84.
[50] Carcangiu ML, Zampi G, Rosai J. Poorly differentiated ("insular") thyroid carcinoma. A reinterpretation of Langhans' "wuchernde Struma". Am J Surg Pathol 1984; 8(9): 655-68.
[51] Albareda M, Puig-Domingo M, Wengrowicz S, *et al.* Clinical forms of presentation and evolution of diffuse sclerosing variant of papillary carcinoma and insular variant of follicular carcinoma of the thyroid. Thyroid 1998; 8(5): 385-91.
[52] Carcangiu ML, Bianchi S. Diffuse sclerosing variant of papillary thyroid carcinoma. Clinicopathologic study of 15 cases. Am J Surg Pathol 1989; 13(12): 1041-9.
[53] Chan JKC, Tsui MS, Tse CH. Diffuse sclerosing variant of papillary thyroid carcinoma. A histological and immunohistochemical study of three cases. Histopathology 1987; 11: 191-201.
[54] Gomez-Morales M, Alvaro T, Munoz M, *et al.* Diffuse sclerosing papillary carcinoma of the thyroid gland: immunohistochemical analysis of the local host immune response. Histopathology 1991; 18(5): 427-33.
[55] Rocha AS, Soares P, Seruca R, *et al.* Abnormalities of the E-cadherin/catenin adhesion complex in classical papillary thyroid carcinoma and in its diffuse sclerosing variant. J Pathol 2001; 194(3): 358-66.
[56] Fusco A, Santoro M, Grieco M, *et al.* RET/PTC activation in human thyroid carcinomas. J Endocrinol Invest 1995; 18(2): 127-9.
[57] Sheils OM, O'Leary JJ, Sweeney EC. Assessment of ret/PTC-1 rearrangements in neoplastic thyroid tissue using TaqMan RT-PCR. J Pathol 2000; 192(1): 32-6.
[58] Basolo F, Giannini R, Monaco C, *et al.* Potent mitogenicity of the RET/PTC3 oncogene correlates with its prevalence in tall-cell variant of papillary thyroid carcinoma. Am J Pathol 2002; 160(1): 247-54.
[59] Giordano TJ, Kuick R, Thomas DG, *et al.* Molecular classification of papillary thyroid carcinoma: distinct BRAF, RAS, and RET/PTC mutation-specific gene expression profiles discovered by DNA microarray analysis. Oncogene 2005; 24(44): 6646-56.
[60] Sugaya R, Ishimaru S, Hosoya T, Saigo K, Emori Y. A Drosophila homolog of human proto-oncogene ret transiently expressed in embryonic neuronal precursor cells including neuroblasts and CNS cells. Mech Dev 1994; 45(2): 139-45.
[61] Romei C, Elisei R. RET/PTC Translocations and Clinico-Pathological Features in Human Papillary Thyroid Carcinoma. Front Endocrinol 2012; 3: 54.
[62] Prescott JD, Zeiger MA. The RET oncogene in papillary thyroid carcinoma. Cancer 2015; doi: 10.1002/cncr.29044. [Epub ahead of print]
[63] Ciampi R, Nikiforov YE. RET/PTC rearrangements and BRAF mutations in thyroid tumorigenesis. Endocrinology 2007; 148(3): 936-41.
[64] Jhiang SM, Sagartz JE, Tong Q, *et al.* Targeted expression of the ret/PTC1 oncogene induces papillary thyroid carcinomas. Endocrinology 1996; 137(1): 375-8.

[65] Fischer AH, Bond JA, Taysavang P, O.Eugene B, Wynford-Thomas D. Papillary thyroid carcinoma oncogene (RET/PTC) alters the nuclear envelope and chromatin structure. Am J Pathol 1998; 153(5): 1443-50.
[66] Zou M, Shi Y, Farid NR. Low rate of ret proto-oncogene activation (PTC/retTPC) in papillary thyroid carcinomas from Saudi Arabia. Cancer 1994; 73(1): 176-80.
[67] Motomura T, Nikiforov YE, Namba H, *et al*. ret rearrangements in Japanese pediatric and adult papillary thyroid cancers. Thyroid 1998; 8(6): 485-9.
[68] Nikiforov YE. RET/PTC Rearrangement in Thyroid Tumors. Endocr Pathol 2002; 13(1): 3-16.
[69] Nikiforov YE, Koshoffer A, Nikiforova M, Stringer J, Fagin JA. Chromosomal breakpoint positions suggest a direct role for radiation in inducing illegitimate recombination between the ELE1 and RET genes in radiation-induced thyroid carcinomas. Oncogene 1999; 18(46): 6330-4.
[70] Thomas GA, Bunnell H, Cook HA, *et al*. High prevalence of RET/PTC rearrangements in Ukrainian and Belarussian post-Chernobyl thyroid papillary carcinomas: a strong correlation between RET/PTC3 and the solid-follicular variant. J Clin Endocrinol Metab 1999; 84(11): 4232-8.
[71] Ito T, Seyama T, Iwamoto KS, *et al*. *In vitro* irradiation is able to cause RET oncogene rearrangement. Cancer Res 1993; 53(13): 2940-3.
[72] Mizuno T, Iwamoto KS, Kyoizumi S, *et al*. Preferential induction of RET/PTC1 rearrangement by X-ray irradiation. Oncogene 2000; 19(3): 438-43.
[73] Nikiforova MN, Stringer JR, Blough R, Medvedovic M, Fagin JA, Nikiforov YE. Proximity of chromosomal loci that participate in radiation-induced rearrangements in human cells. Science 2000; 290(5489): 138-41.
[74] Rabes HM, Demidchik EP, Sidorow JD, *et al*. Pattern of radiation-induced RET and NTRK1 rearrangements in 191 post-chernobyl papillary thyroid carcinomas: biological, phenotypic, and clinical implications. Clin Cancer Res 2000; 6(3): 1093-103.
[75] Wirtschafter A, Schmidt R, Rosen D, *et al*. Expression of the RET/PTC fusion gene as a marker for papillary carcinoma in Hashimoto's thyroiditis. [see comments]. Laryngoscope 1997; 107(1): 95-100.
[76] Sheils O, Smyth P, Finn S, Sweeney EC, O'Leary JJ. RET/PTC rearrangements in Hashimoto's thyroiditis. Int J Surg Pathol 2002; 10(2): 167-8; discussion 8-9.
[77] Elisei R, Romei C, Vorontsova T, *et al*. RET/PTC rearrangements in thyroid nodules: studies in irradiated and not irradiated, malignant and benign thyroid lesions in children and adults. J Clin Endocrinol Metab 2001; 86(7): 3211-6.
[78] Nikiforova MN, Caudill CM, Biddinger P, Nikiforov YE. Prevalence of RET/PTC rearrangements in hashimoto's thyroiditis and papillary thyroid carcinomas. Int J Surg Pathol 2002; 10(1): 15-22.
[79] Di Pasquale M, Rothstein JL, Palazzo JP. Pathologic features of Hashimoto's-associated papillary thyroid carcinomas. Hum Pathol 2001; 32(1): 24-30.
[80] Capella G, Matias-Guiu X, Ampudia X, de Leiva A, Perucho M, Prat J. Ras oncogene mutations in thyroid tumors: polymerase chain reaction- restriction-fragment-length polymorphism analysis from paraffin- embedded tissues. Diagn Mol Pathol 1996; 5(1): 45-52.
[81] Esapa CT, Johnson SJ, Kendall-Taylor P, Lennard TW, Harris PE. Prevalence of Ras mutations in thyroid neoplasia. Clin Endocrinol 1999; 50(4): 529-35.
[82] Cohen Y, Xing M, Mambo E, *et al*. BRAF mutation in papillary thyroid carcinoma. J Natl Cancer Inst 2003; 95(8): 625-7.
[83] Fukushima T, Suzuki S, Mashiko M, *et al*. BRAF mutations in papillary carcinomas of the thyroid. Oncogene 2003; 22(41): 6455-7.
[84] Xu X, Quiros RM, Gattuso P, Ain KB, Prinz RA. High prevalence of BRAF gene mutation in papillary thyroid carcinomas and thyroid tumor cell lines. Cancer Res 2003; 63(15): 4561-7.
[85] Melillo RM, Castellone MD, Guarino V, *et al*. The RET/PTC-RAS-BRAF linear signaling cascade mediates the motile and mitogenic phenotype of thyroid cancer cells. J Clin Invest 2005; 115(4): 1068-81.
[86] Nikiforova MN, Ciampi R, Salvatore G, *et al*. Low prevalence of BRAF mutations in radiation-induced thyroid tumors in contrast to sporadic papillary carcinomas. Cancer Lett 2004; 209(1): 1-6.
[87] Sheu SY, Schwertheim S, Worm K, Grabellus F, Schmid KW. Diffuse sclerosing variant of papillary thyroid carcinoma: lack of BRAF mutation but occurrence of RET/PTC rearrangements. Mod Pathol 2007; 20(7): 779-87.

[88] Lin X, Finkelstein SD, Zhu B, Silverman JF. Molecular analysis of multifocal papillary thyroid carcinoma. J Mol Endocrinol 2008; 41(4): 195-203.
[89] Gandhi M, Evdokimova V, Nikiforov YE. Mechanisms of chromosomal rearrangements in solid tumors: the model of papillary thyroid carcinoma. Mol and Cell Endocrinol 2010; 321(1): 36-43.
[90] Trovisco V, Soares P, Preto A, *et al*. Type and prevalence of BRAF mutations are closely associated with papillary thyroid carcinoma histotype and patients' age but not with tumour aggressiveness. Virchows Arch 2005; 446(6): 589-95.
[91] Chiosea S, Nikiforova M, Zuo H, *et al*. A novel complex BRAF mutation detected in a solid variant of papillary thyroid carcinoma. Endocr Pathol 2009; 20(2): 122-6.

CHAPTER 10

Foods: Functional Foods, Food Additives and Dietetic Supplements

Margarita Lobo[1], Jimena García[2] and Javier Del Pino[1,*]

[1]*Departament of Toxicology and Pharmacology, Veterinary School, Complutense University of Madrid, Madrid, Spain and* [2]*Department of Pharmacology, Health Sciences School, Alfonso X University, Madrid, Spain*

Abstract: Foods are composed of a variety of natural compounds with nutritional effects. However, some of them may also possess anti-nutritional and thyroid toxic effects, such as glucosinolate compounds, which are present in foods derived from higher plants. Currently, functional foods have been incorporated as sources of nutrients to our diet in order to meet certain nutritional requirements not present in conventional food; their effects on the thyroid gland are unknown and should be determined in order to perform a complete risk assessments of these foods. Food supplements, which are used widely by the population in many countries, are another source of nutrients, especially minerals and trace elements such as iodine and zinc that are necessary for the proper functioning of the thyroid gland, but if their use is not controlled they may induce alterations of the thyroid system. Furthermore, many of these dietary supplements also contain plants, algae and soybean in their composition that can exert harmful effects on normal thyroid function. Finally, during food processing different chemical compounds such as nitrate and erythrosine could be used, which could also induce harmful effects on the thyroid system. This chapter will discuss all of the foods and supplements mentioned above and their possible effects on normal thyroid function.

Keywords: Dietetic supplements, food, food additives, functional foods.

INTRODUCTION

Plant foods are mixtures of many substances, and since any substance can be toxic if consumed in large quantities and under certain circumstances, it is not surprising that some plant foods are considered toxic to the thyroid gland. This is the case of many plant foods from the Cruciferae family whose carcinogenic and goitrogenic effects on thyroid gland have been clearly demonstrated in certain populations with a high intake of these foods and lack of iodine in their diet [1].

*Corresponding author Javier Del Pino:** Department of Toxicology and Pharmacology, Complutense University of Madrid, Madrid, Spain; E-mail: jdelpino@pdi.ucm.es

Javier Del Pino, Maria Jesus Diaz and Maria Teresa Frejo (Eds)

Metabolism of cyanogenic plants like cassava, sorghum, bamboo, lima bean, which are important sources of carbohydrates for many populations, releases thiocyanate that has been proved to have goitrogenic properties [2, 3].

Currently there is a significant increase in consumption of new foods called functional foods, especially soy, which could lead to iodine goitrogenic effects due to the fact that elevated soy consumption and diets poor in iodine are associated with alterations in the thyroid [4]. Also, the use of dietary supplements, that are widespread today, can cause thyrotoxicosis since some of them may contain fraudulently added active thyroid hormones besides minerals and dietary elements [5]. Furthermore, plant supplements, which are consumed worldwide, may contain many components that could alter the normal functioning of the thyroid system due to their phytochemical components. Therefore, the increasing use of plant supplements presents a particular challenge to health care of patients due to the high risk of possible of plants with drugs [6].

Food additives used to preserve flavor or enhance taste and appearance could also induce disruption of the thyroid system. Nitrite and nitrate salts are additives used in cured meats such as bacon, sausage and ham avoid the growth of bacteria spores and to add color and flavor [7]. Nitrate salts are natural components of plants, contained in high levels in leafy vegetables such as lettuce and spinach and in some root vegetables such as beets, and are also a contaminant in drinking water [8-10]. Nitrate salts are of particular interest because they cause thyroid cancer by competitively inhibiting thyroid iodine uptake, chronically increasing the production of thyroid stimulating hormone (TSH), causing thyroid cancers in animal models [11]. Dye additive foods such as erythrocin possess a negative effect on thyroid function in some cases partnering with tumors in the thyroid gland [12].

GOITROGENIC COMPOUNDS IN PLANT FOODS

Glucosinolates

Some raw foods have been found present compounds that disrupt thyroid gland functions by interfering with absorption of iodine, which is an essential element during development for maintaining cognitive function and hormonal balance [13]. The decreased iodine uptake causes an increase in thyroid size, leading to goiter [14]. Many foods have been classify as goitrogens such as spinach, yucca, cassava, peanuts, soybeans, strawberries, sweet potatoes, apricots, pears and brassica vegetables including broccoli, Brussels sprouts, cabbage, canola, cauliflower, mustard greens and radishes. Iodine uptake from these plant foods could be inhibited by the goitrogenic substances called glucosinolates (GLS) that are present in them (Fig. **1**) [15].

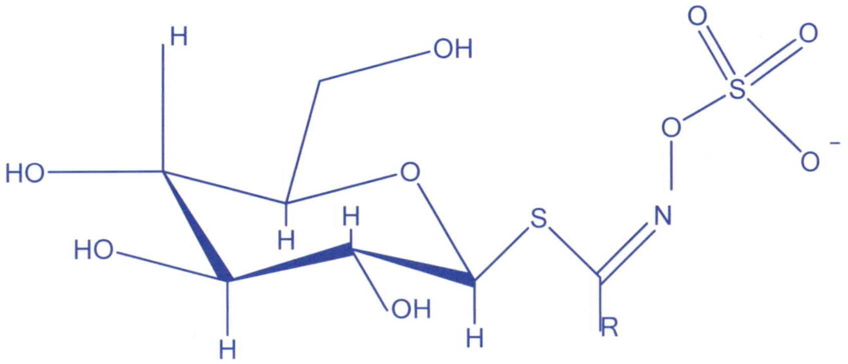

Figure 1: Glucosinolate chemical structure.

Most GLSs are chemically and thermally not alterable and therefore their hydrolysis is principally enzymatic [16]. Enzymatic hydrolysis is carried out by myrosinase, a β-thioglucosidase enzyme that co-occurs in plants with glucosinolates. In intact plant tissues, myrosinase is contained in different compartments of its substrate. After tissue disruption, enzyme and substrate (GLS) come into contact, producing hydrolysis of the thioglucosidic bond, and thereby yielding glucose and an unstable aglycone, thiohydroxamate-O-sulfonate (Fig. **2**). The latter experiences spontaneous reorganization into different possible compounds: isothiocyanates (ITCs), nitriles and elemental sulfur, thiocyanates, epithionitriles, oxazolidine-2-thiones andindolyl compounds. High intake of these plants could induce thyroid toxicity. In this regard, it has been reported that consumption of large amounts of Chinese cabbage (Brassica rapachinensis) could cause myxedema coma [17].

Thiocyanate and nitrile are the products of degradation of isothiocyanate and cause inhibition of iodine incorporation by the thyroid gland which is greater if there is iodine deficiency in the diet [18]. The thiocyanate monovalent anion, which inhibits iodide transport, is not concentrated in the gland and acts by uncoupling oxidative phosphorylation of thyroid gland [19]. Goitrin products of glucosinolate hydrolysis, have been reported to not diminish the ability of the thyroid to incorporate iodine, but rather to block the formation of iodinated amino acids through thyroid peroxidase (TPO) inhibition [20]. Moreover, thyroxine (T4) secretion has been described to be decreased and the stored hormone to be depleted by reduction of re-synthesis [20]. These compounds have been shown to increase TSH secretion that causes a highly vascular hyperplastic thyroid gland, which has a much greater ability to incorporate iodide [20].

However, little information is available about the salubrious and injurious effects of the GLS and their hydrolysis products regarding the dose. Depending on the quantity of these vegetables ingested by humans and animals, some positive or negative metabolic results of these molecules have been reported. In this regard, GLS have been described to be anticarcinogenic with antioxidant and antibiotic activity and to induce phase-II detoxification enzymes [16]. Moreover, indole-3-carbinol (I3C), a hydrolysis product of GLS has been shown to both stimulate and inhibit carcinogenesis [16]. According to these data intake of plant foods, which contain high levels of GLS, could also present different effects on thyroid system depending on the dose. Therefore, further studies are required to clarify these issues.

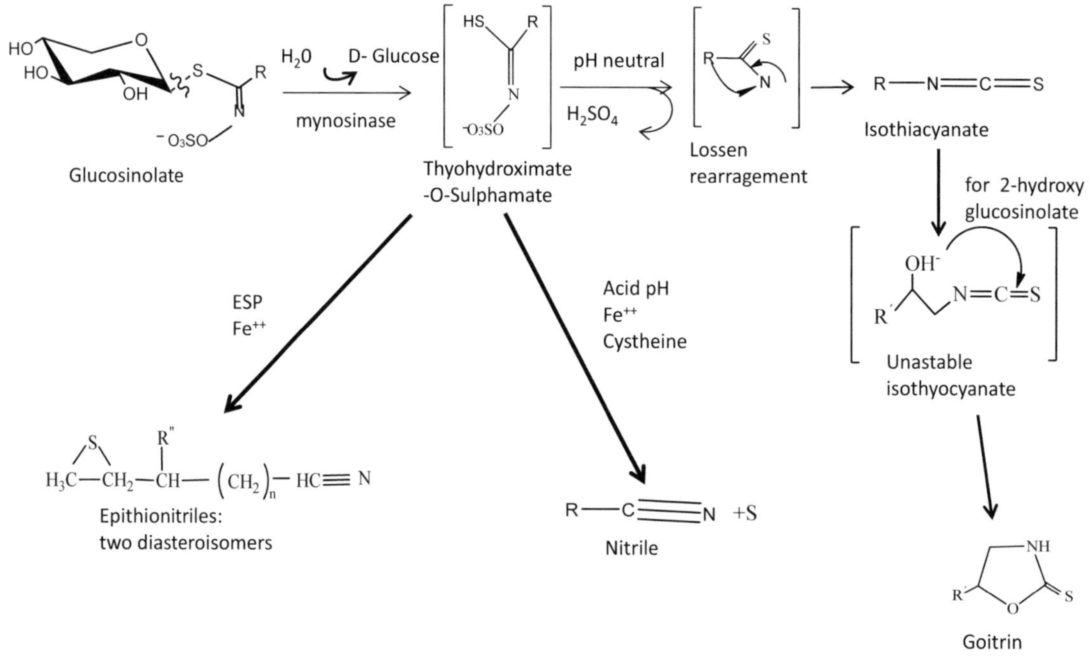

Figure 2: Glucosinolate hydrolysis and formation of GLS-hydrolysis products.

Flavonoids

Flavonoids are natural compounds necessary for plant defense and development that act as pigments [21, 22]. Among flavonoids, flavonols are those contained in greatest amounts in vegetable foods, with quercetin, kaempferol, and myricetin being the three most prevalent [23]. Flavonoids, have been described to be capable of interfering with thyroid hormone homeostasis. The first report describing the antithyroid action of flavonoids was published as early as 1950s, when Moudgal and coworkers [15] reported that rats fed with a diet containing 20 mg of arachidoside and anacardioside, pigments isolated from nuts, developed goiter. These authors showed that flavonoids were able not only of inhibiting thyroid hormone synthesis, but also of decreasing thyroidiodide uptake *in vitro*. An antithyroid effect of millet, which is a staple food consumed by poor populations in many regions of Africa and Asia, has been reported and these effects correlated with the c-glycosyl flavones content, suggesting that flavonoids could exert goitrogenic effects *in vivo* [24]. In addition, it was shown that the staple food pearl millet presents high quantity of apigenin and luteolin, flavonoids able of reducing both organification and discharge of thyroid hormones [25].

The mechanism through which flavonoids could inhibit thyroid hormone synthesis is not well understood. Divi and Doerge [21] assessed the actions of the flavonoids baicalein, biochanin A, catechin, fisetin, flavanone, flavone, kaempferol, morin, myricetin, naringenin, naringin, quercetin and rutin on blockade of TPO. All flavonoids tested excluding flavanone and flavone blocked tyrosine iodination by TPO, but with markedly different potencies. These authors also described that blockade of TPO by fisetin, kaempferol, naringenin, and quercetin, compounds that present a resorcinol moiety, was consistent with the previously observed inhibition with resorcinol and derivatives. Reactive resorcinol radicals inactivate the enzyme through covalent binding to catalytic amino acid radical(s). Due to their blocking effect on TPO activity, these compounds might produce an increase in TSH levels, resulting in thyroid gland growth and goiter, specifically when consumed at high concentrations.

FUNCTIONAL FOODS

Functional foods are foods that have been shown to provide certain specific health effects besides nutritional value, either due to their content of natural nutrients and/or bioactive substances, or due the fact that these substances are added to the food, giving beneficial effect on health. These effects have been demonstrated by scientific studies. Functional foods should be taken as part of the individual's diet, regularly and continuously, to be able to produce the anticipated health effects [26].

Soy Products

Soy foods are functional foods derived from soy proteins and isoflavones and provide health benefits such as easing postmenopausal symptoms in women, reducing the risk of osteoporosis, preventing cardiovascular disease and antimutagenic effects [26, 28]. However, soy contains the flavonoids genistein and daidzein, which have been described to block TPO activity, even in concentrations similar to those found in serum of subjects consuming soy derivatives that could disrupt thyroid hormones levels [29]. It has been shown that soy consumption in humans leads to a transient elevation in TSH levels, with significant correlation between basal levels of daidzein and TSH that suggests an effect of this flavonoid on the HPT axis [30]. Moreover, it has been reported that soy consumption by dogs for 12 months raised serum T4, without alteration in triiodothyronine (T3) levels [30]. The authors suggested that this result could be due to the blockade of 5′-deiodinase activity. Furthermore, a suppressive effect of some flavonoids on thyroid function in rats has been reported [31].

There are some controversial data about this issue in humans. Goiter in infants fed with soy formula was reported, which was usually reversed by changing to cow's milk or iodine-supplemented diets [32]. Hydovitz [33], Shepard and coworkers [34], Ripp [35] and Fort and coworkers [36] conducted retrospective epidemiologic studies on teenagers and children diagnosed with autoimmune thyroid diseases (Hashimoto's thyroiditis or Graves' disease). The children ingesting soy formula during infancy had twice the prevalence of autoimmune disease (31%) compared to healthy siblings (12%) or controls (13%). However, elevated prevalence of autoimmune thyroiditis in children fed with soy formulas reported by Fort and coworkers [36] has been criticized because children put on soy formula could more likely present autoimmune disorders (*e.g.*, food allergies, presence of viral gastroenteritis). These critics could also be questioned because only 0.5%-1.0% of American infants present true allergies, but about 20% are on soy formula. The alternative hypothesis to explain the observations of Fort and coworkers [36] could be the stimulation of immune function by genistein, and possible neoantigen formation through covalent binding of genistein to TPO, increasing the prevalence of autoimmune disease.

Bitto and coworkers [37] showed that genistein intake by climacteric women for 36 months did not significantly affect thyroid function. The same was reported in a study by Bruce and coworkers [38] in which climacteric women consumed soy-derived isoflavones daily for 6 months. However, Ishizuki and coworkers [39] administered 30 g of soybeans to healthy subjects every day for 1 or 3 months and described that some hypometabolic symptoms and goiter appeared in half the subjects taking soybeans for 3 months, but the symptoms disappeared 1 month after the suspension of soybean consumption. The authors suggested that excessive soybean consumption may produce goiter in healthy people, depending on the duration of the treatment. Further studies of autoimmune thyroiditis in children consuming soy formula and in adults under different health conditions are needed to clarify this controversy.

Green and Black Teas

Tea is the main broadly widely consumed beverage in the world, second only to water. Green and black teas reduce the risk of cardiovascular diseases, present anticarcinogenic and neuroprotective effects, and have the potential to cause significant effects on metabolic targets such as satiety, thermogenesis, and fat oxidation among other effects [40-43]. However, Chandra and coworkers [44] reported that green and black tea extracts, present in some functional foods, alter thyroid gland physiology and architecture, with enlargement of the thyroid gland as well as hypertrophy and/or hyperplasia of the thyroid follicles and blockade of TPO and deiodinase type I activities. Thyroidal Na^{+}, K^{+}-ATPase activity was increased, along with a reduction in serum T3 and T4, and an increase in TSH levels. Moreover, Chandra and De [45] showed that the catechin flavonol, present in green and black tea extracts, is able to block TPO activity and decrease both serum T3 and T4 levels, and increase TSH concentration. Genistein and daidzein could also be present in green and black tea extracts and the treatment with them has also been shown to decrease total serum T3 and T4 and increase TSH levels in orchidectomized middle-aged rats [46]. Thus, depending on the dose and time of treatment and species, flavonoids seem to show relevant antithyroid effects, altering biosynthesis, metabolism and transport of thyroid hormones *in vivo* and *in vitro*. However, relevant adverse effects, such as goiter, are not very often described among humans consuming vegetables containing flavonoids.

Seaweed and Other Kelps

Seaweeds present bioactive substances not contained in terrestrial food sources, including different proteins (lectins, phycobiliproteins, peptides, and amino acids), polyphenols, and polysaccharides. Thus, seaweeds are a new source of substances with potential to be used in human health applications. The proposed benefits of seaweeds include cardioprotective potential, antiviral, anticancer and anticoagulant properties as well as the ability to regulate gut and risk factors for obesity and diabetes [47, 48]. Moreover, seaweeds are a notable source of some essential elements such as iron and iodine, but the mineral composition of seaweed is very inconstant because of many exogenous and endogenous factors [49].

However, various reports have described thyroid disruption after seaweed consumption similar to that induced after excessive iodine intake. In this regard, Matola and coworker [50] described a case of thyroid dysfunction after the consumption of a kelp-containing marketed diet in a 45-year-old woman with no preceding thyroid disease. The clinical history was compatible with a case of iodine-induced thyrotoxicosis followed by prolonged inhibition of the sodium-iodide symporter activity as a consequence of excessive iodine ingestion from kelp. Moreover, Crawford and coworkers [51] reported a series of thyroid dysfunction cases in adults related with ingestion of a brand of soy milk produced with kombu (seaweed), and a case of hypothyroidism in a newborn whose mother had been drinking this milk. They also reported two cases of neonatal hypothyroidism linked to maternal composition of seaweed made into soup. These products were found to present high levels of iodine. In addition, short-term dietary supplementation with kelp has been shown to significantly increase both basal and post stimulation TSH. These results corroborate preceding studies on the effects of supplemental iodide given to euthyroid subjects for a similar period [52].

Despite raising awareness of iodine deficiency, the potential toxicity of iodine excess, especially from sources such as seaweed, is less well recognized. These cases highlight the risks of excess iodine intake from dietary sources and support the necessity of monitoring iodine levels in imported foods and commercially available seaweed preparations.

DIETETIC SUPPLEMENTS AND NUTRACEUTICS

Nutraceuticals are generally taken as concentrates of certain nutrients and are presented in pharmaceutical matrix (tablets, pills, suspensions, *etc*.). Thus they do not form part of the diet and do not replace any daily food intake, but exert a reducing role of disease risk, providing certain health benefits. In general, nutraceuticals are taken for a certain time, but not as often as functional food are ingested [53].

Food supplements are defined as "foodstuffs that are concentrated sources of nutrients and other substances with a nutritional or physiological effect, alone or in combination, which are marketed in a way that allow a certain product dosage that should be taken in small unit quantities, whose purpose is to supplement the normal diet" [54]. The difference between food supplement and nutraceutical lies in its method of use. Thus, the food supplements are considered more useful for preventing or treating a nutritional deficit, while nutraceuticals are used for preventing and treating diseases [54].

Although the majority of dietetic supplements and nutraceutics available today on the market containing vitamins, minerals, herbs and amino acids are probably safe, the medical community recommends more studies to evaluate the potential benefits and adverse effects of such products including any impact on thyroid function.

Thyroid Hormones in Nutritional Supplements

Numerous natural products marketed today claim to contain either thyroid extract or substances that have a positive effect on thyroid function or thyroid hormone metabolism, which are also purportedly both safe and beneficial for general health. Researchers have focused on verifying such statements by both analyzing the content of these products and studying their effects on human volunteers.

Csako and coworkers [55] carried out an *in vitro* analysis measuring T4 andT3 levels in three generally available natural hormone preparations, and detected apparent T3 content by high-performance liquid chromatography in two of them. Administration of twice the recommended dose to human volunteers did not lead to clinical consequences, however, the authors recommended against the use of "scientifically unsound and relatively expensive OTC thyroid preparations," with unproven therapeutic efficacy.

Ma and coworkers [56] and Bauer and coworkers [57] described two patient cases aged 38 and 78 years respectively, who developed thyrotoxicosis after ingestion of the OTC dietary supplement Tiratricol. In the first case, it was used as a slimming aid, and in the second, it was given as a health supplement for 'mild anemia'. Taylor and Czarnowski [58] reported signs of hyperthyroidism in a patient after taking a European dietary supplement marketed to increase metabolism, which was initially not reported to her physician as she assumed that it was safe. In all of these cases, symptoms were resolved and thyroid function tests normalized after discontinuation of the preparations.

The presence of active thyroid hormone in food supplements is of great concern, as the use of thyroid hormones, both T4 and T3, should only be carried out under medical supervision and should be reserved for use in patients with an appropriate indication, specifically confirmed hypothyroidism. Dietary supplements and herbs should be strictly regulated for hormonal content and active thyroid hormone must be available only by prescription. In addition, healthcare providers should vigilantly screen all their patients for the use of herbal and dietary supplements and appropriately educate them on the potential drug interactions and side effects that can be associated with the use of such products.

Quercetin

Quercetin is available as a dietary supplement for its antioxidant, antiproliferative and anti-inflammatory properties [59-63]. However, concerns have been raised about the potential toxic effects of excessive intake of quercetin, and several studies have demonstrated that flavonoids, included quercetin, could interfere with thyroid function [64]. Quercetin inhibits thyroid function and decreases the expression of the main thyroid-restricted genes involved in thyroid hormone synthesis [65]. Moreover, Giuliani and coworkers [66] demonstrated that quercetin inhibits thyroid iodine uptake *in vitro* and *in vivo*. These data are relevant given the worldwide diffusion of dietary supplements containing high amounts of quercetin, and they should spur on human studies to better define the anti-thyroid effects of quercetin. There are no studies in humans that confirm these effects. Therefore, to define quercetin as a thyroid endocrine disruptor for humans further studies must be conducted in subjects ingesting quercetin supplements or involved in clinical trials with quercetin. Meanwhile, we also suggest that the use of quercetin in pregnant and lactating women should be avoided, along with its use for patients with hypothyroidism and in candidates for radioiodine administration.

Isoflavones

Many food supplements are marketed today that contain substances (isoflavones) derived from soy to reduce menopause symptomatology, although in comparison to other species, the bioavailability of flavonoids to the human thyroid might be limited [67, 68]. Despite this limited access to the thyroid gland, because these compounds can be consumed in high doses they could lead to thyroid disruption, especially when predisposing factors are present, such as deficiency of iodine, subclinical hypothyroidism or antibodies against thyroid proteins [67, 69]. In these populations, hypothyroidism and subclinical hypothyroid state [70] are most likely to occur (up to 4% and 10%, respectively) [68, 71]. Incidence of chronic autoimmune thyroiditis, the major risk factor for the development of hypothyroid disease in women, elevates with age in women [72].

Isoflavones have a similar chemical structure to T3 and T4, which suggests that they may be active in the thyroid gland (Fig. **3**) [4, 21]. Due to the potential interactions between phytoestrogens and the thyroid gland, it is likely that the thyroid function of hypothyroid individuals ingesting high amounts of phytoestrogen- or goitrogen-rich foodstuffs and supplements may be negatively affected [73]. Indeed, *in vitro* studies showed that the isoflavones genistein, daidzein and biochanin A inhibited thyroperoxidase (TPO) [4]. These compounds acted as alternative substrates for iodination [4, 21]. If blockade of TPO was to take place *in vivo*, concentrations of thyroid hormones would be decreased and potentially stimulate the synthesis of TSH.

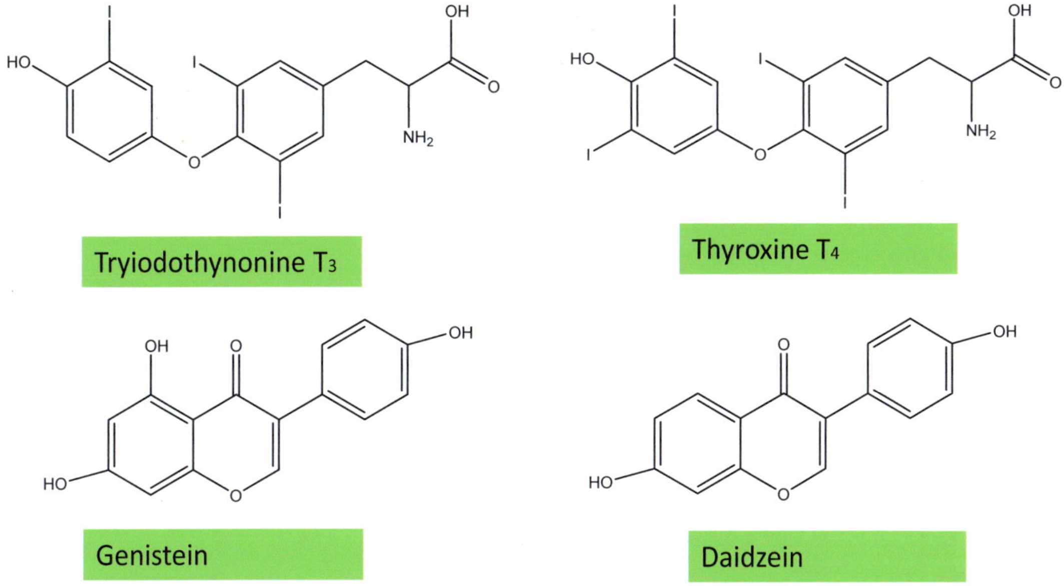

Figure 3: The structural similarity of genistein and daidzein to the thyroid.

Dietary genistein produces a strong stimulation of T-cell- and B-cell-mediated immunity in rats [74, 75], an action found with other estrogenic compounds. Inactivation of TPO by dietary genistein in rats is likely produced through covalent binding of genistein to TPO [21]. This could result in to a new antigenic form of TPO (a neoantigen) that could stimulate recognition by the immune system [75, 76]. Further support for this notion comes from the fact that anti-TPO is the major thyroid autoantigen circulating inhuman serum [77]. Although the origin of thyroid autoimmunity is unknown, the different genistein effects in rats suggests that soy ingestion could cause or exacerbate this illness.

According to these data, climacteric women who ingest large amounts of soy products may be at higher risk of thyroid disruption suggesting the necessity to be aware of, and monitoring for, possible thyroid problems resulting from ingestion of soy products.

Ginkgo Biloba Extract

Ginkgo biloba extract (GBE) is an alcohol distilled of leaves from the Ginkgo biloba tree. The extract is usually dried to a powder and formulated into pills, tablets, or capsules for ingestion. Ginkgo biloba seeds have been used in ancient Chinese medicine to treat pulmonary issues, alcohol abuse, and bladder infections, while ginkgo leaves came into use later to treat skin infections, as well as heart and lung disease [78, 79]. Currently, GBE is a popular herbal supplement that is utilized to improve circulation and brain function and the treatment of tinnitus [80].

Terpene trilactones and flavonol glycosides are usually regarded as the main contributors to the positive biological actions assigned to ginkgo [81], whereas, ginkgolic acids are typically regarded as causing negative biological activities such as cytotoxicity and mutagenicity [82].

Besides its protective health effects, it has been reported that Ginkgo biloba could induce thyroid tumors after long term exposure. In this regard, after three months and two years exposure by gavage to Ginkgo biloba extract in F344/N rats and B6C3F1/N mice, thyroid tumour induction was reported based on increased incidence of thyroid gland follicular cell adenoma [83]. In addition to morphological lesions, TSH levels were elevated. Thyroid follicular cell tumors emerge in rodents from mutations or from disruptions of thyroid and pituitary hormones (*e.g.* increase in TSHa) [84]. Chemicals that lack mutagenic activity and cause thyroid proliferation/tumorogenesis associated to elevations in TSH levels do not always have a similar carcinogenic mechanism in humans [84]. Further studies are necessary to determine if these effects could be also observed in humans and to determine the mechanisms through which ginkgo induces thyroid tumors.

Iodine and Zinc

Iodine deficiency in the population is an emerging concern. Iodine supplementation has been used to prevent iodine diet deficiencies, but chronic overconsumption of iodine reduces organic binding of iodine by the thyroid gland, which results in hypothyroidism and goiter [85]. Besides supplementation, overconsumption of iodine could come through the raising use of iodinated contrast radiologic studies, amiodarone administration, excess seaweed consumption, among other sources [86], which could also induce thyroid disruption.

On the other hand, the use of supplements containing iodine in earlier phases could confuse physicians to perform the ablation of the thyroid gland by radioiodine treatment. It is a standard protocol to induce a reduction in the body's iodine reserves before treatment with radioiodine for thyroid cancer [87]. These patients should avoid an iodine-rich diet, but they often use dietary supplements containing iodine. In a patient who had undergone computed tomographic (CT) scanning with an iodine-rich contrast agent 2 months earlier, it was observed that the level of urinary iodine was elevated to 394 μg per liter (reference range, 42 to 350) [88]. The patient reported they were consuming a large number of supplements, and after several studies measuring the iodine content of the 22 supplements the patient had been taking the selenium supplement was found to be the source of the excess iodine. Once the patient interrupted taking all supplements and maintained a normal diet, his 24-hour iodine excretion returned to normal. Physicians who use radioiodine are conscious that excess exogenous iodine alters the efficacy of iodine-131 therapy. In this patient, excessive iodine ingestion came from an unexpected source of kelp enriched with selenium. Although it is not habitual to evaluate urinary iodine concentrations in patients receiving radioiodine, it would be necessary for physicians to review patient treatments and dietary habits carefully to prevent ingestion of hidden sources of iodine.

Zinc has been reported to be an essential metal needed for proper thyroid hormone metabolism, and zinc deficiency may lead to decreased thyroid hormone levels and resting metabolic rate (RMR) [89]. However, different studies have shown that moderate to excessive Zn intake in humans [90] and animals [91] could disrupt thyroid hormones. In this regard, it was reported that excess Zn in chicks decreased the levels of serum T4 and T3 [91, 92] which could lead to hypothyroidism.

FOOD ADDITIVES

Nitrate

Inorganic nitrates/nitrites are naturally occurring compounds in foods, especially plant foods and vegetables, and are also used as food additives. Major sources of exogenous nitrates exposure are vegetables and drinking water, while exogenous nitrite sources are mainly processed meat and animal food products; more than 80-95 percent of dietary intake of nitrate is attributed to vegetables, especially green leafy vegetables including lettuce and spinach, cabbage, rocket, red beetroot and radish [93]. Drinking water also contains varying contents of nitrate; the acceptable concentrations of nitrate in drinking water, as defined by the World Health Organization (WHO) are <50mg/L and 3 mg/L for nitrate and nitrite respectively and the sum of the ratios of the concentration of each to its guideline value should not exceed 1 [94]. Moreover, the acceptable daily intakes (ADI) of nitrate and nitrite from food sources have been defined to be 3.7 and 0.06 mg/kg respectively by the Scientific Committee on Foods and confirmed by the Joint Food and Agriculture Organization (FAO)/WHO Expert Committee on Food Additives (JECFA) [95].

Inorganic nitrates/nitrites exposure has been suggested to induce thyroid disruption through inhibition of iodide uptake. They competitively bind to the sodium-iodide symporter (NIS) and decrease iodide bioavailability, thyroidal iodide stores and thyroid hormone production and consequently induce release of TSH from the pituitary gland [96]. In this regard, animal studies showed that short-term exposure to high levels of nitrate (1500 and 3000 mg/kg/day of sodium nitrate, ~295 and 590 times of ADI) in the diet interfered with normal iodine thyroid metabolism and had a goitrogenic effect especially in limited iodine diets. Moreover, administration of high doses of nitrate induced histological changes in thyroid follicle and decreased urinary iodine excretion in rats, an observation that suggested that high nitrate exposure could interfere with gastrointestinal iodine absorption *via* inhibition of Na+/K+-ATPase and energy generation for iodide trans-membrane transport, and inhibition of NIS that traps iodine in the gastrointestinal system (Fig. **4**) [97]. In addition, a short-term intervention with high and low concentrations of nitrate in female rat diet, at three dietary iodine levels (0.68, 0.23 and 0.08 mg/kg, as high, medium and low), indicated that only the combined high-nitrate and the low-iodine diet induced hyperplasia, hypertrophy, and follicular colloid depletion, plus decreased iodide uptake, and increased weight of the thyroid gland [97]. It was also reported that chronic exposure to high levels of nitrate leads to development of hypertrophy and goiter. The mechanism could be through chronic stimulation of the thyroid gland by TSH, which has been reported to induce changes in the follicular cells and to induce hypertrophy and hyperplasia [97].

It is notable that in most cases, extremely high-nitrate doses (~10-600 times the ADI) have been reported to induce anti-thyroid effects in animals, indicating no grounds for extrapolation of these findings to humans who are exposed only to acceptable dietary nitrate levels. In this regard, a meta-analysis of epidemiological surveys performed by Bahadoran and coworkers [98] showed no significant association between nitrate exposure and the risk of thyroid cancer, hyper- and hypothyroidism and a significant association was only found between higher exposures to nitrite and the risk of thyroid cancer. Some issues including methodological limitations of the studies such as models used to estimate dietary intake of nitrate/nitrite, lack of homogeneity between the methods of assessment, lack of consideration of varying contents of nitrate/nitrite in raw and cooked foods, a wide variation in nitrate/nitrite exposure, different definitions of exposure in various studies, and different iodine status among populations located in various geographic areas maybe the reasons for the inconsistent findings. Moreover, a positive association between nitrate intake through drinking water and thyroid cancer has been reported recently in women from Iowa [99]. However, the study was perform only in women and included only 40, which limits its conclusions. Finally, a large study conducted by Kilfoy and coworkers [11] evaluated the hypothesis that intake of nitrates is associated with the risk of thyroid cancer, in a prospective cohort study in the USA, analyzing half a million people from 50 to 71 years of age at the beginning of the study. Nitrites from the diet or from nitrate reduction to nitrite through oral bacteria react with amines and amides *in vivo* to form nitrosamines and nitrosamides (collectively known as N-nitroso compounds (NOC), which are potent animal carcinogens and have been reported to induce thyroid tumors [11]. They also investigated the association with consumption of dietary nitrite to examine the hypothesis that dietary precursors of the NOCs may increase the risk of thyroid cancer. They found that a higher intake of nitrates in the diet was associated with an increased risk of thyroid cancer for both papillary and follicular subtypes.

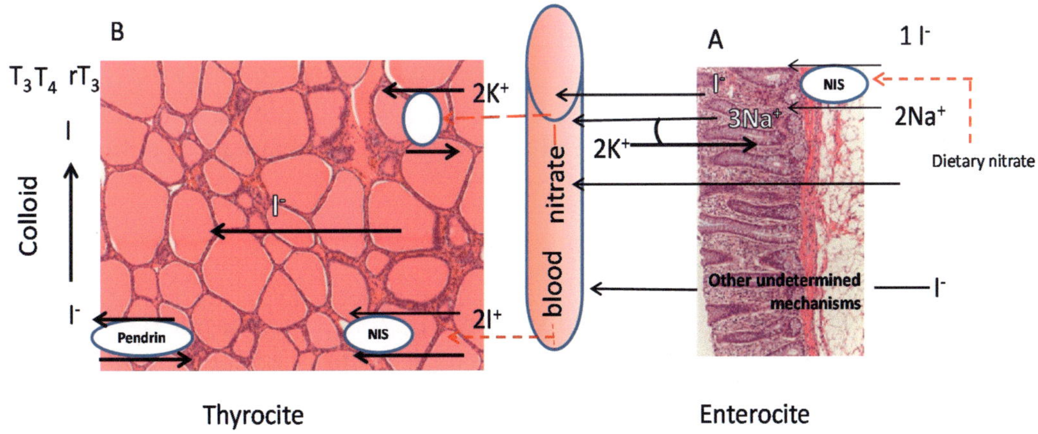

Figure 4: Nitrate/nitrite exposure effects on iodine metabolism. A) Nitrate could disrupt gastrointestinal iodine absorption by iodide trans-membrane transport inhibition through Na+/K+ ATPase blockade, and sodium-iodide symporter (NIS) inhibition, which trap iodine in enterocyte. B) Nitrate could also competitively bind to the NIS, and decrease iodide uptake and thyroidal iodide stores. Dash-lines indicate inhibitory effects. T3, triiodothyronine; T4, thyroxine; rT3, reverse T3; NIS, the sodium iodide synmport; I, iodine.

Reviewing the studies described above, additional research to clarify the association between nitrate/nitrite exposure and thyroid function and the risk of cancer in humans is needed.

Erythrosine

Erythrosine, recognized also as FD&C Red #3, is a xanthene dye presenting four iodine atoms [100]. It was approved for use in 1907. The possible carcinogenic and oncogenic actions of erythrosine are produced by secondary effects on the thyroid and pituitary glands [101]. The ADI for erythrosine was settled by the JEFCA to be 0.1 mg/kg based on erythrosine's NOAEL for thyroid and pituitary effects in humans of 60 mg/day equivalent to 1 mg/kg/day obtained in a 14-day study in human volunteers [102]. The applied uncertainty factor was 10.

TSH synthesized in the pituitary gland controls thyroid structure and function, and stimulates thyroid growth. Tumors can be produced by hyperstimulation of the thyroid through TSH. In this regard, it has been reported that rats fed with 4.0% erythrosine (2464 mg/kg/day dose) in a lifetime study showed inhibition of T4 to T3conversion, leading to in a long-term increased stimulation of the thyroid through TSH. Moreover, elevated incidence of thyroid follicular cell hyperplasia, adenomas and carcinomas was found. According to this data the NOEL was settled at 0.5% of the diet, or 251 mg/kg/day. The mechanisms responsible for the elevated serum reverse T3 seems to be, first, T4 concentration due to 5-monodeiodinase inhibition with subsequent conversion to reverse T3 rather than active T3; and, second, reverseT3 concentration due to 5-monodeiodinase inhibition leading to inability to degrade reverse T3 further to diiodothyronine (T2) [103]. Further studies are required to clarify the mechanism of action and if human exposure could lead to these effects.

CONCLUSION

Thyroid hormones regulate body homeostasis in adults, and during development they have also a key role in body development, especially of the central nervous system. Many foods used in the dairy diet could lead to thyroid disruption. In this regard, consumption of plant foods containing a high quantity of GLS and flavonoids could lead to goitrogenic effects in areas where they are the main sources of carbohydrates and iodine intake in the diet is low. In these regions supplementation with iodine is necessary and reduction in the consumption of these foods and a change in carbohydrate sources to avoid this health problem.

Consumption of some novel foods or food supplements has been related to disruption of the thyroid system, mainly in animal studies. Therefore, further studies are needed to determine if other products could also produce these effects and if they could lead to these effects also in humans. Moreover, studying the factors and predisposing conditions that could lead to these effects and the mechanisms through which these actions are produced is needed to perform a complete risk assessment of these products to avoid health problems in the population, especially in those more susceptible to suffer these effects. Finally different chemical compounds are used during food processing, which could also induce harmful effects on the thyroid system. Thus it is also necessary to perform further studies on the different compounds used during food processing to identify possible substances that could alter thyroid function in humans, and the mechanisms through which these actions may be produced.

CONFLICT OF INTEREST

The author confirms that author has no conflict of interest to declare for this publication.

ACKNOWLEDGEMENTS

We thank the Micros Veterinaria for the pictures of thyrocite and enterocyte.

REFERENCES

[1] Shibamoto T, Bjeldanes LF. Toxinas naturales de los alimentos vegetales. In: Shibamoto T, Bjeldanes LF, Eds. Introducción a la toxicología de los alimentos. Zaragoza, Acribia S.A, 1996; pp. 63-68.

[2] Lindner E. Sustancias tóxicas en alimentos naturales y en los condimentos. In: Lindner E, Ed. Toxicologia de los alimentos. Segunda ed. Zaragoza, Acribia, 1995; pp. 14-30.

[3] Lopez de Cerain A, Gil AG, Bello J. Alimentos con sustancias tóxicas de origen natural: Plantas superiores alimenticias. In: Cameán AM, Repetto M, Eds. Toxicología Alimentaria. Buenos Aires, Diaz de Santos, 2006; pp. 192-209.

[4] Divi R, Chang, Doerge, D. Anti-thyroid isoflavones from soybean: isolation, characterization, and mechanisms of action. BiochemPharmacol 1997; 54: 1087-1096.

[5] Hershman JM. Thyroid Health Supplements Contain Significant Amounts of Thyroid Hormones. ClinThyroidol 2013; 25: 166-167.

[6] Gardiner P, Phillips R, Shaughnessy A. Herbal and dietary supplement-drug interactions in patients with chronic illnesses. Am Fam Physician 2008; 77: 73-78.

[7] Lück E. Chemical preservation of food. Zentralbl Bakteriol Mikrobiol Hyg B 1985; 189(2-3): 299-310.

[8] Nolan B, Hitt K. Vulnerability of shallow ground water and drinking-water wells to nitrate in the. Environ SciTechnol 2006; 40:7834-7840.

[9] Johnson C, Kross B. Continuing importance of nitrate contamination of groundwater and wells in rural areas. Am J Ind Med 1990; 18: 449-456.

[10] Nolan B, Hitt K, Ruddy B. Probability of nitrate contamination of recently recharged groundwaters in the conterminous United State. Environ SciTechnol 2002 36: 2138-2145.

[11] Kilfoy BA, Zhang Y, Park Y, *et al.* Dietary nitrate and nitrite and the risk of thyroid cancer in the NIH-AARP Diet and Health Study. Int J Cancer 2011; 129(1): 160-172.
[12] EFSA Panel on Food Additives and Nutrient Sources added to Food (ANS). Scientific Opinion on the reevaluation of Erythrosine (E 127) as a food additive.EFSA Journal 2011; 9(1): 1854. Available from: http://www.efsa.europa.eu/en/efsajournal/pub/ 1854.htm
[13] Gaitan E. Goitrogens. BaillieresClinEndocrinolMetab. 1988; 2(3): 683-702.
[14] Greer MA. Goitrogenic substances in food.Am J ClinNutr 1957; 5: 440-444.
[15] Moudgal NR, Raghupathy E, Sarma PS. Studies on goitrogenic agents in foods. Journal of Nutrition 1958; 66: 291-303.
[16] Polat U.The Effects on Metabolism of Glucosinolates and Theirs Hydrolysis Products. JBiol Environ Sci 2010; 4(10): 39-42.
[17] Chu M, Seltzer TF. Myxedema Coma Induced by Ingestion of Raw Bok Choy. N Engl J Med 2010; 362(2): 1945-1846.
[18] Erdogan MF. Thiocyanate overload and thyroid disease.Biofactors 2003; 19: 107-111.
[19] Medeiros-Neto G, Knobel M. Iodine deficiency disorders. In: De Groot LJ, Ed. Endocrinology.6th edition. New York, Elsevier, 2010.
[20] Heaney R, Fenwick G. Identifying toxins and their effects: glucosinolates. In: Watson D, Ed. Natural toxicants in food (progress and prospects). Chichester, Ellis Horwood, 1976; pp. 76-109.
[21] Divi RL, Doerge DR. Inhibition of thyroid peroxidase by flavonoids dietary. Chem Res Toxicol 1996; 9: 16-23.
[22] Van der Heide D, Kastelijn J, Schröder-van der J. Flavonoids and thyroid disease. Bio Factors 2003; 19: 113-119.
[23] Yao L, Jiang Y, Shi J, *et al.* Flavonoids in food and their health benefits. Plant Foods Hum Nutr 2004; 59: 113-122.
[24] Gaitan E, Lindsay R, Reichert R, *et al.* Antithyroid and goitrogenic effects of millet: role of C-Glycosyl flavones. J Clin Endocrinol Metab 1989; 68: 707-714.
[25] Sartelet H, Sergha S, Lobstein A, *et al.* Flavonoids extracted from Fonio millet (Digitariaexilis) reveal potent antithyroid properties. Nutrition 1996; 12: 100-106.
[26] Ibanez E, Cifuentes A. Benefits of using algae as natural sources of functional ingredients. J Sci Food Agric 2013; 93: 703-709.
[27] Agyei D. Bioactive Proteins and Peptides from Soybeans. Recent Pat Food Nutr Agric 2015; 29: 29.
[28] Chen KI, Erh MH, Su NW, Liu WH, Chou CC, Cheng K.C. Soyfoods and soybean products: from traditional use to modern applications. Appl Microbiol Biotechnol 2012; 96: 9-22.
[29] Akiyama T, Ishida J, Nakagawa S, Ogawara H, Shibuya M, Fukami Y. Genistein, a specific inhibitor of tyrosine-specific protein kinases. J Biol Chem 1987; 262: 5592-5595.
[30] Cerundolo R, Michel K, Court, MH, *et al.* Effects of dietary soy isoflavones on health, steroidogenesis, and thyroid gland function in dogs. Am J Vet Res 2009; 70: 353-360.
[31] Chang H, Doerge D. Dietary Genistein Inactivates Rat Thyroid Peroxidase *in Vivo* without an Apparent Hypothyroid Effect. ToxicolApplPharmacol 2000; 168(3): 244-252.
[32] Van Wyk J, Arnold F M, Wynn J, Pepper F. The effects of a soybean product on thyroid function in humans. Pediatrics 1959; 24: 752-60.
[33] Hydovitz JD. Occurrence of goiter in an infant on a soy-diet.The New England Journal Medicine 1960; 262: 351-353.
[34] Shepard TH, Pyne GE, Kirschvink JF, McLean M. Soybean goiter. N Engl J Med 1960; 262: 1099-1103.
[35] Ripp JW. Soybean-induced goiter.Am J Dis Child 1961; 102: 106-109.
[36] Fort P, Moses N, Fasano M, Goldberg T, Lifshitz F. Breast and soy-formula feedings in early infancy and the prevalence of autoimmune thyroid disease in. J Am CollNutr 1990; 9: 164-167.
[37] Bitto A, Polito F, Atteritano M, *et al.* Genisteinaglycone does not affect thyroid function: results from a three-year, randomized, double-blind, placebo-controlled trial. J ClinEndocrinolMetabol 2010; 95: 3067-3072.
[38] Bruce B, Messina M, Spiller GA. Isoflavone supplements do not affect thyroid function in iodine-replete postmenopausal women. J Med Food 2003; 6(4): 309-316.
[39] Ishizuki Y. The effects on the thyroid gland of soybeans administered experimentally in healthy subjects. Nippon Naibunpi Gakkai Zasshi 1991; 67(5): 622-629.

[40] Caruana M, Vassallo N. Tea Polyphenols in Parkinson's Disease. Adv Exp Med Biol 2015; 863: 117-137.
[41] Kobalka AJ, Keck RW, Jankun J. Synergistic anticancer activity of biologicals from green and black tea on DU 145 human prostate cancer cells. Cent Eur J Immunol 2015; 40: 1-4.
[42] Vinson JA, Teufel K, Wu N. Green and black teas inhibit atherosclerosis by lipid, antioxidant, and fibrinolytic mechanisms. J Agric Food Chem 2004; 52: 3661-3665.
[43] Westerterp-Plantenga M, Diepvens K, Joosen AM, Berube-Parent S, Tremblay A. Metabolic effects of spices, teas, and caffeine. Physiol Behav 2006; 89: 85-91.
[44] Chandra AK, De N, Choudhury RS. Effect of different doses of unfractionated green and black tea extracts on thyroid physiology. Hum ExpToxicol 2011; 30(8): 884-96.
[45] Chandra AK, De N. Goitrogenic/antithyroidal potential of green tea extract in relationto catechin in rats. Food Chem Toxicol 2010; 48: 2304-2311.
[46] Šošić-Jurjević B, Filipović B, Ajdzanović V, *et al.* Suppressive effects of genistein and daidzein on pituitary-thyroid axis in orchidectomized middle-aged rats. ExpBiol Med 2010; 235: 590-598.
[47] Valverde J, Hayes M, McLoughlin P, Rai DK, Soler-Vila A. Cardioprotective potential of irish macroalgae: generation of glycine betaine and dimethylsulfoniopropionate containing extracts by accelerated solvent extraction. Planta Med 2015; 81: 679-684.
[48] Brown ES, Allsopp PJ, Magee PJ, *et al.* Seaweed and human health. Nutr Rev 2014; 72: 205-216.
[49] Misurcova L, Machu L, Orsavova J. Seaweed minerals as nutraceuticals. Adv Food Nutr Res 2011; 64: 371-390.
[50] Di Matola T, Zeppa P, Gasperi M, Vitale M. Thyroid dysfunction following a kelp-containing marketed diet. BMJ Case Rep 2014; 29: 206-330.
[51] Crawford B, Cowell T, Emder P, *et al.* Iodine toxicity from soy milk and seaweed ingestion. Med J Aust 2010; 193: 413-415.
[52] Clark CD, Bassett B, Burge MR. Effects of kelp supplementation on thyroid function in euthyroid subjects. Endocr Pract 2003; 9: 363-369.
[53] EK K. Nutraceutical-definition and introduction. AAPS Pharm Sci 2003; 5(3): E25.
[54] Mechanick JI, Brett EM, Chausmer AB, Dickey RA, Wallach S. American Association of Clinical Endocrinologists. American association of clinical endocrinologist's medical guidelines for the clinical use of dietary supplements and nutraceuticals.EndocrPract 2003; 9(5): 417-470.
[55] Csako G, Corso D, Kestner J, Bokser A, Kennedy P, Pucino F. Evaluation of two over-the- counter natural thyroid hormone. Ann Pharmacother 1992; 26(4): 492-494.
[56] Ma R, Chan M, Poon W, So W, Chow C. Thyroid dysfunction due to overthe-counter usage of tiratricol. Intern Med J 2008; 38(7): p. 611-612.
[57] Bauer BA B, Elkin P, Erickson D, Klee G, Brennan M. Symptomatic hyperthyroidism in a patient taking the dietary supplement tiratricol. Mayo Clin Proc. 2002; 77(6): p. 587- 590.
[58] Taylor T, Czarnowski C. What caused this case of asymptomatic hyperthyroidism? J FamPract 2009; 58(4): 203-206.
[59] Arts I, Hollman P. Polyphenols and disease risk in epidemiologic studies. Am J ClinNut 2005; 81: 317S-325S.
[60] Boots A, Haenen G, Bast A. Health effects of quercetin: From antioxidant to nutraceutical. Euro J Pharmacol 2008; 585: 325-337.
[61] Gupta S, Kim J, Prasad S, Aggarwa B. Regulation of survival,proliferation, invasion, angiogenesis, and metastasis of tumor cells through modulation of inflammatory pathways by nutraceuticals. Cancer Metastasis Rev 2010; 29: 405-434.
[62] Pandey A, Patnaik R, Muresanu D, Sharma A, Sharma H. Quercetin in hypoxia-induced oxidative stress: novel target for neuroprotection. Int Rev Neurobiol 2012; 102: 107-146.
[63] Russo M, Spagnuolo C, Tedesco I, Bilotto S, Russo G. The flavonoid quercetin in disease prevention and therapy: facts and fancies. BiochemPharmacol 2012; 83: 6-15.
[64] Egert S, Rimbach G. Which Sources of Flavonoids: Complex Diets or Dietary Supplements?.AdvNutr 2011; 2: 8-14.
[65] Giulian C, Saji M, Bucci I, Fiore G, Liberatore M, Singer D, Monaco F, Kohn LD, Napolitano G. Transcriptional regulation of major histocompatibility complex class I gene by insulin and IGF-I in FRTL-5 thyroid. J Endocrinol 2006; 189: 605-615.

[66] Giuliani c, Bucci I, Di Santo S, *et al.* The flavonoid quercetin inhibits thyroid-restricted genes expression. Food ChemToxicol 2014; 66: 23-29.
[67] Duncan A, Underhill K, Xu X, Lavalleu J, Kurzer M. Soy isoflavones exert modest hormonal effects in premenopausal women. J ClinEndocrinolMetab 1999; 84: 192- 197.
[68] Vanderpump M, Tunbridge W. The epidemiology of thyroid diseases. In: Braverman L, Utiger RD, Eds. The Thyroid. Philadelphia, Lippincott-Raven, 1996; pp. 474-482.
[69] HampL R, Ostatnikova D, Celec P, Putz Z, Lapcík O, Matucha P. Shortterm effect of soy consumption on thyroid hormone levels and correlation with phytoestrogen level in healthy subjects. EndocrRegul 2008; 42(2-3): 53-61.
[70] Woeber K. Subclinical thyroid dysfunction. Arch Intern Med 1997; 157: 1065-1068.
[71] Canaris G, Manowitz N, Mayor G, Ridgeway E. The Colorado thyroid disease prevalence study. Arch Intern Med 2000; 160: 526-534.
[72] Mittal N, Hota D, Dutta P, *et al.* Evaluation of effect of isoflavone on thyroid economy & autoimmunity in oophorectomised women: a randomised, double-blind, placebo-controlled trial. Indian J Med Res 2011; 133: 633-40.
[73] Hughes I, Woods HF. Phytoestrogens and Health, Committee on Toxicity of Chemicals in Food. London: UK. 2003. Available from: http://cot.food.gov.uk/sites/default /files/cot/phytoreport0503.pdf
[74] Delclos K, Bucci T, Lomax L, *et al.* Effects of dietary genistein exposure during development on male and female CD (Sprague-Dawley) rats. ReprodToxicol 2001; 15: 647-663.
[75] Zhang Y, Song T, Cunnick J, Murphy P, Hendrich S. Daidzein and genistein glucuronides *in vitro* are weakly estrogenic and activate human natural killer cells at nutritionally relevant concentrations. J Nutr 1999; 129: 399-405.
[76] Dansette P, Bonierbale E, Minoletti C, Beaune P, Pessayre D, Mansuy D. Drug-induced immunotoxicity. Eur J Drug MetabPharmacokinet 1998; 23: 443-451.
[77] McKenzie J, Zakarija M. Thyroid autoimmunity. In: Braverman L, Utiger R, Eds. Philadelphia, Lippincott-Raven, 1996.
[78] MahadyGB. Ginkgo biloba for the prevention and treatment of cardiovascular disease: A review of the literature. J CardiovascNurs 2002; 16: 21-32.
[79] Smith JV, Luo Y. Studies on molecular mechanisms of Ginkgo biloba extract. App. MicrobiolBiotechnol 2004; 64: 465-472.
[80] National Toxicology Program (NTP). Toxicology and carcinogenesis studies of Ginkgo biloba extract in F344/N rats and B6C3F1/N mice (gavage studies). Research Triangle Park, North Carolina, USA 2013.
[81] Van Beek TA, Montoro P. Chemical analysis and quality control of Ginkgo biloba leaves, extracts, and phytopharmaceuticals. J Chromatogr 2009; 1216: 2002-2032.
[82] Westendorf J, Regan J. Induction of DNA strand-breaks in primary rat hepatocytes by ginkgolic acids. Pharmazie 2000; 55: 864-865.
[83] Dunnick JK, Nyska A. The toxicity and pathology of selected dietary herbal medicines.ToxicolPathol 2013; 41(2): 374-386.
[84] Hill RN, Crisp TM, Hurley PM, Rosenthal SL, Singh DV. Risk assessment of thyroid follicular cell tumors. Environ Health Perspect 1998; 106: 447-57.
[85] Baker DH. Iodine toxicity and its amelioration. Exp Biol Med 2004; 229: 473-478.
[86] Leung AM, Braverman LE Iodine-induced thyroid dysfunction. Curr Opin Endocrinol Diabetes Obes 2012; 19: 414-419.
[87] Rosen J, Gardiner P, Sape R, *et al.* Complementary and Alternative Medicine Use Among Patients with Thyroid Cancer. Thyroid 2013; 23(10): 1238-1246.
[88] Arum S, He X, Braverman L. Excess Iodine from an Unexpected Source. N Engl J Med 2009; 360(4): 424-426.
[89] Maxwell C, Volpe SL. Effect of zinc supplementation on thyroid hormone function. A case study of two college females. Ann Nutr Metab 2007; 51: 188-194.
[90] Nishiyama S, Futagoishi-Suginohara Y, Matsukura M, *et al.* Zinc supplementation alters thyroid hormone metabolism in disabled patients with zinc deficiency. J Am Coll Nutr 1994; 13: 62-67.
[91] Dean CE, Hargis BM, Hargis PS. Effects of zinc toxicity on thyroid function and histology in broiler chicks. Toxicol Lett 1991; 57: 309-318.

[92] Kaya S, Kececi T, Haliloglu S. Effects of zinc and vitamin A supplements on plasma levels of thyroid hormones, cholesterol, glucose and egg yolk cholesterol oflaying hens. Res Vet Sci 2001; 71: 135-139.

[93] Hord N, Tang Y, Bryan N. Food sources of nitrates and nitrites: the physiologic. Am J ClinNutr 2009; (90): 1-10.

[94] World Health Organization (OWH). Nitrate and nitrite in drinking-water; Background document for development of WHO Guidelines for Drinking-water Quality. Geneva: Switzerland 2011; Report No: 23.

[95] Opinion of the Scientific Panel on Contaminants in the Food chain on a request from the European Commission to perform a scientific risk assessment on nitrate in vegetables. The EFSA Journal 2008; pp. 1-79.

[96] Bloomfield R, Welsch C, Garner G, Muhrer M. Effect of dietary nitrate on thyroid function. Science 1961; 134: 1690.

[97] Kostogrys R, Pecio A. Nitrate affect thyroid status and serum triacylglycerol in Wistar rats. Pol J Food NutrSci 2006; 15: 71-76.

[98] Bahadoran Z, Parvin M, Asghar G, Kabir, Fereidoun A, Farzad H. Is dietary nitrate/ nitrite exposure a risk factor for development of thyroid ?. Nitric Oxide 2015; 47: 65-76.

[99] Warda M, Kilfoya B, Weyerb P, Anderson K, Folsom A, Cerhand J. Nitrate Intake and the Risk of Thyroid Cancer and Thyroid Disease. Epidemiology 2010; 21(3): 389-395.

[100] Ghorpade V, Deshpande SS, Salunkhe DK. Food colors. In: Maga JA, Tu AT, Eds. Food Additive Toxicology. Marcel Dekker Inc, 1995.

[101] Poulsen E. Case study: erythrosine. Food AdditContam 1993; 10(3): 315-323.

[102] Gardner D, Utiger R, Schwartz S, *et al.* Effects of oral Erythrosine on thyroid function in normal men. ToxicolApplPharmacol. 1986; 91: 299-304.

[103] Capen CC. Toxic Responses of the Endocrine System. In: Curtis D. Klaassen PD, Ed. Toxicology: The Basic Science of Poisons. 7th edition. New York, McGraw-Hill 2007; p. 838-840.

CHAPTER 11

Industrial Chemicals

Maria Teresa Frejo, Maria Jesus Diaz and Javier Del Pino*

Departament of Toxicology and Pharmacology, Veterinary School, Complutense University of Madrid, Madrid, Spain

Abstract: Thyroid hormones (THs) play a key role during development, especially of the Central Nervous System and in adulthood in homeostasis control. They are regulated by the dynamic interrelationships between the hypothalamus, pituitary and thyroid gland. It has been shown that a large number of industrial chemicals could affect the hypothalamic-pituitary-thyroid axis and disrupt the thyroid system, which is a cause of concern, because these alterations could induce severe neurological effects during development as well as alterations in homeostasis. Classically, these chemicals have been identified and classified as toxic agents due to their ability to alter TH levels. However, other mechanisms have been shown to contribute to thyroid system disruption, such as interference with thyroid hormone receptors or enzymes or transporters that play an important role in mediating the action of these hormones. The aim of this chapter is to provide a review of the effects of industrial chemicals on the thyroid system and the mechanisms through which they induce these effects.

Keywords: Acrylamide, benzophenone-2, bisphenol A, dioxins, nonylphenol, octyl methoxycinnamate, PBDEs, perchlorate, perfluorinated chemicals, phthalates, polychlorinated biphenyls, resorcinol, sodium chlorate, thiocyanate, tributyltin.

INTRODUCTION

In the last 50 years, industrial compounds' toxicity and hazards to public health have been shown by clinical studies [1], especially due to their structural similarity to hormones [2-4]. The thyroid system is one of the most affected endocrine systems. Thyroid hormones have a key role in numerous physiological processes such as metabolic regulation, bone remodeling, cardiac function and mental state. So maintaining normal function of the thyroid gland for psychological and physiological well-being is essential [5].

Thyroid hormones are especially important in fetal development, especially in the development of the nervous system, which depends on the normal levels of these

*Corresponding author **Javier Del Pino:** Department of Toxicology and Pharmacology, Complutense University of Madrid, Madrid, Spain; E-mail: jdelpino@pdi.ucm.es

Javier Del Pino, Maria Jesus Diaz and Maria Teresa Frejo (Eds)

hormones, and it has been observed that their deficiency reduces neuronal growth and differentiation in the cerebral cortex, hippocampus and cerebellum [6, 7]. Therefore, an alteration of the thyroid system could have harmful effects on physiology and development of the whole organism.

Thyroid disrupter industrial chemicals include a wide range of chemical structures acting through different mechanisms (Fig. **1**), which have been studied in experimental animals [8, 9]. Moreover, there is also evidence of their effects by alteration of thyroid hormone homeostasis in humans [10, 11]. However, there are a number of uncertainties in the interpretation of study results in animals and in the extrapolation of these results to humans [12, 13] as well as in the variety of mechanisms of action through which alteration in TH levels is caused.

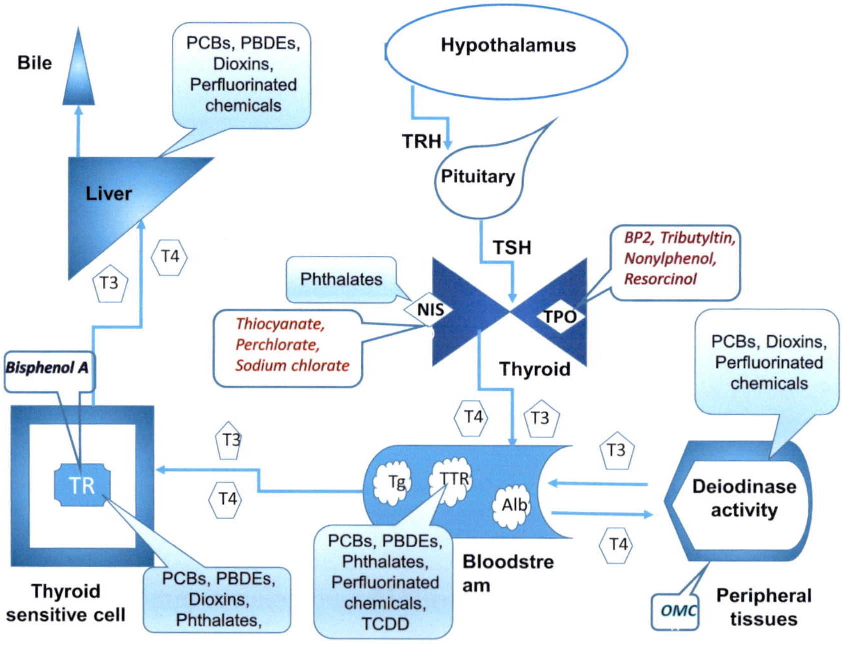

Figure 1: Possible mechanisms of action of industrial chemicals on the hypothalamic–pituitary–thyroid axis. TRH, thyrotropin releasing hormone; TSH, thyroid stimulating hormone; T4, thyroxine; T3, triiodothyronine; TR, thyroid hormone receptor; NIS, the sodium iodide synmporter; TPO, thyroperixidase; Alb, albumin; Tg, thyroxin-binding globulin; TTR, transthyretin; OMC, octylmethoxycinnamate.

The aim of this chapter is to provide a review of the existing data on how industrial chemicals disrupt the thyroid system based on their mechanisms of action in order to highlight the risks inherent to human and animal health due to the short and long term use of these products.

INDUSTRIAL CHEMICALS THAT DISRUPT THE THYROID SYSTEM ONLY THROUGH ONE MECHANISM OF ACTION

Inhibition of Iodide Uptake into the Thyrocyte Cell Membrane by Blocking the NIS Carrier

The first step in the biosynthesis of thyroid hormones is iodide uptake from the bloodstream and its transport against a gradient across the lumen follicular cells by the sodium/iodide symporter (NIS) protein [14]. NIS is capable of carrying other anions besides iodide, such as thiocyanate (SCN), perchlorate (ClO_4-) and sodium chlorate ($NaClO_3$), which inhibit the accumulation of iodine in the thyroid gland by competition with said anion.

Thiocyanate

Although thiocyanate is not an industrial compound itself, cigarette smoke contains cyanide that is metabolized to thiocyanate in the body, which can decrease the absorption of iodine in the thyroid by competitive inhibition of NIS [15]. Blocking the iodide uptake mechanism has a similar effect to iodine deficiency. In this regard, blood levels of thyroxine (T4) and triiodothyronine (T3) are decreased, causing a compensatory increase in the secretion of thyroid-stimulating hormone (TSH) from the pituitary gland, which produces hypertrophy and hyperplasia of the follicular cell with an elevation thyroid weight and development of goiter [16].

On the other hand, newborn babies from mothers who smoked during pregnancy are more likely to have low serum T4 [17], increased levels of TSH, thyroid enlargement [18, 19] and low iodine levels in both mothers and their babies [20]. These effects have been hypothesized to be related to thiocyanate exposure. This is a cause of concern due to the fact that THs are needed for normal neurological development. Further studies are needed to confirm this hypothesis and determine the implication of this compound in thyroid disruption of the smoker population.

Perchlorate

Perchlorates occur both naturally and through manufacturing, used as a rocket propellant, in the preparation of explosives, fireworks, flares, airbag deployment systems, commercial fertilizers and by pharmaceutical industries [21]. Perchlorate is an ion that could affect thyroid function because it competitively inhibits iodine transport in thyroid follicular cells through inhibition of NIS [22, 23]. Therefore, it could induce hypothyroidism in different stages of life [24-26].

Experimental studies in animals provide strong evidence that perchlorates could alter thyroid homeostasis [27]. However, human studies remain controversial. In this regard, Blount and coworkers [28] settled a relationship between the presence of perchlorates in blood and urine, and TSH (positive association) and total T4 (negative association) levels, especially in women with a urinary iodide level of <100 mg/L. In contrast, other studies of perchlorate exposure have not determined a substantial relationship to thyroid parameters. In this sense, no effects on thyroid function including iodide uptake, serum thyroid hormones, TSH and thyroglobulin have been reported in healthy volunteers after 6 months of exposure to perchlorate in doses up to 3 mg/day [29]. Moreover, thyroid gland iodine uptake in workers in an ammonium perchlorate generation plant was negatively correlated with their presence at work [30]. Therefore, it remains doubtful whether environmentally occurring levels of perchlorate have any effects on humans.

Finally, the National Research Council in 2005 concluded that perchlorate exposure could produce TSH and TH disruption followed by hypertrophy and hyperplasia of the follicular cells [31]. Hypothyroidism could be developed only in people who fail to compensate for the perchlorate effect with an increase in iodine uptake. The Committee, based on clinical, occupational, environmental and epidemiological studies, recommended a reference dose of 0.0007 mg/kg/day of iodine, which should protect health in most sensitive populations [31].

Sodium Chlorate ($NaClO_3$)

Sodium chlorate is utilized as an oxidizing agent in dyes, explosives, matches, and leather industries. It is also found as a drinking water disinfection by-product after chlorine dioxide disinfection [32]. It causes thyroid system disruption through inhibition of the sodium/iodide cotransporter. The toxicity data for $NaClO_3$ are reduced and come primarily from subchronic studies. In this regard, Bercz and coworkers [33] described a concentration-dependent reduction in T4 levels in African green monkeys. Moreover, McCauley and coworkers [34] reported thyroid gland colloid depletion after $NaClO_3$ subchronic exposure in rats. Furthermore, in a chronic toxicity study in rats exposed to $NaClO_3$ in drinking water, an increased incidence of follicular cell tumors was reported [35]. In addition, a dose dependent decrease in serum T4 was observed which was higher between PND 4-21, but at 90 days of age T4 levels were similar to controls. Increases in TSH values were higher from 4 and 21 days to 90 days in rats, and they were only observed at high doses. The increase in TSH resulted in a 13% incidence of follicular cell adenomas and carcinomas in males and 9% incidence in females compared to 2% in controls of both genders [35]. According to this data, this compound could induce an alteration in the thyroid system, but the epidemiological studies did not find significant effects in humans [35]. Further studies are required to determine the possible effect of these compounds on the human thyroid system.

Thyroid Peroxidase (TPO) Inhibition

TPO is the main enzyme that participates in the synthesis of thyroid hormones. TPO inhibition leads to disruption of both the iodination of tyrosyl residues in thyroglobulin and the coupling reaction of iodotyrosine to form T4 and T3 [36]. The main chemicals that inhibit TPO include phenols (such as nonylphenol and resorcinol); and various compounds such as benzophenone-2, which is an ingredient used as sunscreen in cosmetics [37], and tributyltin chloride (TBTCL) [38].

Nonylphenol

Nonylphenol is used in several detergents, plastics and pesticides [39]. Schmutzler [40] showed that nonylphenol inhibits the activity of TPO in Human FTC-133 thyroid carcinoma cells stably transfected with a plasmid coding for human TPO with an IC_{50} of 57 µmol/L, similar to that of genistein used as positive control (50 mmol/L). Moreover, Xi and coworkers [41] showed that exposure to nonylphenol altered the structure and function of the thyroid gland in rats. It was administered at three doses for 15 days orally (40, 80 and 200 mg/kg/day) showing that there was an increase in TSH, a decrease of free T3 and T4 and thyroid lesions such as damage to the endoplasmic reticulum and mitochondria.

Resorcinol

Resorcinol (1, 3-dihydroxybenzene, CASRN108-46-3) is a chemical used in products such as pharmaceuticals or dyes like fluorescein [42]. However, it is mainly used for the production of synthetic resins and in the rubber industry in the production of tires (approximately 50%). It is also used for bonding wood in high quality applications (approximately 25%) and is an important chemical intermediate in the manufacture of specialty chemicals [43].

Resorcinol effects on thyroid function have been described by some authors [42, 43] indicating that it decreased T4 and T3 and increased TSH. Paul and coworkers [44] studied the effect of 21 chemical compounds on TPO by high-throughput screening assay and showed that resorcinol inhibits the TPO enzyme. These results were consistent with those found by Doerge and Divi [45], which suggested that TPO catalyzed the oxidation of resorcinol derivatives. Resorcinol derivatives also present the ability to inhibit TPO and goitrogenic responses determined in humans and animals [42]. The widespread nature of resorcinol derivatives in the environment suggests that exposure to these substances could lead to thyroid dysfunction in humans.

Tributyltin

Triorganotins, such as tributyltin chloride (TBTCl), are environmental pollutants commonly found in anti-fouling paints used on ships and other vessels. TBTCl has been reported to inhibit TPO. In this regard, Sharan and coworkers [38] showed that TBTCl (0.5, 5 and 50 μg/kg/day) treatment of male Swiss albino mice during 45 days induced hypothyroidism related to a reduction of the expression level and activity of TPO, which was correlated with decreased levels of both T4 and T3.

Benzophenone-2

Different studies have suggested that certain UV filters used in sunscreen, such as benzophenone-2, could behave as thyroid disruptors. In this regard, Schmutzler and coworkers [46] analyzed the possible adverse effects of benzophenone-2 on the hypothalamic-pituitary-thyroid (HPT) axis, through its action on TPO. They tested, through an *in vitro* assay based on recombinant human TPO (POTrh), whether certain UV filters presented thyroid effects. These UV filters (4-MBC, OMC, BP2 and BP3) were compared to two known antithyroid products: genistein, a goitrogenic synthetic flavonoid (F21388), and bisphenol A (BPA); and 2 TPO inhibitors, propylthiouracil (PTU) and methimazole (MMI). From these compounds, only BP2 showed a potent inhibition of POTrh. Then they analyzed the effect of BP2 and found that inhibition was exerted on POTrh with H_2O_2, but not in the absence of this substrate, like genistein. The dependence on this substrate could be due to the presence of two resorcinol groups in the BP2 molecule, since the latter has demonstrated an inhibitory effect on TPO. No inhibition occurred in the presence of appropriate concentrations of iodide.

To evaluate the *in vivo* effect of BP2 on thyroid function, ovariectomized rats were treated for 5 days with various amounts of BP2, and a decrease in the levels of T4 was found. The increase in TSH was also substantial at these doses, but no decline in T3 was observed. Moreover, BP2 did not induce an interaction in NIS transporter function [47].

Deiodination Inhibition

T4 is mono iodinated by 5'-deiodinase to T3 before interacting with the target cells. Under certain conditions (such as liver and kidney diseases) or exposure to xenobiotics, T4 is transformed by 5'-deiodinase to 3,3',5'-triiodothyronine ("reverse T3"), which is biologically inactive [48].

Octylmethoxycinnamate

Deiodinases enzyme activity has been reported to be affected by octyl methoxycinnamate (OMC), an ultraviolet radiation blocking agent used in sunscreens, causing a decrease in plasma T3 [49]. In this regard, Klammer and coworkers [49] investigated deiodinase activity in ovariectomized rats treated for 5 days with different doses of OMC or 17-β estradiol (E2) as a control. They analyzed thyrotropin-releasing hormone (TRH) expression in the hypothalamus measured by mRNA levels, serum TSH, T3 and T4 levels determined by radioimmunoassay, NIS expression of TSH receptor by Western blot and TPO and 5'-iodothyronine deiodinase type I (DI1) activity. Whereas E2 did not affect serum levels of TSH, T4 or T3, OMC produced a dose-dependent serum decrease in these hormones (TSH 38%, T3 63% and T4 75%). TH receptor expression was not affected by OMC, while in the thyroid, TSH receptor expression (144% over the control group) was stimulated, but not NIS expression.

TPO activity was not changed, but DI1 activity was reduced by OMC (between 64% and 72%, depending on the dose). This effect could be a direct response to the drop in TH levels due to the fact that DI1 expression is stimulated by THs at the transcriptional level through the T3 response element in the promoter of the DI1 gene [50, 51]. These data are similar to those obtained in another experiment, where OMC was administered for 12 weeks to ovariectomized rats, significantly lowering the levels of T4 [52]. However, this research showed that the impact of OMC on hormonal homeostasis is rapid and induces significant changes in the levels of T4 and T3 in a short period of time.

Thyroid Receptor Binding Alteration

The functions of the thyroid hormones in target cells are regulated by three nuclear receptors: T3Rα1, T3Rβ1 and T3Rβ2, which are encoded by two genes, T3Rα and T3Rβ [53]. It has been reported that some industrial chemicals could block the action of THs on their receptors [54].

Bisphenol A

Bisphenol A (4,40-isopropylidenediphenol, BPA), one of the highest volume chemicals produced worldwide, is polymerized to form plastics based on polycarbonate and epoxy resins like some PVC plastics [55]. Moreover, this compound is used in food containers and as dental sealants [56]. The ester bond that allows polymerization of BPA can be broken primarily by exposure to heat releasing free BPA [57]. The known sources and pathways of human exposure to BPA have been recently discussed [58, 59]. In this regard, Howe and coworkers [60] estimated that human ingestion of BPA from food was about 6.6 mg/person/day. However, it is thought that there are other routes of exposure than from foods. Stahlhut and coworkers [61] found a longer than expected retention time for BPA in humans suggesting that the increase was due to non-food sources.

Bisphenol A is considered an endocrine disruptor that could alter thyroid function [62]. Romano [63] postulated that prenatal exposure to BPA may have sex-specific effects on thyroid hormones in infants. They investigated whether maternal urinary BPA concentration during pregnancy was associated with alterations in the concentrations of THs in mothers and the umbilical cord, and with maternal iodine concentration. The study was conducted among pregnant women from 16 and 26 weeks gestation in Cincinnati, Ohio, from 2003 to 2006. No significant differences at 16 weeks of gestation were observed, but at 26 weeks, an association between TSH levels and BPA levels (at 10 times higher than the BPA average) was determined in girls, but not in boys.

In animals, study results are contradictory. In this regard, it was reported that BPA does not induce effects on THs in adult rats and that there were no consistent effects [64-66]. However, Zoeller [56] found that BPA exposure during development in rats produced an endocrine pattern similar to that described in thyroid resistance syndrome. Specifically, T4 levels were increased during development in the offspring of animals treated with BPA, but TSH levels were not different from controls.

The fundamental mechanism of action of BPA is to impair the action of THs by blocking T3 binding to TR, and by enrolling the nuclear corepressor N-CoR to the TR, leading to repression of transcription. Moriyama [67], observed that the activation or repression of T3 genes mediated through TRα1 and TRβ was suppressed in a dose-dependent way by BPA, concluding that this compound is an antagonist of gene expression dependent on T3. However, other studies have indicated that BPA is a weak ligand for this receptor, but its derivatives, tetrabromobisphenol A (TBBPA) and tetrachlorobisphenol A (TCBPA), showed higher affinity for thyroid receptors [68-71]. Moreover, it has been hypothesized, according to the thyroid hormone alteration profile induced by BPA, that this compound is a TRβ antagonist, through which this effect is mediated [72]. If this hypothesis is confirmed, it is probable that BPA could produce similar effects to thyroid resistance syndrome in which the TRβ receptor is deficient and leads to high serum T4 and normal or slightly increased TSH concentrations [73]. On the other hand, there are recent *in vitro* studies showing that BPA is an antithyroid compound in the lack of a canonical Thyroid Response Element (TRE) [56], which suggests that other pathways of TH disruption are present.

Taking all this together, BPA could interfere with thyroid hormone signaling both in animals and humans, but further studies are needed to clarify these data and determine the range of safe doses that do not induce any harmful effect on human health and particularly on the thyroid system.

INDUSTRIAL CHEMICALS THAT DISRUPT THE THYROID SYSTEM THROUGH MORE THAN ONE MECHANISM OF ACTION

Polychlorinated Biphenyls

Polychlorinated biphenyls (PCBs) were discovered in the twentieth century and have been used widely in the industry. Due to their great biological, thermal and chemical stability as well as their high dielectric constant, the PCBs were massively used until the mid-1970s as insulation for electrical equipment such as transformers, switches, capacitors and electronic thermostats, refrigerants and heat transfer agents. For their anti-flammability characteristics, most dielectric oils with PCBs were mainly used in areas of high fire risk, such as industrial plants, in electric traction public transport and in the petrochemical industry. They were also used as dielectric and hydraulic fluids such as oil modifiers and heat exchange fluid and vacuum pumps [74].

Due to the fact that PCBs are compounds resistant to molecular degeneration, they are persistent in the environment [75]. The most contaminated areas of the earth are named "PCB deposits" and include the Baltic Sea, Hudson Bay and the Great Lakes area [75]. In addition to their persistence in the environment, PCBs may undergo a process called biomagnification, which refers to the progressive accumulation of persistent substances from one to other successive trophic levels [76]. They have been removed from industrial use because of their carcinogenic and polluting potentials. Current legislation limits the use of these compounds; for example inside USA their use is only allowed within a "closed system". Their manufacture has been prohibited since 1977 in the United States and since 1983 in Germany. Currently, their use is prohibited in most of the world [74].

PCBs are a large family of compounds that are known as congeners, consisting of two linked phenyl rings and varying degrees of chlorination [77]. There are 209 possible congeners that have been synthesized, but only 50 of them are classified as a threat to the environment [78]. PCBs with higher degree of chlorination at meta- and para- positions are metabolically more persistent and have a similar structure to thyroxine [75]. These compounds are related with thyroid toxicity and are directly responsible for the decrease in circulating levels of THs [79].

The main route of PCB exposure, besides the environmental, is from food, especially fish from contaminated areas [80, 81]. Although, the environment remains an important reservoir of PCBs, as other sources of exposure are buildings constructed before 1980 due to the fact that PCB Aroclor was commonly used in construction [82]. In this regard, Gabrio and coworkers [83] reported that different German school teachers presented PCBs at high blood levels due to inhalation, with the consequent health problems.

The effects of exposure to PCBs on THs in experimental animals have been extensively studied. In this regard, PCB exposure has been shown to induce a decrease in TH levels, especially T4 [84]. Histopathological changes indicative of hyperactivity have been found in the thyroid gland after subcutaneous and oral exposure to PCBs [85]. Moreover, PCBs are metabolized to hydroxylated compounds (OH-PCBs) and they cross the placental barrier in animals. In this sense, Meerts and coworkers [86] studied, in pregnant rats exposed to 4-OH-2,3,3',4',5-pentachlorobiphenyl (4-OH-CB_{107}), the presence of this metabolite in liver, fetal brain and plasma. Their results showed a decrease in T4 both in maternal and fetal blood, and an increase in TSH levels and T4 deiodination to T3 in the fetus. This relationship between thyroid disruption and PCB concentrations has also been found in wild animals. In this regard, a significant decrease of T3 and/or T4 in sea lions, polar bears and seals after PCB exposure has been described [87-90]. In addition, it has been reported that PCB perinatal exposure affected the development of white matter in rat pups imitating some effects of hypothyroidism on white matter, suggesting that PCBs can affect neurological development partly through alteration of THs [91].

Many studies on the effects of exposure to PCBs in human populations have been conducted, and most of them agreed that PCB levels presented in pollution affected thyroid homeostasis [92], decreasing and increasing T4 and TSH respectively, especially in people aged over 60 [79] and pregnant women [93].

PCBs affect thyroid function through different mechanisms:

1. Reduction of the binding ability to thyroid hormone transport proteins in the bloodstream

Halogenated aromatic hydrocarbons are structurally similar to thyroid hormones and therefore can compete with them in binding to TH transport proteins. In this regard, PCB competitively binds to transthyretin (TTR) [94]. By contrast, it has not been shown that these compounds could compete with TH in their binding to thyroxine-binding globulin (TBG) or albumin transport proteins [95-96].

Metabolites and derivatives of these compounds have a higher affinity than their parent compounds, indicating an important role for halogenation and hydroxylation in this effect [75]. In this regard, hydroxylated PCBs have been suggested to be able to specifically inhibit transport of T4 by competitive binding to TTR *in vitro* [97]. In addition, Meerts and coworkers [86] studied the exposure effects to 5 mg/kg of [^{14}C]-labeled or unlabeled 4-OH-CB_{107}, one of the major PCB metabolites detected in blood, on gestation days 10 to 16 in pregnant women and fetus blood. It was found that this metabolite was bound to TTR in mothers and fetuses, decreasing T4 levels in fetal plasma.

2. Increase in hepatic metabolism by regulating glucuronosyltransferases or sulfotransferases that metabolize hormones in the liver

PCBs induce hepatic microsomal enzymes and alter the thyroid system [98]. Hepatic microsomal enzymes play an important role in the metabolism of thyroid hormones because glucuronic acid conjugation by glucuronosyltransferases is the limiting step in biliary excretion of T4, and sulfation or sulfuroconjugation by sulfotransferase is the limiting step in biliary excretion of T3 [99-101]. It has been found that after continuous exposure in rats (2 years duration) to different PCBs, these enzymatic pathways could be induced, which produced thyroid stimulation continued by disruption of the HPT axis [102], resulting in increased circulating TSH levels that led to an increase in the development of tumors derived from follicular cells.

It has been reported that PCBs cause a significant decrease in serum levels of THs due to alterations in thyroid structure, plus induction of uridine diphosphate glucuronyl transferase (UDPGT) and increased removal of T4-glucuronide in bile [103]. In this regard, PCBs have been reported to produce a significant dose-dependent decrease of T4 levels in rats. After removal of PCB from the diet, T4 levels in the blood returned to normal at 35 weeks. These changes in circulating levels of T4 were accompanied by hypertrophy and hyperplasia of the thyroid follicular cell [104].

3. Inhibition or upregulation of deiodinase production that converts T4 to T3

Shimizu and coworkers [105] examined the possible influence of PCBs on thyroid metabolism *in vitro*. They tested deiodinase activity using the microsomal fraction of HEK-293 cells expressing recombinant human iodotyrosine dehalogenase 1 (IYD), and found that hydroxylated PCBs showed an inhibitory action on deiodinase activity. However they observed that hydroxylated chemical compounds, but not halogenated compounds such as bisphenol A or halogenated chemicals without a hydroxyl group like amiodarone, lacked inhibitory activity on deiodinases. Thus, they concluded that the critical structural requirement for the inactivation of deiodinases is a halogenated phenolic ring [106]. These studies are consistent with those made by Butt and coworkers [107] that showed deiodinase activity inhibition *in vitro* and T4 level reduction in liver microsomes after PCB exposure.

4. Action as agonist or antagonist of thyroid hormone receptors

PCBs also alter the expression of TH-responsive genes. OH-PCBs have been reported to inhibit the binding of T3 to TH receptors [71]. Moreover, it has been indicated that the TRβ has little affinity for OH-PCBs in humans [108]. Therefore, the competitive binding of PCBs could be both receptor and compound specific. Moreover, these compounds could block the action of T3 by enhancing the enrollment of transcriptional corepressors and/or the dissociation of coactivators [109]. In this regard, Iwasaki and coworkers [110] reported that 4-OH-PCB was able to inhibit TR/coactivator (SRC-1) complex mediated transactivation, and that this mechanism could explain the inhibition of TR-mediated transcription in the presence of OH-PCB in simian kidney cells. Other potential mechanisms of action may involve crosstalk with other nuclear receptors. In this sense, it has been reported that OH-PCB can partially separate the heterodimer RXR/TR from the T3-responsive element, a mechanism that could be involved in the inhibition of transcription induced by PCBs [111].

Polybrominated Diphenyl Ethers (PBDEs)

Polybrominated diphenyl ethers (PBDEs) are mainly used as flame retardants in different products to delay the ignition and burning of materials [112]. Due to their lipophilicity, PBDEs bioaccumulate, and their levels in human tissues have increased significantly over the last decade [113] including in serum [114], milk [115-119] and umbilical cord [120].

The structure of PBDEs, two halogenated phenyl rings linked by an ether bond, is structurally similar to THs, which suggests potential thyroid toxicity [56]. Recently there have been various studies on the ability of PBDE to disrupt thyroid function in both animals and humans. In this regard, exposure to PBDE has been reported to reduce serum total and free T4 levels and increase serum TSH in rodents [121-124]. These effects depended on the PBDE mixture used. Compounds with fewer bromines had higher activity in reducing the levels of thyroid hormone in serum [125].

There are a few studies of PBDE effects on the thyroid system in humans. Herbstman and coworkers [126], conducted a comprehensive study on mother-infant pairs, measuring exposure to PBDE in the umbilical cord during birth, finding that there was a decrease in the levels of total T4 and free T4 in natural child birthed, but not in caesarean delivered. In addition, in a study with eleven employees of an electronics recycling company, T4 levels were analyzed over 1.5 years. PBDE levels were throughout during the study and there was no characteristic trend over time, with small no relevant changes [127]. However, in another study of 110 men, a significant negative association between TSH and BDE-47 [128] was shown. Therefore, current knowledge on the action of PBDEs on human thyroid function is very limited and further studies to confirm their effects in humans are needed.

Different studies have been performed to determine the mechanisms by which PBDE exposure could lead to TH disruption. These studies show that the mechanisms involved are:

5. Reduction of thyroid hormone binding to transport proteins in the bloodstream

Meerts [129] investigated the interaction of several PBDEs and their role in the binding of T4 to TTR. PBDEs were capable of competing with the T4-TTR binding only after their metabolic conversion in liver microsomes, suggesting the important role of hydroxylation. In this regard, *ex vivo* binding of BDE-47 to plasma TTR has been shown after oral exposure in female rats [130], confirming that PBDE metabolites are transported *in vivo* by TTR.

6. Increase of conjugation and elimination

Rodent studies have shown that the PBDE called DE-71 decreased levels of thyroid hormones and induced UDPGT, pentoxyresorufin (PROD), and ethoxyresorufin-O-deethylase (EROD) liver enzyme activity [131]. Moreover, DE-71 and DE-79 oral treatment for 4 days in weanling rats leads to dose-dependent depletion of T4, which was accompanied by up to four fold induction of UDPGT activity [125].

7. Binding to thyroid hormone receptor and alteration of gene expression

It has also been postulated that some PBDEs or their hydroxylated metabolites could interact directly with TH receptors. In this regard, Marsh and coworkers [132] reported that hydroxylated PBDEs can bind to both TRα and TRβ, but with a notable preference for TRβ. In addition, Kojiba and coworkers [133] assessed the ability of different PBDEs and their metabolites to affect TH receptors through transcription assays using the CHO-K1 cell line. They found that 4-OH-BDE90 has a significant antagonistic action on TRβ1 and TRα1, without apparent differences between the actions on TRα1 or TRβ1.

Several animal studies showed that exposure to PBDEs may decrease circulating levels of vitamin A [134, 135], which is an important co-regulator of gene expression together with the signaling of the THs [136]. Moreover, vitamin A deficiency produced higher sensitivity to low levels of THs in rodents exposed to PBDEs [137]. According to these data Zoller [56] hypothesized that PBDEs could induce their effects on the thyroid system independently through both mechanisms.

Dioxins: 2,3,7,8-tetrachloro-dibenzo-p-dioxin (TCDD)

The polychlorinated dibenzo-p-dioxins (PCDD) and furans (PCDF) are persistent, highly toxic environmental pollutants formed in industrial combustion processes. The most typical prototype of this family is 2,3,7,8-tetrachloro-dibenzo-p-dioxin (TCDD). It has been shown that TCDD given to pregnant rats passed through the placental barrier and was excreted in the milk [138]. It has also been reported that maternal exposure to TCDD (100 ng/kg/day) from 10 to 16 days of gestation caused a decrease in serum levels of T4 in the offspring [139]. Moreover, TCDD exposure has been reported to cause a decrease in T4 and free T4 [140] and to increase TSH [141] as well as to produce thyroid hyperplasia in rats [142].

There are few studies in humans. In a study conducted with children whose mothers were exposed to dioxins in the area of the accident of Seveso (Italy), it was found that these children had very high levels of TSH compared to unexposed mothers [143]. Moreover, in a large study of veterans from Vietnam, it was reported that the group with the highest exposure to TCDD showed a significant increase in TSH levels [144], and a higher prevalence of thyroid diseases [145].

According to different studies the proposed mechanism of action of TCDD is based on:

1. Induction of hepatic UDPGT activity through the aryl hydrocarbon receptor (AhR) and increased T4-glucuronide elimination in bile

TCDD induces UDPGT 1A6 in liver through AhR, increasing glucuronic acid conjugation, which leads to an increased removal of T4 in bile, with decreased concentration in blood. Subsequently, the negative feedback mechanism triggers the release of TSH, leading to elevated serum TSH [141].

2. Alteration in the expression of genes involved in TH synthesis

Katarzynska and coworkers [146] found that TCDD caused up-regulation in gene expression of thyroglobulin and TPO in chickens, although in earlier studies by Pocar and coworkers [147] these effects on gene expression in porcine thyrocytes were not found. However, both studies reveal that TCDD caused a decrease in the regulation of mRNA expression and activity of cathepsin B, the enzyme responsible for thyroglobulin solubilization and subsequent release of thyroid hormones [148], which could explain the decrease in T4 and T3 secretion observed in chickens.

3. Alterations in deiodinase activity

Viluksela [149] investigated the 5'-deiodinases levels I and II (5'-DI and 5'-DII) in rats treated with TCDD, which produced a rapid and dose-dependent decrease in T4 circulation followed by a decrease in the hepatic activity of 5'-DI 1-2 days later and induced an apparent increase in the activity of 5'-DII. Changes in 5'-DI and 5'-DII activity were secondary to a decrease in T4 levels. The 5'-DI activity in thyroid and kidney as well as the T3 circulating levels were unaffected, concluding that TCDD did not have a significant influence on the activity of deiodinases. However, recently Song [150] reported that TCDD decreased the expression of deiodinases in cultured human neuroblastoma SH-SY5Y cells, which could cause a decrease in these enzymes that produces the effect observed on THs. Further studies are require to confirm these data.

Phthalates

Phthalates are a group of chemicals extensively used as emollients and plastic additives both for industrial uses and for consumer products. Despite the fact that certain phthalates were banned such as DEHP for children's toys, several classes of phthalates are still used in cosmetics, paints, food packaging, cleaning agents and medical devices such as tablet coatings, blood bags and tubes [151-153].

Phthalates do not accumulate in the organism and are metabolized and excreted primarily in the urine within hours or a few days, but due to their continued use, they produce continue exposure, especially in certain groups such as newborns and hospital patients with repeated transfusions and dialysis [154, 155].

Experimental studies have found an association between phthalate exposure and alteration of TH levels. Johns [156] investigated the association between exposure to various phthalates and free T4, free T3, TSH and sex hormones in pregnant women. They found an inverse association between mono-3-carboxypropyl phthalate (MCPP) and free T3 and between mono-ethyl phthalate (MEP) and progesterone, concluding that phthalates may be associated with altered levels of thyroid and sex hormones and that the magnitude of these effects depends on the time of exposure during pregnancy. In a study perform in 76 pregnant women, a significant negative association between DBP, phthalate metabolites and total and free T4 concentrations [157] was found. Similarly, a negative association between exposure to di(2-ethylhexyl) phthalate (DEHP) and free total T4 and T3 in adult men has been shown [155]. In addition, Boas and coworkers [158] conducted a study in children, reporting that these are exposed to similar amounts of phthalates as adults, and their exposure was negatively associated with serum levels of T3 and growth factor.

There are a few animal studies on the effects of phthalates on the thyroid system. In this regard, dibutyl phthalate (DBP) was reported to decrease T3 and T4 in a dose-dependent manner in rats [159], and several studies have demonstrated morphological changes in the thyroid after exposure to phthalates [160].

Experimental studies have shown different phthalate mechanisms on thyroid homeostasis, which can be classified into:

1. Interference with NIS activity

Breous [161] showed that diisodecyl phthalate (DIDP), benzyl butyl phthalate (BBP) and dioctyl phthalate (DOP) increased promoter activity of human NIS 2.5, 2.6 and 2.4 times respectively and enhanced expression of the endogenous NIS mRNA.

2. Competitive TTR binding

Ishihara and coworkers [162] investigated the effects of different compounds, including phthalates, on binding to TTR using ([^{125}I] T3), determining that they bind to TTR, but with a potency lower than that of T3, although this should be taken into account.

3. Gene expression alteration

Liu and coworkers [163] conducted a study with Sprague-Dawley rats treated with DEHP at increasing doses for 30 days. Gene expression of thyroid hormone receptors, deiodinases, transthyretin, and liver enzymes was measured; transthyretin protein levels were analyzed. The results showed that DEHP caused histological changes in follicular thyroid and hypertrophy and hyperplasia of epithelial cells. Moreover, DEHP significantly reduced thyroid hormones (T3, T4) and TH receptors, while TSH was not affected.

After exposure to DEHP, thyroid hormone biosynthesis was suppressed through NIS and TPO level reductions. In addition, it also affected deiodinase levels and transthyretin. Levels of TSH receptor (TSHr) were reduced, while the levels of TH receptors were upregulated. The metabolism of thyroid hormones was accelerated due to increased gene expression of liver enzymes (UDPGTs and CYP2B1) by DEHP. Therefore, taken together, the observed results indicate that phthalates may reduce thyroid hormone levels through a wide range of mechanisms of action.

Perfluorinated Chemicals

Perfluorinated compounds are a large family of industrial products, among which perfluorooctane sulfonate (PFOS) and perfluorooctanoic acid (PFOA) are included [164]. They are amphiphilic very stable substances and have high thermal, chemical and biological resistance [165]. Due to these properties, they are used in many industrial products such as cosmetics, textiles, non-stick coatings and waterproofing, stain removers, cleaners, pesticides among others [166].

Various studies have been conducted in humans to determine the association of these compounds with thyroid hormones. In this regard, a large study in 506 employees of a manufacturing firm described negative associations between PFOA and free T4 [167], which indicates that exposure to high levels of PFOA may interfere with the function of the human thyroid. Moreover, in a study of the National Health and Nutrition Examination Survey (NHANES) in the United States, women with high levels of PFOA and men with high levels of PFOS were more prone to thyroid pathologies [168].

In animal studies a decrease in T4 levels after both short-term [169] and long-term PFOS exposure was found [170]. A decrease in T3 levels was reported after PFOA exposure in rats [169] and monkeys [171]. However, a single dose exposure to PFOS has been described to induce a transient increase in free T4 and a decrease of TSH, followed by a decrease in T4 and T3 levels [172]. It has also been shown that perinatal exposure to PFOS decreased serum T4 levels, both in rat dams [173] and in their offspring [174, 175]. Rats exposed in utero and/or lactation to PFOS may present reduced thyroid hormone levels in their offspring [176].

In addition, Coperchini [177] conducted a study to assess the effects of PFOA and PFOS in thyroid cells, for which they used Fisher rat thyroid line-5 (FRTL-5) cells, finding that these compounds produce significant inhibition of cell proliferation, mainly by increased cell death.

The proposed mechanisms of action of perfluorinated compounds are:

1. Increased glucuronic acid conjugation and deiodination

Yu [178] conducted a study administering PFOS in water to Sprague-Dawley rats for 91 consecutive days at three different concentrations (1.7, 5, and 15 mg/L) and analyzed total and free T4 and T3 levels and TSH. The mRNA expression of two isoforms of UGT1A6 and UGT1A1 and DI1 in the liver, was determined. The expression of UGTIA1 in the liver was upregulated, but no effect was observed on UGT1A6 at the two higher doses of 5.0 and 15.0 mg/L of PFOS. PFOS treatment increased DIO1 expression in a dose-dependent manner. These results indicate that increase of T4-glucoroconjugacion *via* UGT1A1 and increased conversion of T4 to T3 *via* DI1 are partly responsible for the effects of PFOS in rat thyroid.

2. Reduced binding ability of THs to thyroid transport protein in the bloodstream

Weiss [179] conducted a study with 24 perfluorinated compounds (PFCs) to examine their binding capacity to TTR. They concluded that the PFCs have only 1/10 binding power to TTR of the natural T4 hormone and are less strongly bound than many other environmental pollutants. However, due to their relatively high concentrations in the environment, PFCs could contribute significantly to the reduction of T4. The results also support the observations that binding to TTR can take place even in the absence of hydrogen bonding interaction with the hydroxyl group from TTR Ser-117 residue.

Acrylamide

Acrylamide is a compound widely used in the chemical industry. Monomers are used for the production of polymers that are employed as flocculants in the wastewater treatment, and as dewatering aids, laminating resins, textile resins, soil stabilizers, gel chromatography and electrophoresis photography [180].

Monomeric forms are well known for their neurotoxic effects, producing neuropathies both at the central and peripheral nervous system in experiments with rats [181]. It has also been observed that the acute and chronic exposure to acrylamide produces neurotoxic effects in exposed workers [180]. Acrylamide has been classified as a likely human carcinogen, although epidemiologic studies in either occupationally exposed workers or the general populations of different countries in which acrylamide is present in some foods and beverages have not found consistent evidence of elevated cancer risk [182]. By contrast, acrylamide has been reported to cause tumors in different organs, among them the thyroid gland in mice and rats [182]. The discrepancy between animal and human studies could be due to the fact that the rodent thyroid is much more active than the human, which makes rodents more susceptible to thyroid tumors than humans [183], thus any extrapolation from rodents data to humans should be made with great care.

Its effects at the level of the thyroid hormones are poorly understood. Lin and coworkers [184] reported a negative association between urinary levels of the acrylamide metabolite N-acetyl-S-(propionamide)-cysteine (AAMA) and free T4 in 793 adolescents and young subjects, especially in women. Moreover, Khan [180] described in Fischer 344 rats after 2 and 15 mg/kg/day for 2 and 7 days oral exposure to acrylamide respectively, that no changes were observed at the lower dose, but in animals treated for 7 days at the higher dose an increase in T4 levels and a decrease in TSH levels were found. In addition, Bowyer and coworkers [185] reported that in Fischer 344 male rats treated with acrylamide (2.5, 10 and 50 mg/kg/day) for 14 days no effect on the HPT axis was found except for a decrease in T4 at the highest dose tested. Furthermore, Hamdy and coworkers [186] reported that Sprague Dawley male rats treated with 10, 15 mg/kg/day body weight of acrylamide for 8 weeks, showed lower T3 and T4 levels than controls. The differences observed between acrylamide actions on T4 could be due to differences in the species, time of exposure or vehicles used.

According to these data, there are few studies on the effects and mechanisms of action of acrylamide on the thyroid system and their results are inconclusive. More studies to obtain conclusive results are needed.

CONCLUDING REMARKS

Humans are continuously exposed to a large number of industrial products, some of which can affect thyroid hormone homeostasis. The primary role of these hormones in nervous system development has led to a growing interest in determining the mechanisms by which these compounds act and the possible additive or synergistic effects that they would have on the metabolism of thyroid hormones, because the population is not only exposed to a single compound, but to many compounds either separately or together throughout their lives. Thus, small changes in thyroid function can have negative results for health. In particular, during development, humans may be vulnerable to even very subtle changes that can cause neurological disorders and cognitive deficits.

On the other hand, the human population is exposed to a very high number of different types of industrial chemicals, but our knowledge about their effects on the thyroid system is limited to a few compounds and even the knowledge of these compounds is in some cases insufficient or contradictory. Therefore further studies are needed to confirm the mechanisms and effects of industrial chemicals described to be thyroid disruptors and determine if other compounds to which the population are exposed could also disrupt the thyroid system in order to establish procedures at the legislative level to adequately protect the health of the population.

CONFLICT OF INTEREST

The author confirms that author has no conflict of interest to declare for this publication.

ACKNOWLEDGEMENTS

None Declared.

REFERENCES

[1] Patrick L. Thyroid disruption: Mechanisms and clinical implications in human health. Altern Med Rev 2009; 14: 326-346.
[2] Woodruff TK, Walker CL. Fetal and early postnatal environmental exposures and reproductive health effects in the female. Fertil Steril 2008; 89: e47-e51.
[3] Lee DH, Lee IK, Jin SH, Steffes M, Jacobs Jr DR. Association between serum concentrations of persistent organic pollutants and insulin resistance among nondiabetic adults: results from the National Health and Nutrition Examination Survey 1999-2002. Diabetes Care 2007; 30: 622-628.
[4] Crews D, McLachlan JA. Epigenetics, evolution, endocrine disruption, health, and disease. Endocrinology 2006; 147: S4-S10.
[5] Boas M, Feldt-Rasmussen U, Main KM. Thyroid effects of endocrine disrupting chemicals. Mol Cell Endocrinol 2012; 355:240–248.
[6] Auso E, Lavado-Autric R, Cuevas E, Del Rey FE, Morreale dE, Berbel P. A moderate and transient deficiency of maternal thyroid function at the beginning of fetal neocorticogenesis alters neuronal migration. Endocrinology 2004; 145: 4037-4047.
[7] Lavado-Autric R, Auso E, Garcia-Velasco JV, *et al.* Early maternal hypothyroxinemia alters histogenesis and cerebral cortex cytoarchitecture of the progeny. J Clin Invest 2003; 111: 1073-1082.
[8] Brucker-Davis F. Effects of environmental synthetic chemicals on thyroid function. Thyroid 1998; 8: 827-856.
[9] DeVito M, Biegel L, Brouwer A, *et al.* Screening methods for thyroid hormone disruptors. Environ Health Perspect 1999; 107: 407-415.
[10] Blount BC, Pirkle JL, Osterloh JD, Valentin-Blasini L, Caldwell KL. Urinary perchlorate and thyroid hormone levels in adolescent and adult men and women living in the United States. Environ Health Perspect 2006; 114: 1865- 1871.
[11] Steinmaus C, Miller MD, Howd R. Impact of smoking and thiocyanate on perchlorate and thyroid hormone associations in the 2001-2002 national health and nutrition examination survey. Environ Health Perspect 2007; 115: 1333- 1338.
[12] Capen CC. Mechanistic data and risk assessment of selected toxic end points of the thyroid gland. Toxicol Pathol 1997; 25: 39-48.
[13] Tabb MM, Kholodovych V, Grun F, Zhou C, Welsh WJ, Blumberg B. Highly chlorinated PCBs inhibit the human xenobiotic response mediated by the steroid and xenobiotic receptor (SXR). Environ Health Perspect 2004; 112: 163- 169.
[14] Atterwill CK, Collins P, Brown CG, Harland RF. The perchlorate discharge test for examining thyroid function in rats. J Pharmacol Meth 1987; 18: 199-203.
[15] Tonacchera M, Pinchera A, Dimida A, *et al.* Relative potencies and additivity of perchlorate, thiocyanate, nitrate, and iodide on the inhibition of radioactive iodide uptake by the human sodium iodide symporter. Thyroid 2004; 14(12): 1012-1019.
[16] Patrick L. Thyroid Disruption: Mechanisms and Clinical Implications in Human Health. Altern Med Rev 2009; 14(4): 326-346
[17] Pearce EN. Iodine in pregnancy: is salt iodization enough? J Clin Endocrinol Metab 2008; 93(7): 2466-2468.

[18] Meberg A, Marstein S. Smoking during pregnancy: effects on the fetal thyroid function. Acta Pediatr Scand 1986; 75: 762-766.
[19] Chanoine JP, Toppet V, Bourdoux P, Spehl M, Delange F. Smoking during pregnancy: a significant cause of neonatal thyroid enlargement. Br J Obstet Gynaecol 1991; 98: 65-68.
[20] Laurberg P, Nøhr SB, Pedersen KM, Fuglsang E. Iodine nutrition in breast-fed infants is impaired by maternal smoking. J Clin Endocrinol Metab. 2004; 89(1): 181-187.
[21] Dasgupta PK, Dyke JV, Kirk AB, Jackson WA. Perchlorate in the United States. Analysis of relative source contributions to the food chain. Environ Sci Technol 2006; 40(21): 6608-6614.
[22] Soldin OP, Braverman LE, Lamm SH. Perchlorate clinical pharmacology and human health: A review. Therap Drug Monit 2001; 23: 316-331.
[23] Clewell RA, Merrill EA, Narayanan L, Gearhart JM, Robinson PJ. Evidence for competitive inhibition of iodide uptake by perchlorate and translocation of perchlorate into the thyroid. Intl J Toxicol 2004; 23: 17-23.
[24] Li Z, Li FX, Byrd D, *et al*. Neonatal thyroxine level and perchlorate in drinking water. J Occup Environ Med 2000; 42: 200-205.
[25] Lamm SH, Braverman LE, Li FX, Richman K, Pino S, Howearth G. Thyroid health status of ammonium perchlorate workers: A cross-sectional occupational health study. J Occup Environ Med 1999; 41: 248-260.
[26] Lamm SH, Doemland M. Has perchlorate in drinking water increased the rate of congenital hypothyroidism? J Occup Environ Med 1999; 41: 409-411.
[27] Jugan ML, Levi Y, Blondeau JP. Endocrine disruptors and thyroid hormone physiology. Biochem Pharmacol 2010; 79 (7): 939-947.
[28] Blount BC, Pirkle JL, Osterloh JD, Valentin-Blasini L, Caldwell KL. Urinary perchlorate and thyroid hormone levels in adolescent and adult men and women living in the United States. Environ Health Perspect 2006; 114 (12): 1865-1871.
[29] Braverman LE, Pearce EN, He X, *et al*. Effects of six months of daily lowdose perchlorate exposure on thyroid function in healthy volunteers. J Clin Endocrinol Metabol 2006; 91(7): 2721-2724.
[30] Braverman LE, He X, Pino S, *et al*. The effect of perchlorate, thiocyanate, and nitrate on thyroid function in workers exposed to perchlorate long-term. J Clin Endocrinol Metab. 2005; 90 (2): 700-706.
[31] National Research Council: Health Implications of Perchlorate Ingestion. Washington, DC, National Academic Press, 2005; pp. 1-260.
[32] Khan MA, Fenton SE, Swank AE, Hester SD, Williams A, Wolf DC. A Mixture of Ammonium Perchlorate and Sodium Chlorate Enhances Alterations of the Pitutary-Thyroid Axis Caused by the Individual Chemicals in Adult Male F344 Rats. Toxicol Pathol 2005; 33: 776-783.
[33] Bercz JP, Jones L, Garner L, Murray D, Ludwig DA, Boston J. Subchronic toxicity of chlorine dioxide and related compounds in drinking water in the nonhuman primate. Environ Health Perspect 1982; 46: 47-55.
[34] McCauley PT, Robinson M, Daniel FB, Olson GR. The effects of subchronic chlorate exposure in Sprague–Dawley rats. Drug Chem Toxicol 1995; 18(2 & 3): 185-199.
[35] Hooth MJ, Deangelo AB, George MH, *et al*. Subchronic Sodium Chlorate Exposure in Drinking Water Results in a Concentration-Dependent Increase in Rat Thyroid Follicular Cell Hyperplasia. Toxicol Pathol 2001; 29 (2): 250-259.
[36] Schmutzler C, Hamann I, Hofmann PJ, *et al*. Endocrine active compounds affect thyrotropin and thyroid hormone levels in serum as well as endpoints of thyroid hormone action in liver, heart and kidney. Toxicology 2004; 205: 95-102.
[37] Crofton KM. Thyroid disrupting chemicals: mechanisms and mixtures. Int J Androl 2008; 31:209-223.
[38] Sharan S, Nikhil K, Roy P. Disruption of thyroid hormone functions by low doses exposure of tributyltin: an *in vitro* and *in vivo* approach. Gen Comp Endocrin 2014; 206: 155-165.
[39] Chen L, Zhou HY, Deng QY. Photolysis of nonylphenol ethoxylates: the determination of the degradation kinetics and the intermediate products. Chemosphere 2007; 68(2): 354-359.
[40] Schmutzler C, Hamann I, Hofmann PJ, *et al*. Endocrine active compounds affect thyrotropin and thyroid hormone levels in serum as well as endpoints of thyroid hormone action in liver, heart and kidney. Toxicology 2004; 205: 95-102.

[41] Xi Y, Li D, San W. Exposure to the endocrine disruptor nonylphenol alters structure and functions of the thyroid glands in rats. Regulatory Peptides 2013; 185: 52-56.

[42] Lynch BS, Delzell ES, Bechtel DH. Toxicology Review and Risk Assessment of Resorcinol: Thyroid Effects. Regul Toxicol Pharmacol 2002; 36: 198-210.

[43] Welsch F. Routes and modes of administration of resorcinol and their relationship to potential manifestations of thyroid gland toxicity in animals and man. Int J Toxicol 2008; 27(1): 59-63.

[44] Paul KB, Hedge JM, Rotroff DM, Hornung MW, Crofton KM, Simmons SO. Development of a thyroperoxidase inhibition assay for high-throughput screening. Chem Res Toxicol 2014; 27 (3): 387-99.

[45] Doerge DR, Divi RL. Porphyrin π-cation and protein radicals in peroxidase catalysis and inhibition by anti-thyroid chemicals. Xenobiotica 1995; 25 (7): 761-767.

[46] Schmutzler C1, Bacinski A, Gotthardt I, *et al.* The UV Filter Benzophenone 2 Interferes with the Thyroid Hormone Axis in Rats and is a Potent *In Vitro* Inhibitor of Human Recombinant Thyroid Peroxidase. Endocrinology 2007; 148 (6): 2835-2844.

[47] Schlecht C, Klammer H, Frauendorf H, Wuttke W, Jarry H. Pharmacokinetics and metabolism of benzophenone 2 in the rat. Toxicology 2008; 245 (1-2): 11-17.

[48] Diamanti-Kandarakis E, Bourguignon JP, Giudice LC, *et al.* Endocrine-Disrupting Chemicals: An Endocrine Society Scientific Statement. Endocr Rev 2009; 30: 293-342.

[49] Klammer H, Schlecht C, Wuttke W, *et al.* Effects of a 5-day treatment with the UV-filter octyl-methoxycinnamate (OMC) on the function of the hypothalamo-pituitary-thyroid function in rats. Toxicology 2007; 238 (2-3): 192-199.

[50] Jakobs TC, Schmutzler C, Meissner J, Köhrle J. The promoter of the human type I 5'-deiodinase gene--mapping of the transcription start site and identification of a DR+4 thyroid-hormone-responsive element. Eur J Biochem. 1997; 247 (1): 288-297.

[51] Toyoda N, Zavacki AM, Maia AL, Harney JW, Larsen PR. A novel retinoid X receptor-independent thyroid hormone response element is present in the human type 1 deiodinase gene. Mol Cell Biol. 1995; 15(9): 5100-5112.

[52] Schmutzler C, Hamann I, Hofmann PJ, *et al.* Endocrine active compounds affect thyrotropin and thyroid hormone levels in serum as well as endpoints of thyroid hormone action in liver, heart and kidney. Toxicology 2004; 205 (1-2): 95-102.

[53] Fraichard A, Chassande O, Plateroti M, *et al.* The T3R alpha gene encoding a thyroid hormone receptor is essential for post-natal development and thyroid hormone production. EMBO J. 1997; 16 (14): 4412-4420.

[54] Duntas LH. Chemical contamination and the thyroid. Endocrine 2015; 48 (1): 53-64

[55] Lewis JB, Rueggeberg FA, Lapp CA, Ergle JW, Schuster GS. Identification and characterization of estrogen-like components in commercial resin-based dental restorative materials. Clin Oral Investig 1999; 3: 107-113.

[56] Zoeller, TR. Environmental chemicals targeting thyroid. Hormones 2010; 9 (1): 28-40.

[57] Kang JH, Kondo F, Katayama Y. Human exposure to bisphenol A. Toxicology 2006; 226 (2-3): 79-89.

[58] Vandenberg LN, Maffini MV, Sonnenschein C, Rubin BS, Soto AM. Bisphenol-A and the great divide: A review of controversies in the field of endocrine disruption. Endocr Rev 2009; 30: 75-95.

[59] Stahlhut RW, Welshons WV, Swan SH. Bisphenol-A data in NHANES suggest longer than expected half-life, substantial nonfood exposure, or both. Environ Health Perspect 2009; 117: 784-789.

[60] Howe SR, Borodinsky L. Potential exposure to bisphenol-A from food-contact use of polycarbonate resins. Food Addit Contam 1998; 15(3): 370-375.

[61] Stahlhut RW, Welshons WV, Swan SH. Bisphenol A data in NHANES suggest longer than expected half-life, substantial nonfood exposure, or both. Environ Health Perspect 2009; 117 (5): 784-789

[62] Rochester JR. Bisphenol A and human health: a review of the literature. Reprod Toxicol 2013; 42: 132-155.

[63] Romano ME, Webster GM, Vuong AM, *et al.* Gestational urinary bisphenol A and maternal and newborn thyroid hormone concentrations: the HOME Study. Environ Res 2015; 138: 453-460.

[64] Nieminen P, Lindström-Seppä P, Mustonen AM, *et al.* Bisphenol A affects endocrine physiology and biotransformation enzyme activities of the field vole (*Microtus agrestis*). Gen Comp Endocrinol. 2002; 126 (2): 183-189.

[65] Nieminen P, Lindström-Seppä P, Juntunen M, *et al. In vivo* effects of bisphenol A on the polecat (*Mustela putorius*). J Toxicol Environ Health A. 2002; 65 (13): 933-945.

[66] Xu X, Liu Y, Sadamatsu M, *et al.* Perinatal bisphenol-A affects the behavior and SCR-1 expression of male pups but does not influence on the thyroid hormone receptors and its responsive gene. Neurosci Res 2007; 58:149-155.

[67] Moriyama K, Tagami T, Akamizu T, *et al.* Thyroid hormone action is disrupted by bisphenol A as an antagonist. J Clin Endocrinol Metab 2002; 87: 5185-5190.

[68] Fini JB, Le Mevel S, Turque N, *et al.* An *in vivo* multiwell-based fluorescent screen for monitoring vertebrate thyroid hormone disruption. Environ Sci Technol 2007; 41(16): 5908-5914.

[69] Hofmann PJ, Schomburg L, Kohrle J. Interference of endocrine disrupters with thyroid hormone receptor-dependent transactivation. Toxicol Sci 2009; 110: 125-137.

[70] Jagnytsch O, Opitz R, Lutz I, Kloas W. 2006. Effects of tetrabromobisphenol a on larval development and thyroid hormone-regulated biomarkers of the amphibian *Xenopus laevis*. Environ Res 2006; 101: 340-348.

[71] Kitamura S, Jinno N, Suzuki T, *et al.* Thyroid hormone-like and estrogenic activity of hydroxylated PCBs in cell culture. Toxicology 2005; 208: 377-387.

[72] Zoeller RT, Bansal, Parris C. Bisphenol-A, an environmental contaminant that acts as a thyroid hormone receptor antagonist *in vitro*, increases serum thyroxine, and alters RC3/neurogranin expression in the developing rat brain. Endocrinology 2005; 146: 607-612

[73] Yen PM. Molecular basis of resistance to thyroid hormone. Trends Endocrinol Metab 2003; 14: 327-333.

[74] Agency for Toxic Substances and Disease Registry (ATSDR): Toxicological Profile for Polychlorinated Biphenyls (PCBs). USA. Department of Health and Human Services 2000; pp: 1-948. Available from: http:// www. atsdr.cdc.gov/ toxprofiles/tp17.pdf.

[75] Langer P. Persistent organochlorinated pollutants (PCB, DDE, HCB, dioxins, furans) and the thyroid-review. Endocr Regul 2008; 42:79-104.

[76] Programme AMAP. AMAP Assessment Report: Arctic Pollution Issues. Arctic Monitoring and Assessment Program (AMAP) Oslo. 1998; XII: 1-859.

[77] McFarland VA, Clarke JU. Environmental occurrence, abundance and potential toxicity of polychlorinated biphenyl congeners: considerations for congener- specific analysis. Environ Health Perspect 1989; 81: 225-239.

[78] Henry TB. Ecotoxicology of polychlorinated biphenyls in fish-a critical review. Crit Rev Toxicol. 2015; 6: 1-19.

[79] Turyk ME, Anderson HA, Persky VW. Relationships of thyroid hormones with polychlorinated biphenyls, dioxins, furans, and DDE in adults. Environ Health Perspect 2007; 115: 1197-1203.

[80] Hanrahan LP1, Falk C, Anderson HA, Draheim L, Kanarek MS, Olson J. Serum PCB and DDE levels of frequent Great Lakes sport fish consumers-a first look. The Great Lakes Consortium. Environ Res 1999; 80: S26-S37.

[81] Hites RA, Foran JA, Carpenter DO, Hamilton MC, Knuth BA, Schwager SJ. Global assessment of organic contaminants in farmed salmon. Science 2004; 303: 226-229.

[82] Herrick RF, McClean MD, Meeker JD, Baxter LK, Weymouth GA. An unrecognized source of PCB contamination in schools and other buildings. Environ Health Perspect 2004; 112(10): 1051-1053.

[83] Gabrio T, Piechotowski I, Wallenhorst T, *et al.* PCB-blood levels in teachers, working in PCB contaminated schools. Chemosphere 2000; 40: 1055-1062.

[84] Hallgren S, Darnerud PO. Polybrominated diphenyl ethers (PBDEs), polychlorinated biphenyls (PCBs) and chlorinated paraffins (CPs) in rats-testing interactions and mechanisms for thyroid hormone effects. Toxicology 2002; 177: 227-243.

[85] Kilic N, Sandal S, Colakoglu N, Kutlu S, Seyran A, Yilmaz B. Endocrine disruptive effects of polychlorinated biphenyls on the thyroid gland in female rats. Tohoku J Exp Med 2005; 206: 327-332.

[86] Meerts IA, Assink Y, Cenijn PH, *et al.* Placental transfer of a hydroxylated polychlorinated biphenyl and effects on fetal and maternal thyroid hormone homeostasis in the rat. Toxicol Sci 2002; 68: 361-371.

[87] Debier C, Ylitalo GM, Weise M, *et al.* PCBs and DDT in the serum of juvenile California sea lions: associations with vitamins A and E and thyroid hormones. Environ Pollut 2005; 134: 323-332.

[88] Skaare JU, Bernhoft A, Wiig O, *et al.* Relationships between plasma levels of organochlorines, retinol and thyroid hormones from polar bears (*Ursus maritimus*) at Svalbard. J Toxicol Environ Health Part A 2001; 62: 227-241.
[89] Chiba I, Sakakibara A, Goto Y, *et al.* Negative correlation between plasma thyroid hormone levels and chlorinated hydrocarbon levels accumulated in seals from the coast of Hokkaido, Japan. Environ Toxicol Chem 2001; 20: 1092-1097.
[90] Sormo EG, Jussi I, Jussi M, Braathen M, Skaare JU, Jenssen BM. Thyroid hormone status in gray seal (*Halichoerus grypus*) pups from the Baltic Sea and the Atlantic Ocean in relation to organochlorine pollutants. Environ Toxicol Chem 2005; 24: 610-616.
[91] Sharlin DS, Bansal R, Zoeller RT. Polychlorinated Biphenyls Exert Selective Effects on Cellular Composition of White Matter in a Manner Inconsistent with Thyroid Hormone Insufficiency. Endocrinology 2006; 147: 846-858.
[92] Boas M, Feldt-Rasmussen U, Skakkebæk NE, Main KM. Environmental chemicals and thyroid function. Eur J Endocrinol 2006; 154: 599-611.
[93] Takser L, Mergler D, Baldwin M, de Grosbois S, Smargiassi A, Lafond J. 2005. Thyroid Hormones in Pregnancy in Relation to Environmental Exposure to Organochlorine Compounds and Mercury. Environ Health Perspect 2005; 113: 1039-1045.
[94] Purkey HE, Palaninathan SK, Kent KC, *et al.* Hydroxylated polychlorinated biphenyls selectively bind transthyretin in blood and inhibit amyloidogenesis: rationalizing rodent PCB toxicity. Chem Biol 2004; 11: 1719-1728.
[95] Van den Berg KJ. Interaction of chlorinated phenols with thyroxine binding sites of human transthyretin, albumin and thyroid binding globulin. Chem Biol Interact 1990: 76: 63-75.
[96] Lans MC, Spiertz C, Brouwer A, Koeman JH. Different competition of thyroxine binding to transthyretin and thyroxine-binding globulin by hydroxy- PCBs, PCDDs and PCDFs. Eur J Pharmacol 1994; 270: 129-136.
[97] Darras VM. Endocrine disrupting polyhalogenated organic pollutants interfere with thyroid hormone signalling in the developing brain. Cerebellum 2008; 7(1): 26-37.
[98] Vansell NR1, Muppidi JR, Habeebu SM, Klaassen CD. Promotion of thyroid tumors in rats by pregnenolone-16a-carbonitrile (PCN) and polychlorinated biphenyl (PCB). Toxicol Sci 2004; 81: 50-59.
[99] Vansell NR, Klaassen CD. Increased biliary excretion of thyroxine by microsomal enzyme inducers. Toxicol Appl Pharmacol 2001; 176: 187-194.
[100] Shelby MK1, Cherrington NJ, Vansell NR, Klaassen CD. Tissue mRNA expression of the rat UDP-glucuronosyltransferase gene family. Drug Metab Disp 2003; 31: 326-333.
[101] Dunn RT, Klaassen CD. Thyroid hormone modulation of rat sulphotransferase mRNA expression. Xenobiotica 2000; 30: 345-357.
[102] Vansell NR, Klaassen CD. Increase in rat liver UDP-glucuronosyltransferase mRNA by microsomal enzyme inducers that enhance thyroid hormone glucuronidation. Drug Metabol Disp 2002; 30: 240-246.
[103] Collins WT, Capen CC. Ultrastructural and functional alterations of the rat thyroid gland produced by polychlorinated biphenyls compared with iodide excess and deficiency and thyrotropin and thyroxine administration. Virchow Arch B Cell Pathol 1980; 33: 213-231.
[104] Capen CC, Marti SL. The effects of xenobiotics on the structure and function of thyroid follicular and C-cells. Toxicol Pathol 1989; 17 (2): 266-293.
[105] Shimizu R, Yamaguchi M, Uramaru N, *et al.* Structure-activity relationships of 44 halogenated compounds for iodotyrosine deiodinase-inhibitory activity. Toxicology 2013; 314: 22-29.
[106] Shimizu R. Iodotyrosine Deiodinase, a Novel Target of Environmental Halogenated Chemicals for Disruption of the Thyroid Hormone System in Mammals. Biol Pharm Bull 2014; 37 (9): 1430-1434.
[107] Butt CM, Wang D, Stapleton HM. Halogenated phenolic contaminants inhibit the *in vitro* activity of the thyroid-regulating deiodinases in human liver. Toxicol Sci 2011; 124: 339-347.
[108] Cheek AO, Kow K, Chen J, McLachlan JA. Potential mechanisms of thyroid disruption in humans: interaction of organochlorine compounds with thyroid receptor, transthyretin, and thyroid-binding globulin. Environ Health Perspect 1999; 107: 273-278.
[109] Moriyama K, Tagami T, Usui T, *et al.* Antithyroid drugs inhibit thyroid hormone receptor-mediated transcription. J Clin Endocrinol Metab 2007; 92: 1066-1072.

[110] Iwasaki T, Miyazaki W, Takeshita A, Kuroda Y, Koibuchi N. Polychlorinated biphenyls suppress thyroid hormone-induced transactivation. Biochem Biophys Res Commun 2002; 299: 384-388.

[111] Miyazaki W, Iwasaki T, Takeshita A, Kuroda Y, Koibuchi N. Polychlorinated biphenyls suppress thyroid hormone receptor-mediated transcription through a novel mechanism. J Biol Chem 2004; 279: 18195-18202.

[112] Frederiksen M, Vorkamp K, Thomsen M, Knudsen LE. Human internal and external exposure to PBDEs - a review of levels and sources. Int J Hyg Environ Health 2008; 212: 109-134.

[113] McDonald TA. A perspective on the potential health risks of PBDEs. Chemosphere 2002; 46: 745-755.

[114] Sjödin A, Jones RS, Focant JF, *et al.* Retrospective time-trend study of polybrominated diphenyl ether and polybrominated and polychlorinated biphenyl levels in human serum from the United States. Environ Health Perspect 2004; 112: 654-658.

[115] Haraguchi K, Koizumi A, Inoue K, *et al.* Levels and regional trends of persistent organochlorines and polybrominated diphenyl ethers in asian breast milk demonstrate pops signatures unique to individual countries. Environ Int 2009; 35: 1072-1079.

[116] She J, Holden A, Sharp M, Tanner M, Williams-Derry C, Hooper K. Polybrominated diphenyl ethers (PBDEs) and polychlorinated biphenyls (PCBs) in breast milk from the Pacific Northwest. Chemosphere 2007; 67: S307-317.

[117] Jaraczewska K, Lulek J, Covaci A, *et al.* Distribution of polychlorinated biphenyls, organochlorine pesticides and polybrominated diphenyl ethers in human umbilical cord serum, maternal serum and milk from Wielkopolska region, Poland. Sci Total Environ 2006; 372: 20-31.

[118] Inoue K, Harada K, Takenaka K, *et al.* Levels and concentration ratios of polychlorinated biphenyls and polybrominated diphenyl ethers in serum and breast milk in Japanese mothers. Environ Health Perspect 2006; 114: 1179-1185.

[119] Schecter A, Pavuk M, Papke O, Ryan JJ, Birnbaum L, Rosen R. Polybrominated diphenyl ethers (PBDEs) in U.S. mothers' milk. Environ Health Perspect 2003; 111: 1723-1729.

[120] Herbstman JB, Sjodin A, Apelberg BJ, *et al.* Birth delivery mode modifies the associations between prenatal polychlorinated biphenyl (PCB) and polybrominated diphenyl ether (PBDE) and neonatal thyroid hormone levels. Environ Health Perspect 2008; 116: 1376-1382.

[121] Szabo DT, Richardson VM, Ross DG, Diliberto JJ, Kodavanti PR, Birnbaum LS. Effects of perinatal PBDE exposure on hepatic Phase I, Phase II, Phase III, and deiodinase 1 gene expression involved in thyroid hormone metabolism in male rat pups. Toxicol Sci 2009; 107: 27-39.

[122] Tseng LH, Li MH, Tsai SS, *et al.* Developmental exposure to decabromodiphenyl ether (PBDE 209): Effects on thyroid hormone and hepatic enzyme activity in male mouse offspring. Chemosphere 2008; 70: 640-647.

[123] Darnerud PO, Aune M, Larsson L, Hallgren S. Plasma PBDE and thyroxine levels in rats exposed to bromkal or BDE-47. Chemosphere 2007; 67: S386-392.

[124] Stoker TE, Laws SC, Crofton KM, Hedge JM, Ferrell JM, Cooper RL. Assessment of de-71, a commercial polybrominated diphenyl ether (PBDE) mixture, in the edsp male and female pubertal protocols. Toxicol Sci 2004; 78: 144-155.

[125] Zhou T, Ross DG, DeVito MJ, Crofton KM. Effects of short-term *in vivo* exposure to polybrominated diphenyl ethers on thyroid hormones and hepatic enzyme activities in weanling rats. Toxicol Sci 2001; 61: 76-82.

[126] Herbstman JB, Sjödin A, Apelberg BJ, *et al.* Birth delivery mode modifies the associations between prenatal polychlorinated biphenyl (PCB) and polybrominated diphenyl ether (PBDE) and neonatal thyroid hormone levels. Environ Health Perspect 2008; 116: 1376-1382.

[127] Julander A, Karlsson M, Hagstrom K, *et al.* Polybrominated diphenyl ethers - plasma levels and thyroid status of workers at an electronic recycling facility. Int Arch Occup Environ Health 2005; 78: 584-592.

[128] Hagmar L, Bjork J, Sjodin A, Bergman A, Erfurth EM. Plasma levels of persistent organohalogens and hormone levels in adult male humans. Arch Environ Health 2001; 56: 138-143.

[129] Meerts IA, van Zanden JJ, Luijks EA, *et al.* Potent competitive interactions of some brominated flame retardants and related compounds with human transthyretin *in vitro*. Toxicol Sci 2000; 56: 95-104.

[130] Hallgren S, Darnerud PO. Polybrominated diphenyl ethers (PBDEs), polychlorinated biphenyls (PCBs) and chlorinated paraffins (CPs) in ratstesting interactions and mechanisms for thyroid hormone effects. Toxicology 2002; 177; 227-243.

[131] Stoker TE, Laws SC, Crofton KM, Hedge JM, Ferrell JM, Cooper RL. Assessment of DE-71, a commercial polybrominated diphenyl ether (PBDE) mixture, in the EDSP male and female pubertal protocols. Toxicol Sci 2004; 78: 144-155.

[132] Marsh G, Bergman A, Bladh LG, Gillner M, Jakobsson E. Synthesis of p-hydroxybromodiphenyl ethers and binding to the thyroid hormone receptor. Organohalogen Compd 1998; 37: 305-308.

[133] Kojima H, Takeuchi S, Uramaru N, Sugihara K, Yoshida T, Kitamura S. Nuclear hormone receptor activity of polybrominated diphenyl ethers and their hydroxylated and methoxylated metabolites in transactivation assays using Chinese hamster ovary cells. Environ Health Perspect 2009; 117: 1210-1218.

[134] Hallgren S, Sinjari T, Hakansson H, Darnerud PO. Effects of polybrominated diphenyl ethers (PBDEs) and polychlorinated biphenyls (PCBs) on thyroid hormone and vitamin A levels in rats and mice. Arch Toxicol 2001; 75: 200-208.

[135] Ellis-Hutchings RG, Cherr GN, Hanna LA, Keen CL. Polybrominated diphenyl ether (PBDE)-induced alterations in vitamin A and thyroid hormone concentrations in the rat during lactation and early postnatal development. Toxicol Appl Pharmacol 2006; 215: 135-145.

[136] Tagami T, Yamamoto H, Moriyama K, *et al*. The retinoid x receptor binding to the thyroid hormone receptor: Relationship with cofactor binding and transcriptional activity. J Mol Endocrinol 2009; 42: 415-428.

[137] Ellis-Hutchings RG, Cherr GN, Hanna LA, Keen CL. The effects of marginal maternal vitamin A status on penta-brominated diphenyl ether mixture-induced alterations in maternal and conceptal vitamin A and fetal development in the Sprague Dawley rat. Birth Defects Res B Dev Reprod Toxicol 2009; 86: 48-57.

[138] Kakeyama M, Tohyama C. Developmental neurotoxicity of dioxin and its related compounds. Ind Health 2003; 41(3): 215-230.

[139] Seo BW, Li MH, Hansen LG, Moore RW, Peterson RE, Schantz SL. Effects of gestational and lactational exposure to coplanar polychlorinated biphenyl (PCB) congeners or 2,3,7,8-tetrachlorodibenzo-p-dioxin (TCDD) on thyroid hormone concentrations in weanling rats. Toxicol Lett 1995; 78: 253-262.

[140] Viluksela M1, Raasmaja A, Lebofsky M, Stahl BU, Rozman KK. Tissue-specific effects of 2,3,7,8-tetrachlorodibenzo-p-dioxin (TCDD) on the activity of 5'-deiodinases I and II in rats. Toxicol Lett 2004; 147(2): 133-142.

[141] Nishimura N, Miyabara Y, Sato M, Yonemoto J, Tohyama C. Immuno-histochemical localization of thyroid stimulating hormone induced by a low oral dose of 2,3,7,8-tetrachlorodibenzo-p-dioxin in female Sprague–Dawley rats. Toxicology 2002; 171: 73-82.

[142] Nishimura N, Yonemoto J, Miyabara Y, Sato M, Tohyama C. Rat thyroid hyperplasia induced by gestational and lactational exposure to 2,3,7,8-tetrachlorodibenzo-p-dioxin. Endocrinology 2003; 144: 2075-2083.

[143] Baccarelli A, Giacomini SM, Corbetta C, *et al*. Neonatal thyroid function in Seveso 25 years after maternal exposure to dioxin. PLoS Med 2008; 29; 5(7): e161. doi: 10.1371/journal.pmed.0050161.

[144] Pavuk M, Schecter AJ, Akhtar FZ & Michalek JE. Serum 2,3,7,8-tetrachlorodibenzo-p-dioxin (TCDD) levels and thyroid function in Air Force veterans of the Vietnam War. Ann Epidemiol 2003; 13: 335-343.

[145] Spaulding SW. The possible roles of environmental factors and the aryl hydrocarbon receptor in the prevalence of thyroid diseases in Vietnam era veterans. Curr Opin Endocrinol Diabetes Obes 2011; 18(5): 315-20.

[146] Katarzy´nska D, Hrabia A, Kowalik K, Sechman A. Comparison of the *in vitro* effects of TCDD, PCB 126and PCB 153 on thyroid-restricted gene expression and thyroid hormone secretion by the chicken thyroid gland. Environ Toxicol Pharmacol 2015; 39 (2): 496-503.

[147] Pocar P, Klonisch T, Brandsch C, *et al*. AhR-agonist-induced transcriptional changes of genes involved in thyroid function in primary porcine thyrocytes. Toxicol Sci 2006; 89(2): 408-414.

[148] Friedrichs B, Tepel C, Reinheckel T, *et al*. Thyroid functions of mouse cathepsins B, K, and L. J. Clin Invest 2003; 111: 1733-1745.

[149] Viluksela M, Raasmaja A, Lebofsky M, Stah BU, Rozman KK. Tissue-specific effects of 2,3,7,8-tetrachlorodibenzo-p-dioxin (TCDD) on the activity of 5'-deiodinases I and II in rats. Toxicol Lett 2004; 147(2): 133-142.

[150] Song M, Song MK, Choi HS, Ryu JC. Monitoring of deiodinase deficiency based on transcriptomic responses in SH-SY5Y cells. Arch Toxicol 2013; 87: 1103-1113

[151] Sathyanarayana S, Karr CJ, Lozano P, *et al.* Baby care products: possible sources of infant phthalate exposure. Pediatrics 2008; 121: e260–e268.

[152] Schettler T. Human exposure to phthalates *via* consumer products. Int J Androl 2006; 29: 134-139.

[153] Wormuth M, Scheringer M, Vollenweider M, Hungerbuhler K. What are the sources of exposure to eight frequently used phthalic acid esters in Europeans? Risk Anal 2006; 26: 803-824.

[154] Becker K, Seiwert M, Angerer J, *et al.* DEHP metabolites in urine of children and DEHP in house dust. Int J Hyg Environ Health 2004; 207: 409-417.

[155] Meeker JD, Calafat AM, Hauser R. Di(2-ethylhexyl) phthalate metabolites may alter thyroid hormone levels in men. Environ Health Perspect 2007; 115: 1029-1034.

[156] Johns LE, Ferguson KK, Soldin OP, *et al.* Urinary phthalate metabolites in relation to maternal serum thyroid and sex hormone levels during pregnancy: a longitudinal analysis. Reprod Biol Endocrinol 2015; 13: 4. doi: 10.1186/1477-7827-13-4.

[157] Huang PC, Kuo PL, Guo YL, Liao PC, Lee CC. Associations between urinary phthalate monoesters and thyroid hormones in pregnant women. Hum. Reprod 2007; 22: 2715-2722.

[158] Boas M, Frederiksen H, Feldt-Rasmussen U, *et al.* Childhood Exposure to Phthalates: Associations with Thyroid Function, Insulin-like Growth Factor I, and Growth. Environ Health Perspect 2010; 118 (10): 1458-1464.

[159] O'Connor JC, Frame SR, Ladics GS. Evaluation of a 15-day screening assay using intact male rats for identifying antiandrogens. Toxicol Sci 2002; 69: 92-108.

[160] Howarth JA, Price SC, Dobrota M, Kentish PA, Hinton RH. Effects on male rats of di-(2-ethylhexyl) phthalate and di-n-hexylphthalate administered alone or in combination. Toxicol Lett 2001; 121: 35-43.

[161] Breous E, Wenzel A, Loos U. The promoter of the human sodium/iodide symporter responds to certain phthalate plasticisers. Mol Cell Endocrinol 2005; 244: 75-78.

[162] Ishihara A, Nishiyama N, Sugiyama S, Yamauchi K. The effect of endocrine disrupting chemicals on thyroid hormone binding to Japanese quail transthyretin and thyroid hormone receptor. Gen Comp Endocrinol 2003; 134(1): 36-43.

[163] Liu C, Zhao L, Wei L, Li L. DEHP reduces thyroid hormones *via* interacting with hormone synthesis-related proteins, deiodinases, transthyretin, receptors, and hepatic enzymes in rats. Environ Sci Pollut Res Int 2015; 28:28.

[164] Lau C, Anitole K, Hodes C, Lai D, Pfahles-Hutchens A, Seed J. Perfluoroalkyl acids: A review of monitoring and toxicological findings. Toxicol Sci 2007; 99(2): 366-394.

[165] Biffinger JC, Kim HW, DiMagno SG. (2004). The polar hydrophobicity of fluorinated compounds. Chembiochem 2004; 5: 622-627.

[166] Kissa E. In Fluorinated Surfactants and Repellents. Marcel Dekker Inc., New York. 2001

[167] Olsen GW, Zobel LR. Assessment of lipid, hepatic, and thyroid parameters with serum perfluorooctanoate (PFOA) concentrations in fluorochemical production workers. Int Arch Occup Environ Health 2007; 81: 231-246.

[168] Melzer D, Rice N, Depledge MH, Henley WE, Galloway TS. Association between serum perfluorooctanoic acid (PFOA) and thyroid disease in the U.S. National Health and Nutrition Examination Survey. Environ Health Perspect 2010; 118: 686-692.

[169] Martin MT, Brennan RJ, Hu W, *et al.* Toxicogenomic study of triazole fungicides and perfluoroalkyl acids in rat livers predicts toxicity and categorizes chemicals based on mechanisms of toxicity. Toxicol Sci 2007; 97: 595-613.

[170] Yu WG, Liu W, Jin YH. Effects of perfluorooctane sulfonate on rat thyroid hormone biosynthesis and metabolism. Environ Toxicol Chem 2009; 28: 990-996.

[171] Seacat AM, Thomford PJ, Hansen KJ, *et al.* Sub-chronic dietary toxicity of potassium perfluorooctanesulfonate in rats. Toxicology 2003; 183: 117-131.

[172] Chang SC, Thibodeaux JR, Eastvold ML, *et al.* Thyroid hormone status and pituitary function in adult rats given oral doses of perfluorooctanesulfonate (PFOS). Toxicology 2008; 243: 330-339.

[173] Thibodeaux JR, Hanson RG, Rogers JM, *et al.* Exposure to perfluorooctane sulfonate during pregnancy in rat and mouse. I: maternal and prenatal evaluations. Toxicol Sci 2003; 74: 369-381.
[174] Lau C, Thibodeaux JR, Hanson RG, *et al.* Exposure to perfluorooctane sulfonate during pregnancy in rat and mouse. II: postnatal evaluation. Toxicol Sci 2003; 74: 382-392.
[175] Luebker DJ, York RG, Hansen KJ, Moore JA, Butenhoff JL. Neonatal mortality from in utero exposure to perfluorooctanesulfonate (PFOS) in Sprague-Dawley rats: dose-response, and biochemical and pharamacokinetic parameters. Toxicology 2005; 215: 149-169.
[176] Yu WG, Liu W, Jin YH, *et al.* Prenatal and postnatal impact of perfluorooctane sulfonate (PFOS) on rat development: a cross-foster study on chemical burden and thyroid hormone system. Environ Sci Technol 2009; 43: 8416-8422.
[177] Coperchini F, Pignatti P, Lacerenza S, *et al.* Exposure to perfluorinated compounds: *in vitro* study on thyroid cells. Environ Sci Pollut Res Int. 2015; 22(3): 2287-2294.
[178] Yu, WG, Liu W, Jin YH. Effects of perfluorooctane sulfonate on rat thyroid hormone biosynthesis and metabolism. Environ Toxicol Chem 2009; 28: 990-996.
[179] Weiss JM, Andersson PL, Lamoree MH, Leonards PE, Van Leeuwen SP, Hamers T. Competitive binding of poly- and perfluorinated compounds to the thyroid hormone transport protein transthyretin. Toxicol Sci 2009; 109: 206-216.
[180] Khan MA, Davis CA, Foley GL, Friedman MA, Hansen LG. Changes in thyroid gland morphology after acute acrylamide exposure. Toxicol Sci 1999; 47(2): 151-157.
[181] Crofton KM, Padilla S, Tilson HA, Anthony DC, Raymer JH, MacPhail RC. The impact of dose rate on the neurotoxicity of acrylamide: the interaction of administered dose, target tissue concentrations, tissue damage, and functional effects. Toxicol Appl Pharmacol 1996; 139(1): 163-176.
[182] Rice JM. The carcinogenicity of acrylamide. Mutat Res 2005; 580(1-2): 3-20.
[183] Meek M, Bucher J, Cohen S, *et al.* A framework for human relevance analysis of information on carcinogenic modes of action. Crit Rev Toxicol 2003; 33: 591-653.
[184] Lin CY, Lin LY, Chen YC, *et al.* Association between measurements of thyroid function and the acrylamide metabolite N-Acetyl-S-(propionamide)-cysteine in adolescents and young adults. Environ Res. 2015; 136: 246-252.
[185] Bowyer JF, Latendresse JR, Delongchamp RR, *et al.* The effects of subchronic acrylamide exposure on gene expression, neurochemistry, hormones, and histopathology in the hypothalamus-pituitary-thyroid axis of male Fischer 344 rats. Toxicol Appl Pharmacol 2008; 230(2): 208-215
[186] Hamdy SM, Bakeer HM, Eskander EF, Sayed ON. Effect of acrylamide on some hormones and endocrine tissues in male rats. Hum Exp Toxicol 2012; 31(5): 483-491.

Subject Index

N

O

P

R

S

T

U

V

Y

Z

Made in the USA
Las Vegas, NV
04 November 2026

57425094R10138